Clinical Trials
in Ovarian Cancer

Clinical Trials in Ovarian Cancer

Christine S. Walsh, MD, MS

Rutgers University Press Medicine
New Brunswick, Camden, and Newark, New Jersey, and London

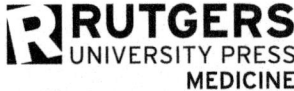
UNIVERSITY PRESS
MEDICINE

Kel McGowan
Executive Editor for Clinical Health and Medicine

This publication was supported in part
by the Eleanor J. and Jason F. Dreibelbis Fund.

Library of Congress Cataloging-in-Publication Data

Names: Walsh, Christine S., 1972– author.
Title: Clinical trials in ovarian cancer / Christine S. Walsh.
Description: New Brunswick, New Jersey : Rutgers University Press, [2017] |
    Includes bibliographical references and index.
Identifiers: LCCN 2016032168 | ISBN 9780813586472 (pbk.: alk. paper) |
    ISBN 9780813586489 (ePub) | ISBN 9780813586496 (Web PDF)
Subjects: | MESH: Ovarian Neoplasms—therapy | Clinical Trials, Phase III
    as Topic
Classification: LCC RC280.O8 | NLM WP 322 | DDC 616.99/465— dc23
LC record available at https://lccn.loc.gov/2016032168

A British Cataloging-in-Publication record for this book is available from
the British Library.

Copyright © 2017 by Christine Walsh

All rights reserved
No part of this book may be reproduced or utilized in any form or by any
means, electronic or mechanical, or by any information storage and retrieval
system, without written permission from the publisher. Please contact
Rutgers University Press, 106 Somerset Street, New Brunswick, NJ 08901.
The only exception to this prohibition is "fair use" as defined by U.S.
copyright law.

Visit our website: www.rutgersuniversitypress.org
Manufactured in the United States of America

This book is dedicated to all women with ovarian cancer and to the health care professionals and scientists who partner with these women to improve outcomes through the identification of better treatment strategies through the clinical trials process.

Contents

List of Tables ix
Preface and Acknowledgments xi

1 Early Stage Epithelial Ovarian Cancer   1
   GOG 7601 (Young, NEJM 1990)   *1*
   GOG 7602 (Young, NEJM 1990)   *5*
   GICOG Trials (Bolis, Ann Oncol 1995)   *9*
   GOG 95 (Young, JCO 2003)   *15*
   ICON1/ACTION Combined Analysis (Trimbos, JNCI 2003)   *19*
   ACTION (Trimbos, JNCI 2003; Trimbos, JNCI 2010)   *24*
   ICON1 (Colombo, JNCI 2003)   *32*
   GOG 157 (Bell, Gynecol Oncol 2006)   *37*
   GOG 157 Exploratory Analysis (Chan, Gynecol Oncol 2010)   *43*

2 Advanced Stage Epithelial Ovarian Cancer: Adjuvant Chemotherapy   46
   GOG 47 (Omura, Cancer 1986)   *46*
   GOG 52 (Omura, JCO 1989)   *50*
   GOG 97 (McGuire, JCO 1995)   *53*
   GOG 111 (McGuire, NEJM 1996)   *57*
   GOG 104 (Alberts, NEJM 1996)   *62*
   ICON2 (Lancet 1998)   *66*
   GOG 132 (Muggia, JCO 2000)   *70*
   Danish Netherlands Trial (Neijt, JCO 2000)   *75*
   OV-10 (Piccart, JNCI 2000)   *80*
   GOG 114 (Markman, JCO 2001)   *86*
   ICON3 (Lancet 2002)   *90*
   GOG 158 (Ozols, JCO 2003)   *95*

AGO/OVAR-3 (du Bois, JNCI 2003) *100*
SCOTROC—Scottish Randomised Trial in Ovarian Cancer
   (Vasey, JNCI 2004) *105*
GOG 172 (Armstrong, NEJM 2006) *109*
GOG 182/ICON5 (Bookman, JCO 2009) *114*
JGOG 3016 (Katsumata, Lancet 2009; Katsumata,
   Lancet Oncol 2013) *119*
MITO-2 (Pignata, Oncology 2009; Pignata, JCO 2011) *126*
AGO-OVAR9 (du Bois, JCO 2010) *132*
OV16 (Hoskins, JNCI 2010) *137*
ICON7 (Perren, NEJM 2011; Oza, Lancet Oncol 2015) *145*
GOG 218 (Burger, NEJM 2011) *151*
MITO-7 (Pignata, Lancel Oncol 2014) *157*

3 Advanced Stage Epithelial Ovarian Cancer: Timing of Surgery and Interval Cytoreduction — 162

EORTC-GCG 55865 (van der Burg, NEJM 1995) *162*
GOG 152 (Rose, NEJM 2004) *168*
EORTC 55971 (Vergote, NEJM 2010) *174*
CHORUS (Kehoe, Lancet 2015) *178*

4 Epithelial Ovarian Cancer: Maintenance Therapy — 186

GOG 178/SWOG 9701 (Markman, JCO 2003) *186*
GOG 175 (Mannel, Gynecol Oncol 2011) *193*

5 Recurrent Epithelial Ovarian Cancer — 200

Topotecan Versus Paclitaxel (ten Bokkel, JCO 1997) *200*
Doxil Study 30-49 (Gordon, JCO 2001; Gordon,
   Gyn Onc 2004) *207*
ICON4/AGO-OVAR 2.2 (Parmar, Lancet 2003) *217*
AGO-OVAR, NCIC CTG, EORTC GCG Trial
   (Pfisterer, JCO 2006) *222*
Gemcitabine Versus PLD (Mutch, JCO 2007) *228*
OVA-301 (Monk, JCO 2010) *235*
CALYPSO (Pujade-Lauraine, JCO 2010) *242*
OCEANS (Aghajanian, JCO 2012) *249*
AURELIA (Pujade-Lauraine, JCO 2014) *256*

Abbreviations 263
References 267
Index 295

List of Tables

1.1 GOG 7601 *4*
1.2 GOG 7602 *8*
1.3 GICOG Trial 1 *13*
1.4 GICOG Trial 2 *14*
1.5 GOG 95 *18*
1.6 ICON1/ACTION Combined Analysis *22*
1.7 ACTION *28*
1.8 ACTION Long-Term Follow-up *31*
1.9 ACTION Long-Term Follow-up, Grade 3 Tumors *31*
1.10 ICON1 *35*
1.11 GOG 157 *41*
1.12 GOG 157 Exploratory Analysis *45*
2.1 GOG 47 *49*
2.2 GOG 52 *52*
2.3 GOG 97 *56*
2.4 GOG 111 *61*
2.5 GOG 104 *65*
2.6 ICON2 *69*
2.7 GOG 132 *73*
2.8 Danish Netherlands Trial *78*
2.9 OV-10 *84*
2.10 GOG 114 *89*
2.11 ICON3 *93*
2.12 GOG 158 *98*
2.13 AGO/OVAR-3 *104*
2.14 SCOTROC *108*
2.15 GOG 172 *113*
2.16 GOG 182/ICON5 *118*

2.17 JGOG 3016 *124*
2.18 MITO-2 *130*
2.19 AGO-OVAR9 *136*
2.20 OV16 *143*
2.21 ICON7 *149*
2.22 GOG 218 *155*
2.23 MITO-7 *160*
3.1 EORTC-GCG 55865 *166*
3.2 GOG 152 *172*
3.3 EORTC 55971 *177*
3.4 CHORUS *184*
4.1 GOG 178/SWOG 9701 *190*
4.2 GOG 175 *198*
5.1 Topotecan Versus Paclitaxel *205*
5.2 Doxil Study 30-49 *213*
5.3 ICON4/AGO-OVAR 2.2 *221*
5.4 AGO-OVAR, NCIC, CTG EORTC GCG Trial *226*
5.5 Gemcitabine Versus PLD *232*
5.6 OVA-301 *240*
5.7 CALYPSO *247*
5.8 OCEANS *254*
5.9 AURELIA *261*

Preface and Acknowledgments

I first met Dana Dreibelbis at the 2014 Annual Meeting of the American Society of Clinical Oncology. Rutgers University Press offered me the opportunity to edit a short clinical book as part of a new publishing initiative. I immediately knew that I wanted to put together a book that summarizes the seminal clinical trials that have shaped the practice of gynecologic oncology.

Clinical trials have been instrumental in creating our current clinical practice paradigms. A clinician taking care of a woman with gynecologic cancer needs to understand this history in order to deliver evidence-based care. In some cases, clinical trials findings result in clear establishment of standard of care therapy. In other cases, optimal treatment regimens are not yet defined, but clinical trials provide data to inform the clinician regarding treatment options and ongoing controversies.

The clinical trials history of any field is vast, making it difficult and time-consuming for any individual to collect and synthesize. Currently, a textbook focused on clinical trials in gynecologic oncology does not exist. Clinical trials are discussed in general textbooks but often within lengthy chapters that cover many other topics. There is no standardized formatting and the reader must wade through the text in order to find relevant information.

The concept for this textbook is to provide a concise, user-friendly reference that focuses solely on clinical trials in gynecologic oncology. The text is formatted in a standardized fashion so the reader can rapidly find relevant information. The seminal phase III trials that have shaped the field are outlined in a standard format to include the details on the rationale for the trial, the patient population studied, treatment details of the experimental arms, assessments, endpoints, statistical considerations, results, conclusions and further commentary. Standardized tables highlight the salient and relevant results by summarizing patient characteristics, treatment delivery, efficacy and toxicities from each seminal phase III trial. The full reference and PMID number are provided for each study so that the reader can easily find the original text and reference for further reading. A list of the abbreviations used in the text is provided at the end of the book for the reader's convenience.

This text focuses on the seminal phase III clinical trials that have been conducted in patients with epithelial ovarian cancer and represents the first in a series of books. Similar textbooks outlining clinical trials in other gynecologic malignancies such as uterine and cervical cancer are forthcoming. I am so appreciative to Dana Dreibelbis and the rest of the staff at RUP for giving this series of textbooks the opportunity to exist.

The care of women with gynecologic malignancies is shaped through the rich history of clinical trials. There is no one-size-fits-all approach when it comes to making treatment decisions. Rather, there are a varied number of treatment options for various clinical scenarios and clinicians often need to make treatment recommendations based on nuances such as individual patient and tumor characteristics as well as treatment side effect profiles. I hope you will find this book to be a useful reference to easily find information regarding the efficacy as well as toxicity profiles of various treatment regimens.

CHAPTER 1

Early Stage Epithelial Ovarian Cancer

Approximately 30% of epithelial ovarian cancers are diagnosed at an early stage and can be completely resected at the time of surgery. GOG 7601 defined low-risk tumors that include stage IA and IB, grade 1 cancer, where adjuvant chemotherapy can be safely omitted. High-risk early-stage ovarian cancers include stage I, grade 3; stage IC; clear cell; and stage II cancers. In this high-risk subgroup, the GICOG and GOG 95 trials demonstrated a lower risk of recurrence with the administration of platinum-based adjuvant chemotherapy. The ACTION and ICON1 trials demonstrated improved overall survival with platinum chemotherapy (mostly carboplatin) compared to observation but suggested that the benefit does not apply to patients who had complete surgical staging. GOG 157 showed no difference in survival between 3 and 6 cycles of carboplatin and paclitaxel, but an exploratory analysis suggested a benefit for 6 cycles with serous histologies.

GOG 7601 (Young, NEJM 1990)

REFERENCE

- Young RC, et al. Adjuvant therapy in stage I and stage II epithelial ovarian cancer. Results of two prospective randomized trials. *N Engl J Med*. 1990;322(15):1021-1027. PMID: 2181310. (Young et al. 1990)

TRIAL SPONSORS

- Ovarian Cancer Study Group (Mayo Clinic, MD Anderson Hospital and Tumor Institute, National Cancer Institute, Roswell Park Memorial Institute)
- Gynecologic Oncology Group (GOG)

RATIONALE FOR TRIAL
- Survival rates vary among patients with early-stage epithelial ovarian cancer. The 5-year survival ranges from 50% to 70% for patients with stage I ovarian cancer. The 5-year survival ranges from 38% to 60% for patients with stage II ovarian cancer.
- Pathologic factors such as cell type and grade only partially account for the variable survivals.
- Earlier studies have demonstrated the importance of thorough surgical staging in order to balance prognostic factors among treatment groups.
- GOG 7601/7602 studies were performed to evaluate the impact of adjuvant therapy following surgical resection and comprehensive staging on outcomes of patients with early-stage epithelial cancer. Because the entire abdomen is at risk for metastatic disease, these trials included only those patients with a standardized and comprehensive surgical exploration in order to determine the true benefit of adjuvant therapy.
- GOG 7601 evaluated patients with lower-risk disease classified as stage IA and IB and grade 1 or grade 2 epithelial ovarian cancer.
- GOG 7602 evaluated patients with higher-risk disease classified as stage I, grade 3 or any stage II epithelial ovarian cancer.

PATIENT POPULATION
- N=92.
- Enrollment started in 1976 by the Ovarian Cancer Study Group and in 1978 by the Gynecologic Oncology Group. Enrollment ended in October 1984.

Inclusion Criteria
- Patients with stage IA and IB and grade 1 or grade 2 epithelial ovarian cancer after complete surgical staging were enrolled.
- Staging was performed through a vertical incision and included total abdominal hysterectomy, bilateral salpingo-oophorectomy, and partial infracolic omentectomy. The tumor capsule was evaluated for rupture, excrescences, and adhesions requiring sharp dissection. Ascitic fluid was examined for malignant cells. In the absence of ascites, separate 250-mL saline washings were obtained from the pelvis and both abdominal gutters. Suspicious lesions were biopsied. Random biopsies of the pelvic peritoneum, cul-de-sac peritoneum, right and left abdominal gutter peri-

toneum, and the undersurface of the right diaphragm were obtained. Pelvic and para-aortic lymph nodes were palpated and sampled.
- Adequate bone marrow, renal, and liver function.

TREATMENT DETAILS

Arm 1
- No further treatment.

Arm 2
- Melphalan 0.2 mg/kg orally daily for 5 days, repeated every 4 to 6 weeks for 12 cycles or 18 months, whichever came first.

ASSESSMENTS
- Before 1983, noninvasive staging procedures such as chest radiography, intravenous pyelography, and lymphangiography were utilized.
- When clinically indicated, pelvic ultrasonography, barium enema, pelvic and abdominal computed tomography (CT) scanning, and proctosigmoidoscopy were performed.
- Patients free of recurrent disease 18 months after study entry underwent routine surgical reexploration.
- Symptomatic patients underwent earlier exploration unless there was documented recurrent disease on noninvasive study.
- At reexploration, all patients underwent peritoneal washings as well as biopsies of the right and left paracolic gutters, cul-de-sac, lateral pelvic wall, small bowel mesentery, and omentum.
- Biopsies were also performed of adhesions and known sites of prior disease. Results have been previously published (Walton et al. 1987).

ENDPOINTS
- Survival.

STATISTICAL CONSIDERATIONS

Stratification Factors
- Cell type.
- Histologic grade.

Sample Size
- Target sample size of 110 patients. Accrual was terminated after 8 years of enrollment at 74% of the goal because the observed rate of relapse was so low that it ruled out the possibility of eventually detecting a moderate difference between the 2 groups.

Statistical Tests
- Method of Kaplan and Meier was used to calculate life-table properties of survival and disease-free survival (Kaplan and Meier 1958).
- Log-rank test was used to compare survival distributions (Mantel 1966).
- Cox proportional hazards regression was used to compare survival after adjusting for baseline characteristics and to investigate the prognostic significance of baseline variables.

Table 1.1 Results of GOG 7601

Treatment arm	No further treatment N=38 evaluable	Melphalan N=43 evaluable	Statistics
Patient characteristics			
Median age	50 years	40 years	
Residual tumor	0%	0%	
Stage Ia_i	94.7%	93.0%	
Stage Ib_i	5.3%	7.0%	
Serous	31.6%	14.0%	
Endometrioid	13.2%	18.6%	
Mucinous	28.9%	35.0%	
Clear cell	2.6%	11.6%	
Other	23.7%	20.9%	
Grade 1	36.8%	44.2%	
Grade 2	13.2%	16.3%	
Reclassified as LMP	39.5%	27.9%	
Efficacy			
Recurrences	N=4	N=1	
Deaths:			
Ovarian cancer, primary	N=3	N=1	
Ovarian cancer, secondary	N=1	N=0	
Complication	N=0	N=1 (aplastic anemia)	
Other	N=0	N=0	
5-year disease-free survival	91%	98%	P=NS
5-year overall survival	94%	98%	P=NS
Toxicity			
Myelosuppression	Not applicable	79%	
Aplastic anemia		N=1, occurred 6 years after treatment	

NS, not significant.

- Methods described by Simon were used to calculate confidence limits (Simon 1986).

CONCLUSION OF TRIAL

- Patients with a diagnosis of stage Ia_i or Ib_i disease after comprehensive surgical staging have an excellent 5-year survival rate of >90%. Adjuvant therapy with oral melphalan did not improve outcomes. In light of the toxicity and risk of second cancers, the identification of a group of patients in whom adjuvant therapy can be withheld represents a significant finding.

COMMENTS

- Clear cell tumors had poorer outcomes. When considering patients who had central pathology review, 38% (3 of 8) of patients with clear cell tumors relapsed compared to 3% (2 of 63) of patients with other histologic tumor types.
- Ovarian tumors of borderline malignancy have a more indolent course than invasive tumors (Scully 1977; Bjorkholm et al. 1982). The 5-year survival was unchanged when patients with borderline tumors were excluded from the analysis (exact survival numbers are not provided in the manuscript).

GOG 7602 (Young, NEJM 1990)

REFERENCE

- Young RC, et al. Adjuvant therapy in stage I and stage II epithelial ovarian cancer. Results of two prospective randomized trials. *N Engl J Med.* 1990;322(15):1021-1027. PMID: 2181310. (Young et al. 1990)

TRIAL SPONSOR

- Ovarian Cancer Study Group (Mayo Clinic, MD Anderson Hospital and Tumor Institute, National Cancer Institute, Roswell Park Memorial Institute)
- Gynecologic Oncology Group (GOG)

RATIONALE FOR TRIAL

- GOG 7601/7602 were performed to evaluate the impact of adjuvant therapy following surgical resection and comprehensive staging on outcomes of patients with early-stage epithelial cancer.

- GOG 7601 evaluated patients with lower-risk disease: stage IA and IB and grade 1 or grade 2 epithelial ovarian cancer.
- GOG 7602 evaluated patients with higher-risk disease: stage I grade 3 or any stage II epithelial ovarian cancer.

PATIENT POPULATION
- N = 145.
- Enrollment started in 1976 by the Ovarian Cancer Study Group and in 1978 by the Gynecologic Oncology Group. Enrollment ended in November 1986.

Inclusion Criteria
- Stage I, grade 3 or stage II epithelial ovarian cancer.
- Staging was performed through a vertical incision and included total abdominal hysterectomy, bilateral salpingo-oophorectomy, and partial infracolic omentectomy. The tumor capsule was evaluated for rupture, excrescences, and adhesions requiring sharp dissection. Ascitic fluid was examined for malignant cells. In the absence of ascites, separate 250-mL saline washings were obtained from the pelvis and both abdominal gutters. Suspicious lesions were biopsied. Random biopsies of the pelvic peritoneum, cul-de-sac peritoneum, right and left abdominal gutter peritoneum, and the undersurface of the right diaphragm were obtained. Pelvic and para-aortic lymph nodes were palpated and sampled.
- Adequate bone marrow, renal, and liver function.

TREATMENT DETAILS

Arm 1
- Melphalan 0.2 mg/kg orally daily for 5 days, repeated every 4 to 6 weeks for 12 cycles or 18 months, whichever came first.

Arm 2
- Intraperitoneal ^{32}P at a dose of 15 mCi of chromic phosphate (dose was 7.5 mCi before 1979).

ASSESSMENTS
- Noninvasive staging procedures: chest radiography, intravenous pyelography, and lymphangiography (before 1983).
- When clinically indicated: pelvic ultrasonography, barium enema, pelvic and abdominal CT scanning, and proctosigmoidoscopy.

- Patients free of recurrent disease 18 months after study entry underwent routine surgical reexploration.
- Symptomatic patients underwent earlier exploration unless there was documented recurrent disease on noninvasive study.
- At reexploration, all patients underwent peritoneal washings as well as biopsies of the right and left paracolic gutters, cul-de-sac, lateral pelvic wall, small bowel mesentery, and omentum. Biopsies were also performed of adhesions and known sites of prior disease. Results have been previously published (Walton et al. 1987).

ENDPOINTS
- Survival.

STATISTICAL CONSIDERATIONS

Stratification Factors
- Cell type.
- Histologic grade.
- Stage.
  - Group A: stage Ia_i or Ib_i disease with poorly differentiated histologic grades and those with stage Ib_{ii} or Ib_{ii} disease.
  - Group B: stage IIa or IIb disease.
  - Group C: stage Ic or IIc disease or any patient with detectable disease.

Sample Size
- The target sample size of 142 was achieved.

Statistical Tests
- Method of Kaplan and Meier was used to calculate life-table properties of survival and disease-free survival (Kaplan and Meier 1958).
- Log-rank test was used to compare survival distributions (Mantel 1966).
- Cox proportional hazards regression was used to compare survival after adjusting for baseline characteristics and to investigate the prognostic significance of baseline variables.
- Methods described by Simon were used to calculate confidence limits (Simon 1986).

CONCLUSION OF TRIAL
- In a higher-risk group of patients with early-stage epithelial ovarian cancer, the 5-year survival was approximately 80% and did not differ

Table 1.2 Results of GOG 7602

Treatment arm	Melphalan N=68 evaluable	^{32}P N=73 evaluable	Statistics
Patient characteristics			
Median age	51 years	52 years	
Residual tumor	2.9%	5.5%	
Stage Ia$_i$	4.4%	1.4%	
Stage Ia$_{ii}$	16.2%	23.3%	
Stage Ib$_{ii}$	7.4%	0%	
Stage Ic	11.8%	9.6%	
Stage IIa	0%	6.9%	
Stage IIb	44.1%	46.6%	
Stage IIc	16.2%	12.3%	
Serous	13.2%	26.0%	
Endometrioid	22.1%	26.0%	
Mucinous	19.1%	13.7%	
Clear cell	19.1%	13.7%	
Other	26.4%	20.5%	
Grade 1	25.0%	28.8%	
Grade 2	26.8%	27.4%	
Grade 3	14.7%	15.1%	
Reclassified as LMP	14.7%	19.2%	
Efficacy			
Recurrences	N=13	N=14	
Deaths			
Ovarian cancer, primary	N=10	N=12	
Ovarian cancer, secondary	N=0	N=2	
Complication	N=2	N=0	
Other	N=3	N=2	
5-year survival	81%	78%	
Toxicity			
Myelosuppression	74%		
GI toxicity	16%		
Death, pre-leukemia	N=2		
Abdominal pain, mild-moderate		21%	
Abdominal pain, severe		6%	
Surgery, bowel obstruction		6%	

LMP, low malignant potential.

between adjuvant oral melphalan and intraperitoneal ^{32}P. Given the 20% recurrence rate, adjuvant therapy should be administered to this group of patients, and ^{32}P is preferred over melphalan because of its limited toxicity and no known risk of leukemia.

COMMENTS

- Clear cell tumors had poorer outcomes. When considering patients who had central pathology review, 35% (9 of 26) of patients with clear cell tumors relapsed compared to 15% (16 of 107) of patients with other histologic tumor types.
- Melphalan use was associated with risk of myeloproliferative disorders and acute leukemia. These complications are uncommon but a known catastrophic risk (Reimer et al. 1977; Greene et al. 1982).
- The 5-year survival of 80% in this trial is substantially better than the previously reported 5-year survival rates of 40% to 60% in other trials. While the comprehensive surgical staging mandated in this trail may have identified a group with better prognosis, it is impossible to know what impact this had on survival within this trial.
- The majority of recurrences were distant (32%) or abdominal (39%), confirming prior observations that the entire abdominal cavity is at risk of recurrence.
- ^{32}P was considered the preferred adjuvant treatment arm from this trial. Given the evidence of efficacy of platinum-containing regimens in advanced ovarian cancer (Decker et al. 1982; Levin and Hryniuk 1987; Neijt et al. 1987), the GOG has designed a replacement trial comparing intraperitoneal ^{32}P with 3 cycles of cyclophosphamide and cisplatin (GOG 95).
- Patients with borderline tumors were evenly distributed between treatment arms, and the comparisons of therapeutic efficacy were not affected by the exclusion of these patients in the analysis.

GICOG Trials (Bolis, Ann Oncol 1995)

REFERENCE

- Bolis G, et al. Adjuvant treatment for early epithelial ovarian cancer: results of two randomised clinical trials comparing cisplatin to no further treatment or chromic phosphate (32P). G.I.C.O.G.: Gruppo Interregionale Collaborativo in Ginecologia Oncologica. *Ann Oncol.* 1995;6(9):887-893. PMID: 8624291. (Bolis et al. 1995)

TRIAL SPONSOR
- Gruppo Interregionale Collaborativo in Oncologico Ginecologia (GICOG), Italy

RATIONALE FOR TRIAL
- Postoperative therapy for early stage ovarian cancer is controversial.
- Approximately 30% of patients die of disease despite appropriate surgery.
- There is a small subset of patients with early-stage ovarian cancer who require no further treatment after surgery (stage IA, grade 1), but there is a lack of consensus about whether other early-stage patients benefit from postoperative adjuvant therapy (NIH consensus conference . . . 1995).
- Three different adjuvant treatment approaches have been used—including abdominopelvic radiotherapy, intraperitoneal radioactive chromic phosphate (^{32}P), and chemotherapy—but most trials have lacked adequate sample size and power to detect significant differences among the treatment groups (Smith et al. 1975; Dembo et al. 1979; Hreshchyshyn et al. 1980; Gronroos et al. 1984; Klaassen et al. 1988; Young et al. 1990; Vergote et al. 1992; Redman et al. 1993).
- This report is of 2 multicenter randomized trials from Italy to determine the efficacy of cisplatin in adjuvant treatment of early-stage ovarian cancer.

PATIENT POPULATION
- N=271 enrolled in 2 randomized trials.
- Enrollment from March 1983 to October 1990.
- Enrollment per FIGO 1976 staging criteria.

Inclusion Criteria
- Trial 1: stage IA and stage IB, grade 2 or 3 early ovarian cancer.
- Trial 2: stage Ia_{ii}, Ib_{ii}, Ic early ovarian cancer.
- No prior therapy except surgery.
- Age <75 years.
- No previous or simultaneous cancers.
- Adequate bone marrow, liver, and renal function.
- No concomitant diseases precluding the use of trial treatments.
- Randomization within 42 days of initial surgery.

TREATMENT DETAILS

Surgical Staging
- Vertical incision to completely visualize abdominal cavity.
- Abdominal hysterectomy, bilateral salpingo-oophorectomy, and infracolic omentectomy.
- Pelvic and para-aortic lymph node addressed by palpation and biopsied (selective when suspicious).
- Random biopsies of liver, diaphragm, pelvic, and abdominal peritoneal surfaces.
- Cytologic examination of pelvic and abdominal free fluid or washings.

Trial 1
- Arm 1: no further therapy.
- Arm 2: cisplatin 50 mg/m^2 every 28 days for 6 cycles.

Trial 2
- Arm 1: ^{32}P.
- Arm 2: cisplatin 50 mg/m^2 every 28 days for 6 cycles.
- Note that from February 1988 to January 1989, there was a shortage of ^{32}P, and all patients enrolled during this time frame received cisplatin. Because randomization was not possible, the principal analysis was removed from all patients enrolled during this period.

Cisplatin Administration (Trials 1 and 2)
- Antiemetic prophylaxis with metoclopramide and/or dexamethasone and/or benzodiazepines.
- Hydration with normal saline 500 mL over 1 hour prior to cisplatin and 2 L of normal saline (with 40 mEq potassium chloride) over 6 hours after cisplatin infusion.
- Postponed for up to 2 weeks if serum creatinine >2 mg/100 mL or 24-hour creatinine clearance was below 50 mL/min. Discontinued if values persisted beyond 4 weeks.

^{32}P Administration (Trial 2)
- 7 to 109 mCi-260-370 MBq.
- Injected into the abdomen in 2 L normal saline.

ASSESSMENTS
- Presurgical staging procedures.
  - Chest radiography, intravenous pyelography, and lymphangiography.
  - If indicated: pelvic ultrasonography, pelvic and abdominal CT scan, barium enema, and proctosigmoidoscopy.

- Toxicity recorded according to World Health Organization recommendations (Miller et al. 1981).
- Followed every 3 months for 2 years and every 6 to 12 months thereafter.
- CT scans, chest x-rays, and ultrasounds assessments were done when clinically indicted.
- CA125 had been used on a routine basis since 1987 but was not used as proof or recurrence in the absence of other positive findings.

ENDPOINTS

- Overall survival.
- Relapse-free survival.

STATISTICAL CONSIDERATIONS

- Kaplan-Meier curves used to describe survival curves (Kaplan and Meier 1958).
- Cumulative incidence was calculated to describe the pattern of different relapses (Gelman et al. 1990).
- Log-rank test and Cox proportional hazards regression model were used to test the significance of chemotherapy effect (Cox 1972; Peto and Peto 1972).
- Cox analysis with backward selection procedure was used to select among baseline covariates, including age, grade, histotype, and surgical vs clinical nodal assessment.
- A global test of heterogeneity comparing a model with covariates plus the factor of interest to one with only covariates was used to test the prognostic role of categorical variables with more than 2 levels (Cox 1972).
- Cutoff date for analysis was December 1993: median follow-up time was 76 months, and maximum observation time was 121 months.

CONCLUSION OF TRIAL

- This is the first trial to demonstrate a reduced relapse rate with use of adjuvant cisplatin chemotherapy in patients with early-stage ovarian cancer. The impact of cisplatin use on survival remains unclear.

COMMENTS

- Cisplatin was dosed at 50 mg/m^2 in both trials, and this is not considered a suboptimal dose.

Table 1.3 Results of GICOG Trial 1

Treatment arm	Observation N=44	Cisplatin N=41	Statistics
Patient characteristics			
Age <45	21.4%	21.9%	
Age 45-55	30.9%	30.7%	
Age >55	57.6%	46.3%	
Stage I	100%	100%	
Serous	30.9%	43.9%	
Endometrioid	23.8%	17.1%	
Mucinous	16.7%	26.8%	
Clear cell	23.8%	9.8%	
Other	4.8%	2.4%	
Grades 1-2	76.2%	58.5%	
Grade 3	23.8%	41.5%	
Lymph nodes			
Clinical assessment	57.1%	65.8%	
Surgical assessment	42.9%	34.1%	
Treatment delivery			
No dose modification	NA	92%	
Efficacy			
Recurrences	35%	17%	
Pelvis only	14%	6%	
Nodes only	3%	3%	
Abdominal	18%	8%	
5-year DFS	65%	83%	HR 0.48 (0.20-1.14)
Deaths	18%	12%	
Ovarian cancer	18%	7%	
Other causes	0%	5%	
5-year OS	82%	88%	HR 1.15 (0.44-2.98)
Toxicity			
Nausea/vomiting	Not reported	>66%	

DFS, disease-free survival; HR, hazard ratio; NA, not applicable; OS, overall survival.

- At time of recurrence, patients initially treated with adjuvant cisplatin had a greater risk of dying compared to the patients initially treated with ^{32}P or observation. This suggests that these patients might have a more virulent disease or resistance to chemotherapy. Two trials are evaluating the question of immediate platinum therapy vs delaying

Table 1.4 Results GICOG Trial 2

Treatment arm	^{32}P N=79	Cisplatin N=82	Statistics
Patient characteristics			
Age <45	24.0%	22.1%	
Age 45-55	44.0%	37.7%	
Age >55	32.0%	40.3%	
Stage I	100%	100%	
Serous	38.7%	40.3%	
Endometrioid	25.3%	25.4%	
Mucinous	9.3%	13.0%	
Clear cell	20.0%	20.8%	
Other	6.7%	2.6%	
Grades 1-2	72.0%	71.4%	
Grade 3	28.0%	28.6%	
Lymph nodes			
Clinical assessment	45.3%	55.8%	
Surgical assessment	54.7%	44.2%	
Treatment delivery			
No dose modification	Not reported	92%	
Could not be implanted	15 of 75 eligible	N/A	
Efficacy			
Recurrences	34%	15%	
Pelvis only	16%	7%	
Nodes only	3%	0%	
Abdominal	15%	8%	
5-year DFS	65%	85%	HR 0.42 (0.22-0.80)
Deaths	21%	19%	
Ovarian cancer	21%	16%	
Other causes	0%	3%	
5-year OS	79%	81%	0.72 (0.37-1.43)
Toxicity			
Nausea/vomiting	Not reported	>66%	

DFS, disease-free survival; HR, hazard ratio; OS, overall survival.

platinum therapy to the time of relapse (Trimbos 1991; Ghersi et al. 1992).
- Lymphadenectomy did not appear to play an important prognostic role in these trials.

- These 2 trials demonstrate the cisplatin is active, even when used at low doses. The authors conclude that in non-high-risk patients, treatment should only be administered at the time of relapse (stage IA, grade 1). Whether or not adjuvant chemotherapy should be administered for stage IC disease is still unclear.

GOG 95 (Young, JCO 2003)

REFERENCE

- Young RC, Brady MF, Nieberg RK, et al. Adjuvant treatment for early ovarian cancer: a randomized phase III trial of intraperitoneal ^{32}P or intravenous cyclophosphamide and cisplatin—a gynecologic oncology group study. *J Clin Oncol.* 2003;21(23):4350-4305. PMID: 14645424. (Young et al. 2003)

TRIAL SPONSORS

- Gynecologic Oncology Group (GOG)
- North Central Cancer Treatment Group (NCCTG)
- Southwest Oncology Group (SWOG)

RATIONALE FOR TRIAL

- Among patients with early-stage ovarian cancer, approximately 20% with stage I and 50% with stage II will die of recurrent disease.
- Trials conducted by the GOG and others defined a subset of patients (stage IA and IB, grade 1) who have >90% chance for long-term survival without additional treatment beyond surgery (Dembo et al. 1979; Klaassen et al. 1988; Young et al. 1990; Vergote et al. 2001).
- For higher-risk patients with early disease, platinum or platinum/^{32}P combinations have demonstrated modest benefit, but no trial has been definitive (Vergote et al. 1992; Bolis et al. 1995).
- The GOG began a randomized trial in 1986 to compare ^{32}P with cyclophosphamide and cisplatin in patients with early-stage ovarian cancer and a high risk for recurrence. This manuscript summarizes the mature results of the trial with a median follow-up of 10 years.

PATIENT POPULATION

- N=251 enrolled.
- Accrual between 1986 and 1994.

Inclusion Criteria
- Early-stage ovarian cancer after definitive surgery and no macroscopic residual disease.
- Stage IA or IB (grade 3), stage IC or II (any grade), or any stage I or II with clear cell histology.
- Adequate bone marrow, renal, and hepatic function.
- Surgical staging was generally done through a vertical midline incision and included a total abdominal hysterectomy, bilateral salpingo-oophorectomy, partial infracolic omentectomy, and resection of all gross disease. The tumor capsule was examined for rupture, excrescences, or any adhesions requiring sharp dissection. Peritoneal fluid volume was estimated and aspirated, or separate washings from the pelvis, paracolic gutter, and infradiaphragmatic areas were sent. All peritoneal surfaces (including the undersurfaces of both diaphragms, serosa, and mesentery) were to be visually inspected and palpated for evidence of implants. If there was no visible metastatic disease, biopsies of the cul-de-sac, vesico-uterine peritoneum, bilateral pelvic side walls, paracolic gutters, undersurface of the diaphragm, and sampling of the pelvic and para-aortic lymph nodes were performed.

Exclusion Criteria
- Borderline or low malignant potential tumors were excluded.

TREATMENT DETAILS

Arm 1: intraperitoneal ^{32}P
- Single dose of 15 mCi intraperitoneal ^{32}P.
- Before administration of ^{32}P, ^{99}m technetium or radio-opaque contrast material was used to evaluate the adequacy of intraperitoneal distribution. Those with inadequate distribution were not treated.

Arm 2: Cyclophosphamide and Cisplatin
- Cyclophosphamide 1 g/m^2.
- Cisplatin 100 mg/m^2.
- Three cycles every 21 days.

ASSESSMENTS
- Not specified in manuscript.

ENDPOINTS
- Not specified in manuscript.

STATISTICAL CONSIDERATIONS

Sample Size

- Planned sample size was 200 patients until at least 28 deaths were reported in the ^{32}P arm.
- Assuming a proportional hazards model, the planned sample size would provide greater than 80% chance of detecting a true treatment effect, improving the 5-year survival rate from 80% to 90% with a type I error of 0.05 for a 1-tail log-rank test.

Statistical Tests

- Kaplan-Meier used to estimate cumulative survival function (Kaplan and Meier 1958).
- Proportional hazards model used to estimate the crude and adjusted hazards ratios (Cox 1972).
- Cumulative or marginal incidence of recurrence used to estimate the probability of recurrence in the presence of competing risks (Gaynor et al. 1993). This is the preferred method when there are competing risks. Methods that treat noncancer deaths as censored survival times tend to overestimate the probability of recurrence.

CONCLUSION OF TRIAL

- In early-stage epithelial ovarian cancer at high risk for recurrence, there was no difference in survival between adjuvant ^{32}P or cyclophosphamide (C) and cisplatin (P), (CP). However, there was lower cumulative recurrence with CP, making this the preferred adjuvant therapy for this patient population.

COMMENTS

- Ten-year probability of recurrence varied by stage.
  - 27% risk for stage I.
  - 44% risk for stage II.
- Ten-year survival rate for all patients on this trial was 68%.
- Other prognostic indicators:
  - Presence of ascites was associated with a higher risk of recurrence after adjusting for stage and grade.
  - Clear cell histology had a relapse rate similar to grade 1 tumors in this trial.
- While both therapies were well tolerated, there were difficulties with ^{32}P administration.

Table 1.5 Results of GOG 95

Treatment arm	^{32}P N=110	Cyclophosphamide+ Cisplatin (CP) N=119	Statistics
Patient characteristics			
Age <49	30.9%	24.3%	
Age 50-69	52.7%	60.5%	
Age >70	16.4%	15.1%	
Stage IA	8.2%	13.4%	
Stage IB	0.9%	2.5%	
Stage IC	61.8%	52.9%	
Stage IIA	3.6%	8.4%	
Stage IIB	2.7%	6.7%	
Stage IIC	22.7%	16.0%	
Serous	22.7%	18.5%	
Endometrioid	26.4%	27.7%	
Mucinous	10.9%	16.0%	
Clear cell	23.6%	21.0%	
Other	16.3%	16.7%	
Grade 1	25.5%	25.2%	
Grade 2	23.6%	27.7%	
Grade 3	27.3%	26.1%	
Clear cell	23.6%	21.0%	
Treatment delivery			
Did not receive treatment	N=10	N=1	
Efficacy			
10-year recurrence rate	35%	28%	29% lower with CP (NS)
Overall survival			17% lower with CP (NS)
Toxicity			
Leukopenia	0%	69.5%	
Granulocytopenia	0%	65.0%	
Thrombocytopenia	0%	8.5%	
Gastrointestinal	4.0%	11.9%	
Renal	0%	1.7%	

CP, cyclophosphamide+cisplatin; NS, not significant.

- ○ 7% had inadequate distribution.
- ○ 3% had small bowel perforation.
- Although there is no difference in survival between treatment arms, the lower recurrence with chemotherapy and the difficulties with ^{32}P administration make chemotherapy the preferred treatment regimen. These data are consistent with those of 2 prior prospective trials.

- The Norwegian Radium Hospital trial compared ^{32}P to cisplatin in 347 patients with completely resected stage I to III ovarian cancer. There was no difference in 5-year disease-free survival. Late bowel complications occurred more frequently with ^{32}P (9% vs 2%) (Vergote et al. 1992).
  - An Italian multicenter trial compared ^{32}P to cisplatin in patients with stage IA_{ii}, IB_{ii}, and IC ovarian cancer. The 5-year disease-free survival rate was better with cisplatin (85% vs 65%, $P=.008$). There was no difference in overall survival (Bolis et al. 1995).
- Putting this trial in the context of the ACTION and ICON1 trials (Colombo et al. 2003; Trimbos et al. 2003a; Trimbos et al. 2003b), data support the use of platinum-based chemotherapy for high-risk stage I and II ovarian cancer. Whether surgical staging will allow for exclusion of adjuvant chemotherapy requires further study.
- While this trial advocates for the use of cisplatin and cyclophosphamide, better adjuvant therapy is required. In this trial, only 65% of stage I and 52% of stage II patients are expected to be alive and free of recurrent ovarian cancer.

ICON1/ACTION Combined Analysis (Trimbos, JNCI 2003)

REFERENCE

- Trimbos JB, et al. International Collaborative Ovarian Neoplasm trial 1 and Adjuvant ChemoTherapy in Ovarian Neoplasm trial: two parallel randomized phase III trials of adjuvant chemotherapy in patients with early-stage ovarian carcinoma. *J Natl Cancer Inst.* 2003a;95(2):105-112. PMID: 12529343. (Trimbos et al. 2003a)

TRIAL SPONSORS

- European Organization of Research and Treatment in Cancer (EORTC)
- Adjuvant ChemoTherapy in Ovarian Neoplasm Trial (ACTION)
- International Collaborative Ovarian Neoplasm (ICON1)

RATIONALE FOR TRIAL

- The question of adjuvant therapy to improve survival in women with early-stage ovarian cancer has not been reliably answered to date.
- Patients with well or moderately differentiated early-stage ovarian cancer (stages I-IIA) may be treated with surgery alone.

- However, because the 5-year survival rate has been reported to be as low as 50% based on stage and grade of the tumor, various trials have investigated the use of adjuvant chemotherapy to improve survival outcomes.
- Whole abdominal radiation with intraperitoneal radioactive chromic phosphate (Richardson et al. 1985).
- GOG trial of observation vs melphalan (Young et al. 1990) included only 46 patients. No difference was found in the 2 arms.
- Italian trial of observation vs cisplatin included only 83 patients (Bolis et al. 1995). Cisplatin improved disease-free survival (hazard ratio [HR], 0.35; 95% confidence interval [CI], 0.14-0.89) but did not impact overall survival (HR, 1.15; 95% CI, 0.44-2.98).
- Scandinavian study of observation vs carboplatin included only 162 patients (Trope et al. 2000). No difference was found in the 2 arms.
- This was a preplanned combined analysis of 2 parallel, randomized controlled trials that compared platinum-based adjuvant chemotherapy with observation after surgery for early-stage ovarian cancer.
  - ICON1: International Collaborative Ovarian Neoplasm 1.
  - ACTION: Adjuvant ChemoTherapy in Ovarian Neoplasm.

PATIENT POPULATION
- N=925; 477 in ICON1 and 448 in ACTION.
- Enrollment between November 1990 and January 2000.

Eligibility for ACTION
- High-risk early-stage ovarian cancer, defined as FIGO stage IA and IB with grade 2 or 3 tumor; all grades of FIGO stages IC to IIA; all clear cell carcinomas.
- Strict guidelines given for comprehensive surgical staging.

Eligibility for ICON1
- All patients with histologically confirmed epithelial ovarian cancer were eligible if the clinician was uncertain whether or not the patient would benefit from immediate adjuvant chemotherapy. Patients of all stages were potentially eligible, but the majority who were enrolled had stage I or II disease.
- Guidelines for surgical staging: total hysterectomy, bilateral salpingo-oophorectomy, and omentectomy (total supracolonic omentectomy if grossly involved or removal of the distal 2 cm if grossly normal).

TREATMENT DETAILS

Arm 1: Observation
- Patients received chemotherapy at the time of confirmed recurrence.

Arm 2: Chemotherapy
- ACTION: At least 4 cycles of platinum-based regimen.
  - Single-agent carboplatin.
  - Single-agent cisplatin.
  - Combination carboplatin.
  - Combination cisplatin.
- ICON1: 6 courses of platinum-based adjuvant chemotherapy.
  - CAP: cyclophosphamide (C) + doxorubicin/Adriamycin (A) + cisplatin (P).
  - Single-agent carboplatin.
  - Other regimens that included platinum at a predefined minimum dose.

ASSESSMENTS
- Confirmation of recurrence.
  - ACTION: cytologic or histologic confirmation.
  - ICON1: clinical, radiologic, or histologic diagnosis.

ENDPOINTS
- Overall survival for both studies (primary endpoint).
- Recurrence-free survival for both studies.

STATISTICAL CONSIDERATIONS
- Analyzed by intention-to-treat basis.
- All statistical tests were 2-sided.
- Stratified log-rank test (by trial) used to compare survival between treatment arms.
- Log-rank statistics used to calculate hazard ratios.
- Kaplan-Meier curves to compare survival curves.
- Exploratory subgroup analyses were performed to determine whether the effect of chemotherapy was different based on age, tumor stage, histologic cell type, and cell differentiation.
- χ^2 test for interaction or trend was used to compare differences in relative effect size.

Table 1.6 Results of ICON1/ACTION Combined Analysis

Treatment arm	Observation N=460	Platinum based N=465	Statistics
Patient characteristics			
Age <55	51%	50%	
Age 55-65	32%	27%	
Age >65	17%	23%	
Stage I	<1%	2%	
Stage IA	38%	36%	
Stage IB	9%	10%	
Stage IC	45%	45%	
Stage II	6%	7%	
Stage III	1%	<1%	
Missing	N=2	N=1	
Serous	31%	36%	
Endometrioid	29%	21%	
Mucinous	20%	20%	
Clear cell	13%	15%	
Other	6%	7%	
Missing	N=14	N=20	
Grade 1	23%	22%	
Grade 2	46%	47%	
Grade 3	32%	32%	
Unknown grade	N=16	N=19	
Treatment delivery			
Single-agent carboplatin		57%	
Combination cisplatin		27%	
Not received		6%	
Combination carboplatin		6%	
Single-agent cisplatin		3%	
CAP		2%	
Missing		N=40	
Efficacy			
5-year OS	74%	82%	HR 0.67 (0.50-0.90)
5-year RFS	65%	76%	HR 0.64 (0.50-0.82)
Toxicity	Not reported	Not reported	

CAP, cyclophosphamide+Adriamycin/doxorubicin+cisplatin; HR, hazard ratio; OS, overall survival; RFS, recurrence-free survival.

- Systematic review of literature to identify all similarly performed trials in early-stage ovarian cancer comparing platinum-based chemotherapy to observation.
  - Pooled hazard ratio calculated to represent the overall risk of an event on immediate chemotherapy vs an event during observation.
  - χ^2 test for heterogeneity was used to test for statistical heterogeneity in all trials.

CONCLUSION OF TRIAL

- The combined analysis of the ICON1 and ACTION trials demonstrates that platinum-based adjuvant chemotherapy improves overall survival and recurrence-free survival at 5 years in patients with early-stage ovarian cancer.

COMMENTS

- There was no evidence that the effect of adjuvant chemotherapy was any different for any subgroups analyzed.
  - Subgroup analysis for staging completeness could not be done because information about surgical staging was not collected in ICON1.
  - Definitive conclusions are limited by small numbers within the subsets.
- Kaplan-Meier survival curves demonstrate an early and sustained separation of the curves for both overall survival (OS) and recurrence-free survival (RFS).
- The results of both individual trials are similar to one another, with both demonstrating a benefit from adjuvant chemotherapy administration (Colombo et al. 2003; Trimbos et al. 2003b).
- Overall survival.
  - ACTION: HR, 0.69 (0.44-1.08).
  - ICON1: HR, 0.66 (0.45-0.97).
- Recurrence-free survival.
  - ACTION: HR, 0.63 (0.44-0.92).
  - ICON1: HR, 0.65 (0.46-0.91).
- Systematic review of the literature identified 8 randomized trials comparing adjuvant chemotherapy to observation in early-stage ovarian cancer.
  - Four trials used melphalan or other non-platinum-based chemotherapy and were of limited relevance to clinical practice at the time (Hreshchyshyn et al. 1980; Krafft et al. 1980; Sigurdsson et al. 1982; Young et al. 1990).

- ○ Four trials, including ACTION and ICON1, were analyzed to provide a pooled estimate of the impact of platinum-based adjuvant chemotherapy (Bolis et al. 1995; Trope et al. 2000; Colombo et al. 2003; Trimbos et al. 2003b).
- ○ Pooled HR for OS: 0.72 (0.55-0.94; $P = .17$).
- ○ Pooled HR for RFS: 0.66 (0.53-0.83; $P < .001$).
- ○ No evidence for heterogeneity between the trials.
- Only one-sixth of the patients in this trial were optimally staged.
- While some might use this trial to justify the administration of platinum-based chemotherapy to the majority of patients with early-stage ovarian cancer, some might argue that evidence to support the use of adjuvant chemotherapy in optimally staged patients is lacking.
- Approximately 20% to 25% of patients with incompletely staged early ovarian cancer will have occult stage III disease (Piver et al. 1978; Piver 1982; Young et al. 1983; Helewa et al. 1986). This might explain the beneficial effect seen with adjuvant chemotherapy in the ICON1/ACTION trials.
- This trial suggests that single-agent carboplatin may be the treatment of choice for early-stage ovarian cancer.
- Strengths of the combined analysis include the large number of patients included as well as the consistent results across the 2 trials.

ACTION (Trimbos, JNCI 2003; Trimbos, JNCI 2010)

REFERENCES

- Trimbos JB, et al. Impact of adjuvant chemotherapy and surgical staging in early-stage ovarian carcinoma: European Organisation for Research and Treatment of Cancer-Adjuvant ChemoTherapy in Ovarian Neoplasm trial. *J Natl Cancer Inst*. 2003b;95(2):113-125. PMID: 12529344. (Trimbos et al. 2003b)
- Trimbos B, et al. Surgical staging and treatment of early ovarian cancer: long-term analysis from a randomized trial. *J Natl Cancer Inst*. 2010;102(13):982-987. PMID: 20445161. (Trimbos et al. 2010)

TRIAL SPONSORS

- European Organization for Research and Treatment of Cancer (EORTC)
- Adjuvant ChemoTherapy in Ovarian Neoplasm (ACTION)

RATIONALE FOR TRIAL
- Approximately 10% to 50% of patients with early-stage ovarian cancer treated with surgery have a recurrence. This high recurrence rate has led to various attempts to use adjuvant treatment.
- A GOG trial randomized patients with stage IA or IB and grade 1 or 2 ovarian cancer to observation or oral melphalan following surgery. There was no survival difference, and although the number of patients in the trial was too small to draw definitive conclusions, the authors advocated for withholding chemotherapy for patients with comprehensively staged, low-grade, early-stage ovarian cancer (Young et al. 1990).
- An Italian study randomized patients with early stage-ovarian cancer to observation or cisplatin chemotherapy after surgery. Chemotherapy led to a decrease in recurrence-free survival (HR, 0.35; 95% CI, 0.14-0.89) but no difference in overall survival (HR, 1.15; 95% CI, 0.44-2.98). Salvage therapy was more effective in patients in the observation arm. The authors advocated for deferring chemotherapy until the time of recurrence (Bolis et al. 1995).
- A Scandinavian study randomized 162 patients with early-stage ovarian cancer to observation or carboplatin following surgery. There was no difference in disease-specific survival (HR, 0.94; 95% CI, 0.37-2.36) or overall survival (HR, 0.98; 95% CI, 0.52-1.83) (Trope et al. 2000).
- All prior randomized trials of adjuvant chemotherapy in early-stage ovarian cancer have lacked statistical power to demonstrate an impact on survival. Prior trials have not accounted for the adequacy of surgical staging. Approximately 24% of non–optimally staged patients with early-stage ovarian cancer have occult stage III disease (Young et al. 1983; Helewa et al. 1986; Soper et al. 1992; Schueler et al. 1998).
- The ACTION trial was a phase III trial conducted to test the efficacy of adjuvant chemotherapy on survival in patients with early-stage ovarian cancer with an emphasis on the extent of surgical staging.

PATIENT POPULATION
- N=448.
- Enrollment between November 1990 and January 2000 from 40 centers in 9 European countries.

Inclusion Criteria
- Epithelial ovarian cancer.
  - FIGO stages IA-IB, grades 2-3

- All stages IC and IIA.
  - All stages I to IIA with clear cell histology.
- Surgical treatment.
  - Total abdominal hysterectomy, bilateral salpingo-oophorectomy, surgical staging.
  - Conservative surgery consisting of unilateral salpingo-oophorectomy and surgical staging permitted for stage IA cancers (Zanetta et al. 1997; Morice et al. 2001).
  - Surgical staging had to consist of at least careful inspection and palpation of peritoneal surfaces, biopsies of suspicious lesions.
- Staging categories.
  - Optimal: inspection and palpation of all peritoneal surfaces, biopsies of any suspicious lesions, peritoneal washings, infracolic omentectomy, peritoneal washings, blind biopsies (from the pouch of Douglas, bladder, pelvic sidewalls, paracolic gutters, right hemidiaphragm), iliac and periaortic lymph node sampling.
  - Modified: anything between optimal and minimal staging.
  - Minimal: inspection and palpation of all peritoneal surfaces and the retroperitoneal area, biopsies of any suspicious lesions for metastases, peritoneal washings, and infracolic omentectomy.
  - Inadequate: less than minimal staging but at least careful inspection and palpation of all peritoneal surfaces and the retroperitoneal area, biopsies of any suspicious lesions for metastases.

Exclusion Criteria
- Prior or concomitant second malignancy.
- WHO performance status greater than 3.
- Prior treatment with chemotherapy or radiation therapy.
- Expected inadequacy of follow-up.
- Interval of more than 6 weeks between surgery and randomization.

TREATMENT DETAILS

Arm 1: Observation
- After surgery, no treatment until recurrence.

Arm 2: Chemotherapy
- At least 4 courses of a platinum-based regimen following surgery, but 6 courses were recommended.
- Allowed regimens.
  - Single-agent platinum of cisplatin 75 mg/m^2.

- ◦ Single-agent platinum of carboplatin 350 mg/m^2.
- ◦ Combination platinum-based regimens.
- Dose modifications for drug toxicity.
- Each center had to define its adjuvant chemotherapy regimen and stay with that regimen for the duration of the trial.

Treatment After Recurrence
- Confirmed cytologically or histologically.
- Had to be the same chemotherapy regimen utilized by the center in the adjuvant treatment arm.

ASSESSMENTS
- No details in manuscript.

ENDPOINTS
- Overall survival (primary endpoint).
- Recurrence-free survival.

STATISTICAL CONSIDERATIONS

Stratification Factors
- Institution.
- FIGO stage.
- Grade of tumor differentiation.

Sample Size
- Sample size was set arbitrarily to at least 1000 patients to account for the long life expectancy of patients with early-stage ovarian cancer and the small expected improvement in survival with chemotherapy.
- Interim analyses were performed at fixed intervals.
- Consideration was given to stopping the trial if the P value for the comparison of survival between treatment arms fell below .01.
- The committee closed the study in 2000 before the target accrual was achieved because patient accrual took longer than expected.

Statistical Tests
- Kaplan-Meier method for time-to-event analysis.
- Log-rank test to compare survival.
- Cox proportional hazards regression model to analyze prognostic factors.

Table 1.7 Results of ACTION Trial

Treatment arm	Observation N=224	Chemotherapy N=224	Statistics
Patient characteristics			
Median age (range)	55 (22-77)	54 (18-84)	
Stage IA	33%	35%	
Stage IB	8%	8%	
Stage IC	51%	50%	
Stage IIA	7%	7%	
Missing	1%	0%	
Serous	33%	37%	
Endometrioid	32%	19%	
Mucinous	16%	19%	
Clear cell	12%	17%	
Other/unknown	7%	6%	
Grade 1	12%	12%	
Grade 2	51%	50%	
Grade 3	35%	35%	
Unknown grade	2%	3%	
Optimal staging	34%	34%	
Modified staging	30%	31%	
Minimal staging	27%	24%	
Inadequate staging	9%	11%	
Missing information	1%	0%	
Treatment delivery			
Cisplatin + cyclophosphamide	N/A	47%	
Single-agent carboplatin	N/A	33%	
Protocol violations	13 received chemo	14 had no chemo	
Efficacy (2003)			
No recurrence	73%	82%	
Recurrence			
Locoregional recurrence	9%	6%	
Extrapelvic recurrence	13%	9%	
Combined recurrence	5%	3%	
5-year overall survival	78%	85%	HR 0.69 (0.44-1.08)
Optimally staged			No difference
Non-optimally staged			HR 1.75 (1.04-2.95)
5-year recurrence-free survival	68%	76%	HR 0.63 (0.43-0.92)
Optimally staged			HR 1.14 (0.54-2.39)
Non-optimally staged			HR 1.78 (1.15-2.77)

Table 1.7 Results of ACTION Trial *(continued)*

Treatment arm	Observation N=224	Chemotherapy N=224	Statistics
Efficacy (2010, long-term follow-up)			
Recurrences	38.8%	27.2%	
10-year cancer-specific survival	76%	82%	HR 0.73 (0.48-1.13)
Optimally staged	89%	85%	HR 1.58 (0.61-4.08)
Non-optimally staged	69%	80%	HR 0.58 (0.35-0.95)
10-year recurrence-free survival	62%	70%	HR 0.64 (0.46-0.89)
Optimally staged	72%	78%	HR 0.73 (0.38-1.42)
Non-optimally staged	56%	65%	HR 0.60 (0.41-0.87)
Toxicity			
Not reported			

HR, hazard ratio.

- χ^2 test for interaction to compare difference in relative size of treatment effects between subgroups of staging performance.
- In the 2010 publication of long-term follow up, the median follow-up was 10.1 years (with a cutoff date of May 23, 2008). The analysis was repeated using cancer-specific survival to reduce the bias of deaths from causes other than ovarian cancer (this risk increases with the duration of follow-up).
- Cancer-specific survival was measured from date of randomization to date of death from ovarian cancer. Data were censored at time of last known date alive for patients who had died of causes other than ovarian cancer.
- Recurrence-free survival was measured from date of randomization to date of first documented date of recurrence or death from any cause.

CONCLUSION OF TRIAL

- With 5.5 years of follow-up: In patients with early stage ovarian cancer, adjuvant chemotherapy improved recurrence-free survival. The benefit was limited to patients with nonoptimal staging (ie, patients with more risk of undiagnosed residual disease). In this cohort of patients, of whom two-thirds had undergone nonoptimal surgical staging, there was no difference in overall survival observed.

- With 10.1 years of follow-up: Long-term analyses supported the original conclusions of the trial but now show that optimal surgical staging is associated with improved overall survival. The benefit to adjuvant chemotherapy was limited to patients with nonoptimal surgical staging.

COMMENTS

- Prognostic factors for recurrence-free and overall survival included
  - Staging adequacy
  - Tumor grade
- This study did not find stage to be a prognostic factor. Stage IC disease was not associated with a higher risk of recurrence or death compared to moderately or poorly differentiated stage IA and IB disease. This might be important to consider when defining high-risk early-stage ovarian cancer.
- Of the 448 patients, 151 had optimal staging.
  - Among patients in the observation arm, nonoptimal staging was associated with worse overall survival (HR, 2.31; 95% CI, 1.08-4.96) and recurrence-free survival (HR, 1.82; 95% CI, 1.02-3.24) compared to patients undergoing optimal staging.
  - Among patients receiving adjuvant chemotherapy, there was no difference in overall or recurrence-free survival.
- Because this study demonstrated that the poorer prognosis of non–optimally staged patients could be corrected by administration of adjuvant chemotherapy, chemotherapy may have its impact on treating small-volume occult implants and metastases.
- There was a difference in salvage rates in patients treated for recurrent disease.
  - In non–optimally staged patients, the salvage rates after observation and chemotherapy were similar (70% and 64%).
  - In optimally staged patients, salvage chemotherapy was more successful after observation than after adjuvant chemotherapy (75% and 46%).
  - If this were a reproducible finding in other studies, these data would provide support to postponing chemotherapy until time of recurrence, as long as optimal surgical staging had been performed.
- Adjuvant chemotherapy is effective in patients with occult residual disease (due to nonoptimal surgical staging).

ACTION

Table 1.8 ACTION Trial: Efficacy at Long-Term Follow-Up

Efficacy (2010, long-term follow-up)	Optimal	Nonoptimal	Statistics
10-year cancer-specific survival			
Observation	89%	69%	HR 3.28 (1.47-7.33)
Chemotherapy	85%	80%	HR 1.27 (0.62-2.58)
10-year recurrence-free survival			
Observation	72%	56%	HR 1.91 (1.17-3.11)
Chemotherapy	78%	65%	HR 1.64 (0.91-2.93)

HR, hazard ratio.

Table 1.9 ACTION Trial: Efficacy at Long-Term Follow-Up, Limited to Grade 3 Tumors

Efficacy (2010, long-term follow-up)	Observation	Chemotherapy	Statistics
Limited to grade 3 tumors			
10-year cancer-specific survival			
Optimally staged	85%	69%	HR 2.58 (0.66-9.99)
Non-optimally staged	56%	77%	HR 0.40 (0.19-0.81)
10-year recurrence-free survival			
Optimally staged	64%	49%	HR 1.25 (0.53-2.95)
Non-optimally staged	52%	55%	HR 0.58 (0.33-1.02)

HR, hazard ratio.

- Interpretation of results from this study should include consideration for the smaller sample sizes when performing subgroup analyses.
- In long-term analysis, optimal surgical staging was associated with better survival (Table 1.8).
- While the trial makes conclusions about surgical staging procedures and survival, the trial was not originally designed to look at this question.
- In long-term analysis limited to the grade 3 tumors, administration of chemotherapy after optimal staging does not improve outcomes (Table 1.9). This may be due to the tendency for these tumors to metastasize earlier (Young et al. 1983).
- Design of this study permits no clear-cut guidelines for the treatment of all early-stage ovarian cancers. However, the authors conclude that these data support the recommendation that all patients with nonoptimal staging be offered restaging or adjuvant chemotherapy if restaging is not feasible. They further conclude that this trial provides convincing

evidence to withhold chemotherapy for optimally staged patients, including those with grade 3 tumors, and cite evidence that 20% of long-term survivors of ovarian cancer will develop secondary malignancies as a result of treatment with platinum-based chemotherapy (Travis et al. 1996).

ICON1 (Colombo, JNCI 2003)

REFERENCE

- Colombo N, et al. International Collaborative Ovarian Neoplasm trial 1: a randomized trial of adjuvant chemotherapy in women with early-stage ovarian cancer. *J Natl Cancer Inst.* 2003;95(2):125-132. PMID: 12529345. (Colombo et al. 2003)

TRIAL SPONSORS

- Three parallel trials.
  - Istituto Mario Negri in Milan, Italy.
  - Swiss Group for Clinical Cancer Research (SAAK) in Bern, Switzerland.
  - Clinical Trials Unit of the Medical Research Council (MRC CTU), Cancer Division, London, United Kingdom.

RATIONALE FOR TRIAL

- Early-stage ovarian cancer represents approximately 30% of ovarian cancers. While early-stage ovarian cancer has a better prognosis than stage III and IV disease, 50% will recur (Bjorkholm et al. 1982; Dent et al. 2000).
- Low-risk early-stage ovarian cancer is cured with surgery alone, but there is no clear consensus on what represents low-risk disease.
- No randomized trial has demonstrated a survival advantage of adjuvant therapy in early-stage ovarian cancer after surgery, including those using intraperitoneal radiation therapy, systemic chemotherapy, or abdominal and pelvic radiation therapy (Hreshchyshyn et al. 1980; Krafft et al. 1980; Sigurdsson et al. 1982; Sevelda et al. 1987; Klaassen et al. 1988; Young et al. 1990; Vergote et al. 1992; Chiara et al. 1994; Bolis et al. 1995; Fyles et al. 1998; Trope et al. 2000).
- This trial was designed to answer whether immediate adjuvant chemotherapy after surgery would improve outcomes in patients with early-stage epithelial ovarian cancer.

PATIENT POPULATION
- N = 477 enrolled.
- Enrollment between August 1991 and January 2000 from 84 centers in 5 countries (United Kingdom, Ireland, Brazil, Switzerland, and Italy).
- Anticipating the need for a large number of patients to demonstrate improved outcomes (with low rates of recurrence and death in early-stage ovarian cancer), the eligibility criteria were kept as simple as possible.
  - A patient was eligible if the clinician was unsure whether the patient required immediate chemotherapy and the patient had histologically confirmed epithelial ovarian cancer.
  - Patient fit to receive chemotherapy.
  - No prior malignant disease (except nonmelanoma skin cancer) and no prior radiation therapy or chemotherapy.

TREATMENT DETAILS

Surgery
- All visible tumor had to be removed.
- Thorough surgical staging with total abdominal hysterectomy, bilateral salpingo-oophorectomy, and omentectomy, where appropriate, were recommended as the minimum procedures.

Arm 1: Observation

Arm 2: Chemotherapy
- Recommended: 6 cycles of single-agent carboplatin or CAP (cyclophosphamide + doxorubicin + cisplatin), although other platinum-containing regimens (combination carboplatin or single-agent cisplatin) were allowed.
- Recommended dose of carboplatin.
  - Single-agent: area under the curve (AUC) 5 mg/mL.
  - Combination: AUC 4 mg/mL.
  - AUC method of Calvert (Calvert et al. 1989) where GFR is measured glomerular filtration rate.
- Recommended dose of cisplatin.
  - Single agent: 70 mg/m^2.
- Recommended dose of CAP.
  - Cyclophosphamide 500 mg/m^2.
  - Doxorubicin 50 mg/m^2.
  - Cisplatin 50 mg/m^2.
- Type of planned chemotherapy regimen had to be registered prior to randomization.

ASSESSMENTS
- Follow-up data.
  - Collected 6 and 12 months after randomization and yearly thereafter.
  - Information collected on patients' vital and disease status and treatment for recurrence.

ENDPOINTS
- Overall survival, defined as time from randomization to time of death from any cause (primary endpoint).
- Recurrence-free survival, defined as time to clinically defined recurrence or death from any cause.

STATISTICAL CONSIDERATIONS

Stratification Factors
- Center.
- FIGO stage.
- Degree of tumor differentiation.

Sample Size
- Sample size calculation was complicated by the fact that survival was likely to vary with tumor stage and the difficulty in estimating the proportions of patients with each stage.
- Trial originally planned to include 2000 patients to have 90% power to detect and absolute increase in 5-year survival of 7% (from 60% to 67%) at 2-sided α of 0.05.
- Single independent data monitoring committee would monitor combined data from both ICON1 and ACTION trials (Trimbos et al. 2003a). Trial would not be stopped unless the results were extremely positive—that is, $P<.001$.
- During the trial, the data-monitoring committee noted that survival was better than anticipated and that accrual was slow. The sample size across both trials was reduced to 900 patients. In a combined analysis, this would provide 90% power to detect an improvement in 3-year survival of 6% (from 85% to 91%) at a 2-sided α of 0.05.

Statistical Tests
- Kaplan-Meier curves for OS and RFS.
- Mantel-Cox version of log-rank test to compare survival curves.
- Stratified log-rank test to allow for differences across the 2 randomizing centers.

Table 1.10 Results of ICON1

Treatment arm	Observation N=236	Chemotherapy N=241	Statistics
Patient characteristics			
Median age	55	56	
No residual	99%	99%	
≤2 cm residual	<1%	1%	
Stage I	2%	4%	
Stage IA	41%	37%	
Stage IB	11%	11%	
Stage IC	39%	41%	
Stage II	6%	6%	
Stage III	2%	1%	
Serous	29%	35%	
Endometrioid	25%	20%	
Mucinous	24%	21%	
Clear cell	16%	14%	
Other	5%	10%	
Grade 1	32%	31%	
Grade 2	40%	42%	
Grade 3	28%	27%	
Treatment delivery			
Single-agent carboplatin		87%	
Combination cisplatin		11%	
Combination carboplatin		2%	
Single-agent cisplatin		<1%	
Unspecified chemotherapy		<1%	
No chemotherapy		N=12 (6%)	
Chemotherapy	N=6		
6 cycles per protocol		49%	
6 cycles with modifications		31%	
<6 cycles of chemo		15%	
Efficacy			
5-year overall survival	70%	79%	HR 0.66 (0.45–0.97)
5-year recurrence-free survival	62%	73%	HR 0.65 (0.46–0.91)
Toxicity	Not reported	Not reported	

HR, hazard ratio.

CONCLUSION OF TRIAL
- In women with early-stage ovarian cancer, administration of adjuvant chemotherapy improved 5-year overall survival (70% vs 79%) and 5-year recurrence-free survival (62% vs 73%).

COMMENTS
- ICON1 and ICON2 were initiated at the same time with simple eligibility criteria so that all patients with epithelial ovarian cancer could be considered for entry into one of these trials: ICON1 for early-stage disease and ICON2 for advanced stage disease.
  - The clinician was asked whether the patient required immediate chemotherapy.
  - If the clinician was uncertain, then they were asked to consider enrollment to ICON1 with randomization to observation vs immediate chemotherapy.
  - If the clinical was certain, then they were asked to consider enrollment to ICON2 with randomization to CAP (cyclophosphamide+doxorubicin+cisplatin) vs single-agent carboplatin (International Collaborative Ovarian Neoplasm 1998).
- ICON1 is the largest trial performed to date in early-stage ovarian cancer and provides evidence that adjuvant platinum-based chemotherapy delays recurrence and improves survival in a broad spectrum of patients with early-stage epithelial ovarian cancer.
- While the inclusion criteria for ICON1 were broad with no restrictions on stage or grade, 90% of patients had stage I to IC disease and likely representative of patients seen in clinical practice.
- When ICON1 was launched, there was limited literature to support the use of adjuvant chemotherapy in these patients.
  - Three small, randomized trials compared observation to immediate treatment following surgery for early-stage ovarian cancer (Hreshchyshyn et al. 1980; Krafft et al. 1980; Young et al. 1990).
  - Two small, randomized trials were inconclusive when comparing delayed to immediate platinum-based chemotherapy in patients with early-stage ovarian cancer (Bolis et al. 1995; Trope et al. 2000).
  - A meta-analysis of these trials supports the use of platinum-based chemotherapy in early-stage ovarian cancer (O'Brien and Fleming 1979).
- Limitations to ICON1

- ○ This was an open study that is subject to ascertainment bias. However, the primary endpoint of overall survival is less likely to have been affected by bias. Ascertainment of recurrence was by radiographic criteria, and all patients were followed on the same radiographic assessment timeline, regardless of treatment arm. This also minimizes the likelihood of ascertainment bias.
  - ○ There was a small amount of crossover among the groups. However, the authors predict that the crossover would diminish the possibility of observing an effect and that the benefit of adjuvant chemotherapy was, if anything, underestimated in this trial.
- Given that the majority of patients in this trial received single-agent carboplatin, this should be considered the treatment of choice for patients with early-stage epithelial ovarian cancer.

GOG 157 (Bell, Gynecol Oncol 2006)

REFERENCE
- Bell J, et al. Randomized phase III trial of three versus six cycles of adjuvant carboplatin and paclitaxel in early stage epithelial ovarian carcinoma: a Gynecologic Oncology Group study. *Gynecol Oncol.* 2006;102(3):432-439. PMID: 16860852. (Bell et al. 2006)

TRIAL SPONSOR
- Gynecologic Oncology Group (GOG)

RATIONALE FOR TRIAL
- Approximately 30% of ovarian cancers present at early stage and can be completely resected at the time of initial surgery.
- The question about need for adjuvant therapy for early-stage epithelial ovarian cancer has been the subject of numerous clinical trials in the prior 20 years.
- Patients with stage IA or IB disease and favorable histology have excellent survival of greater than 90% at 6 years after surgical staging only. Adjuvant chemotherapy is considered unnecessary for these patients if a thorough surgical staging has been performed (Young et al. 1990).
- A subgroup of patients with early-stage ovarian cancer have significant 5-year recurrence rates of approximately 25% to 45% and require adjuvant chemotherapy. These patients include

- ○ Stage IA or IB with unfavorable histology, including grade 3 or clear cell.
  - ○ Stage IC.
  - ○ Stage II.
- The optimal adjuvant chemotherapy regimen for these high-risk, early-stage epithelial ovarian cancer patients remains unknown. However, the following series of trials led the GOG to select platinum-based chemotherapy as standard treatment for these patients.
  - ○ An earlier GOG trial demonstrated similar survival rates of approximately 80% at 6 years with either intraperitoneal ^{32}P or oral melphalan (Young et al. 1990).
  - ○ A subsequent GOG study compared intraperitoneal ^{32}P with 3 cycles of cisplatin plus cyclophosphamide. The recurrence rate was 31% lower on the cisplatin regimen, but this was not a statistically significant finding (Young et al. 2003).
  - ○ A multicenter Italian trial compared intraperitoneal ^{32}P to cisplatin in stage IC ovarian cancer and found cisplatin to significantly reduce the relapse rate by 61% (Bolis et al. 1995).
- Carboplatin and paclitaxel is the standard adjuvant chemotherapy regimen for advanced stage ovarian cancer (Alberts et al. 1992; McGuire et al. 1996). This led to the selection of these drugs for this trial.
- The optimal duration of chemotherapy is unknown.
  - ○ In advanced ovarian cancer, 3 trials comparing 5 to 6 cycles with 8 to 12 cycles of cisplatin-based chemotherapy demonstrated no benefit beyond 6 cycles (Bertelsen et al. 1999).
  - ○ In early-stage ovarian cancer, the GOG has historically used 3 cycles of chemotherapy as standard treatment.
- This study was designed to compare recurrence rates with 3 vs 6 cycles of carboplatin and paclitaxel chemotherapy in patients with surgically resected early-stage ovarian cancer.

PATIENT POPULATION

- N=457 enrolled, 427 eligible.
- Enrollment between March 1995 and May 1998.

Inclusion Criteria

- Early-stage epithelial ovarian cancer.
  - ○ Stages: IA grade 3 or clear cell, stage IB grade 3 or clear cell, stage IC, and stage II.

- Staging operation with completely resected tumor.
  - Required procedures included total hysterectomy, bilateral salpingo-oophorectomy, resection of all gross disease, aspiration of free peritoneal fluid, peritoneal washings for cytology, infracolic omentectomy, selective bilateral pelvic and para-aortic node dissections, peritoneal biopsies from 4 pelvic locations and bilateral paracolic areas, and right diaphragm cytology or biopsy.
- Surgical reports, pathology reports, and representative pathology materials were reviewed centrally to confirm eligibility.
- No prior treatment except surgery.
- Adequate bone marrow, renal, and hepatic function.
- GOG performance status less than 3 (listed as less than 4 in the manuscript, but this is likely an error).
- Entered in the trial within 6 weeks following staging laparotomy.

Exclusion Criteria
- Borderline or low malignant potential tumors were ineligible.

TREATMENT DETAILS

- Randomized to 3 or 6 cycles of chemotherapy.
- Chemotherapy details.
  - Paclitaxel 175 mg/m^2 by 3-hour infusion.
  - Carboplatin AUC 7.5 by 30-minute infusion.
  - Treatment was administered every 21 days.
  - Standard paclitaxel premedications included dexamethasone, diphenhydramine, and cimetidine.
- Treatment modifications designed to maximize dose intensity.
- Minimum blood counts for treatment.
  - ANC (absolute neutrophil count) 1500 cells/mm^3.
  - Platelets of 100,000 cells/mm^3.
- Treatment modifications were instituted sequentially.
  - Course delay.
  - Dose reduction (only if delay more than 2 weeks).
  - Filgrastim (only if recurrent delays or neutropenic complications after dose reduction).

ASSESSMENTS

- Toxicity assessed by standard GOG toxicity criteria.
- Weekly blood counts.

- Physical exam prior to each treatment, then every 3 months for 2 years, every 6 months for 3 years, then every year.

ENDPOINTS

- Primary endpoint was recurrence rate. Recurrence was defined as any clinical or radiographic evidence of new tumor.
- Time at risk of recurrence. Assessed from the date of registration to the date of recurrence or to the date of last contact if no recurrence was observed.

STATISTICAL CONSIDERATIONS

Sample Size
- Sample size of 330 patients.
  - Calculated to provide an 85% chance of identifying a 50% reduced risk of recurrence with a 1-tailed α of 0.05. This is comparable to increasing the expected percentage of patients who are recurrence free at 4 years from 80.6% to 89.8%.
  - Interim analysis was to be conducted when at least 35 recurrences were noted in order to rule out an extreme difference in the recurrence rate between the groups.
  - Data were considered to be mature for results release when at least 21% of the eligible patients had experienced a recurrence.
  - To account for a possible loss of statistical power if patients randomized to 6 cycles did not receive all 6 cycles, the statistical design allowed for an increase in the minimum required number of events necessary for study maturity by increasing either the targeted accrual or the postaccrual follow-up period (Lachlin and Foulkes 1986).

Statistical Tests
- Proportional hazards model was used to compare recurrence rates, adjusted for FIGO stage and histologic grade.
- The cumulative incidence of cancer recurrence was estimated using a procedure that treats non-cancer-related death as a competing risk (Pepe and Mori 1993).

CONCLUSION OF TRIAL

- Six cycles of adjuvant chemotherapy does not significantly reduce the cancer recurrence rates compared to 3 cycles of chemotherapy in patients with high-risk, early-stage ovarian cancer. The additional cycles of chemotherapy significantly increased toxicity.

Table 1.11 Results of GOG 157

Treatment arm	CP × 3 cycles N=213	CP × 6 cycles N=214	Statistics
Patient characteristics			
Age <50	32.4%	33.6%	
Age 50-70	53.5%	49.5%	
Age >70	14.1%	16.8%	
Stage I	66.2%	71.0%	
Stage II	33.8%	29.0%	
Serous	24.9%	20.6%	
Endometrioid	21.6%	27.6%	
Mucinous	5.6%	8.9%	
Clear cell	32.9%	28.0%	
Other	15.0%	14.9%	
Grade 1	12.7%	15.9%	
Grade 2	23.5%	22.9%	
Grade 3	31.0%	33.2%	
Treatment delivery			
Completed regimen	95.8%	82.7%	
Reason for stopping			
Progression	0.5%	1.9%	
Death	0.5%	0.5%	
Toxicity	2.8%	12.6%	
Patient refused	0.5%	1.4%	
Other	0.0%	0.9%	
Efficacy			
5-year recurrence rate	25.4%	20.1%	HR 0.76 (0.51-1.13)
Complete staging	23%	20%	HR 0.79
Incomplete staging	Not reported	Not reported	HR 0.66
5-year survival rate	81%	83%	HR 1.02 (0.66-1.57)
Toxicity			
Grade 3/4 neurotoxicity	2%	11%	$P<.01$
Grade 4 granulocytopenia	52%	66%	$P<.01$
Grade 2-4 anemia	32%	48%	$P<.01$

CP, carboplatin+paclitaxel; HR, hazard ratio.

COMMENTS
- After adjusting for FIGO stage and tumor grade, the recurrence risk was 24% lower in patients receiving 6 cycles of chemotherapy (HR, 0.76; 95% CI, 0.51-1.13).
- A large number of patients had incomplete or inadequately documented staging procedures (58 in the 3-cycle arm and 68 in the 6-cycle arm).
- The 5-year cumulative recurrence risk was 22% for patients with complete staging and 26% for patients without (not statistically significant).
- The estimated benefit of 6 cycles was slightly less for patients who had complete staging (HR, 0.79) compared to those with incomplete or incompletely documented staging (HR, 0.66). However, there is not significant evidence of heterogeneity in the treatment effect.
- Cumulative incidence of recurrence within 5 years for different subgroups, irrespective of treatment regimen:
  - Stage I, complete staging: 18%.
  - Stage II, complete staging: 31%.
  - Stage I, incomplete staging: 20%.
  - Stage II, incomplete staging: 40%.
- One patient developed myelodysplastic syndrome 3.5 years after study entry. Due to a prior report of a dose-response relationship between platinum-based chemotherapy and secondary leukemia (Travis et al. 1999), limiting therapy to the fewest effective number of cycles should be considered.
- Patients with early epithelial ovarian cancer appear to have a similar risk of recurrence, regardless of the type of adjuvant therapy received. Across different trials, the 5-year disease-free rate is
  - GOG 157 (this trial): 75% to 80%.
  - After 12 cycles of melphalan or intraperitoneal ^{32}P (Young et al. 1990): 78% to 80%.
  - After 3 cycles of cisplatin and cyclophosphamide (Young et al. 2003): 79%.
  - After 6 cycles of cisplatin (Vergote et al. 1992): 79%.
  - After ^{32}P (Vergote et al. 1992): 82%.
  - After any platinum-based chemotherapy (Trimbos et al. 2003a): 76%.
- Approximately 15% to 30% of patients with early epithelial ovarian cancer have resistance to chemotherapy. This poses the question as to whether withholding postoperative chemotherapy until recurrence would result in acceptable overall survival while sparing the majority of patients who do not need chemotherapy from unnecessary toxicity.

- ○ This question was studied in the ACTION trial in which patients were randomized to either 4 or more cycles of adjuvant chemotherapy or observation (Trimbos et al. 2003b).
- ○ ACTION showed a significant improvement in 5-year recurrence-free survival in patients receiving chemotherapy (76% vs 68%; $P=.02$) but no difference in overall survival (85% vs 78%; $P=.10$).
- Patients who had suboptimal surgical staging and randomized to observation had significantly worse recurrence-free survival (78% vs 65%; $P=.009$) and overall survival (84% vs 75%; $P=.03$).
- In patients who had optimal surgical staging, there was no difference in recurrence-free survival (83% vs 80%) or overall survival (87% vs 89%). However, this represents only 34% of the overall patient population in the trial, and the numbers may be too small to draw definitive conclusions.
- Retrospective studies suggest that withholding adjuvant treatment for patients with unstaged low-risk early ovarian cancers results in a higher rate of cancer recurrence compared to patients who have surgically documented stage I disease (Le et al. 2002).
- The ACTION trial suggest that high-risk stage I patients who have undergone complete surgical staging may have the option to delay chemotherapy until cancer recurrence without significantly compromising survival (Trimbos et al. 2003).
- GOG 157 suggests that after complete surgical staging, patients with high-risk, early-stage ovarian cancer could be treated with 3 cycles of adjuvant carboplatin and paclitaxel chemotherapy, and 3 additional cycles would provide only a marginal reduction in the risk of recurrence while increasing toxicity.
- The risk of recurrent cancer in this patient population appears to be relatively unchanged over the years, and future studies should investigate combination chemotherapy, biological modifiers, and molecular targets.

GOG 157 Exploratory Analysis (Chan, Gynecol Oncol 2010)

REFERENCE

- Chan JK, et al. The potential benefit of 6 vs. 3 cycles of chemotherapy in subsets of women with early-stage high-risk epithelial ovarian cancer: an exploratory analysis of a Gynecologic Oncology Group study. *Gynecol Oncol*. 2010;116(3):301-306. PMID: 19945740. (Chan et al. 2010)

RATIONALE FOR STUDY

- This was an exploratory analysis of GOG 157 to determine whether any subgroups were more likely to benefit from 6 vs 3 cycles of adjuvant chemotherapy.

CONCLUSIONS

- This exploratory analysis suggests that patients with early-stage, high-risk ovarian cancer and serous histology benefit from 6 compared to 3 cycles of adjuvant paclitaxel and carboplatin chemotherapy. The additional chemotherapy reduced the risk of recurrence but did not influence overall survival.

COMMENTS

- Early-stage epithelial ovarian cancer represents a heterogeneous group of tumors.
- The results of this study are consistent with prior studies that demonstrate higher response rates to chemotherapy of serous compared to clear cell cancers.
    - Pectasides (Pectasides et al. 2006): 81% vs 54% response rates for serous vs clear cell.
    - Sugiyama (Sugiyama et al. 2000): 72.5% vs 11.1% response rates for serous vs clear cell.
- This exploratory study was not planned during the design of the original trial, and the trial was not adequately powered for subset analyses. This leaves open the possibility that these results are generated by chance. A test of homogeneity showed that there is no statistically significant evidence that the treatment effect varies across histologies.
- It is possible that more cycles of chemotherapy delayed recurrence rather than prevented relapse and improved survival.

Table 1.12 Results of GOG 157 Exploratory Analysis

Treatment Arm	CP × 3 cycles N=213	CP × 6 cycles N=214	Statistics
Efficacy			
5-year RFS			
Age ≤ 55			HR 0.73 (0.38, 1.39)
Age > 55			HR 0.69 (0.42, 1.15)
Performance status 0			HR 0.98 (0.58, 1.63)
Performance status 1-2			HR 0.49 (0.27, 0.90)
Stage IA or IB			HR 0.74 (0.25, 2.21)
Stage IC			HR 0.75 (0.41, 1.36)
Stage II			HR 0.76 (0.42, 1.39)
Serous	60.4%	82.7%	HR 0.33 (0.14, 0.77)
Non-serous	78.6%	78.7%	HR 0.94 (0.60, 1.49)
Endometrioid			HR 1.07 (0.47, 2.44)
Clear cell			HR 0.90 (0.43, 1.91)
Mucinous			HR 1.68 (0.30, 9.29)
Other			HR 0.74 (0.28, 1.93)
Grade 1			HR 0.36 (0.09, 1.45)
Grade 2			HR 0.67 (0.30, 1.49)
Grade 3			HR 0.78 (0.42, 1.45)
No ascites			HR 0.83 (0.52, 1.33)
Ascites			HR 0.56 (0.27, 1.15)
No tumor rupture			HR 0.60 (0.37, 0.99)
Tumor rupture			HR 1.03 (0.53, 1.97)
Cytology negative			HR 0.67 (0.42, 1.08)
Cytology positive			HR 0.85 (0.42, 1.70)
5-year OS			
Serous	73.2%	85.6%	P=0.19
Non-serous	84.1%	83.0%	

CP, carboplatin+paclitaxel; HR, hazard ratio; OS, overall survival; RFS, recurrence-free survival.

CHAPTER 2

Advanced Stage Epithelial Ovarian Cancer
Adjuvant Chemotherapy

The standard of care adjuvant chemotherapy regimen for advanced ovarian cancer evolved from cyclophosphamide + doxorubicin/Adriamycin + cisplatin (CAP) (GOG 47) to cyclophosphamide + cisplatin (CP) (GOG 52) to paclitaxel + cisplatin (TP) (GOG 111, OV-10) to paclitaxel + carboplatin (TC) (Danish Netherlands Trial, GOG 158, AGO/OVAR-3). However, outcomes may be similar with single-agent platinum therapies (GOG 132, ICON2) or with the exclusion of paclitaxel (ICON3). Outcomes are improved but toxicities are increased with intraperitoneal cisplatin administration (GOG 104, GOG 114, GOG 172). Outcomes appear to be improved with dose density (JGOG 3016) but are not improved with dose intensity (GOG 97) or weekly administration (MITO-7). Addition of a third drug to the paclitaxel and carboplatin backbone does not improve overall survival (GOG 182/ICON5, AGO-OVAR9, OV16, ICON7, GOG218), but the substitution of a different drug for paclitaxel does not compromise outcomes (SCOTROC, MITO-2).

GOG 47 (Omura, Cancer 1986)

REFERENCE
- Omura GA, et al. A randomized trial of cyclophosphamide and doxorubicin with or without cisplatin in advanced ovarian carcinoma. *Cancer.* 1986;57(9):1725-1730. PMID: 3513943. (Omura et al. 1986)

TRIAL SPONSOR
- Gynecologic Oncology Group (GOG)

RATIONALE FOR TRIAL

- The combination of doxorubicin and cyclophosphamide resulted in a better response rate than melphalan in patients with bulky disease (32% vs 20%). However, overall survival was not improved (Omura et al. 1983).
- Cisplatin was found to be a highly active agent in ovarian cancer.
- This trial was performed to determine whether the addition of cisplatin to doxorubicin and cyclophosphamide would improve results.

PATIENT POPULATION

- N = 516, of which 440 were evaluable.
- Enrolled between June 1979 and March 1982.
- Stage IV or suboptimal stage III (defined as residual lesions greater than 3 cm) primary ovarian cancer or recurrent ovarian cancer equivalent to suboptimal stage III or stage IV.

TREATMENT DETAILS

Arm 1: CA (Cyclophosphamide + doxorubicin).
- Cyclophosphamide 500 mg/m^2.
- Adriamycin (doxorubicin) 50 mg/m^2.
- Administered every 3 weeks × 8 courses over 6 months.

Arm 2: CAP (Cyclophosphamide + doxorubicin + Cisplatin).
- Cyclophosphamide 500 mg/m^2.
- Adriamycin (doxorubicin) 50 mg/m^2.
- Cisplatin 50 mg/m^2.
- Administered every 3 weeks × 8 courses over 6 months.

Additional Treatment Details
- Complete responders underwent second-look laparotomy.
- If no evidence of disease or all disease resected, patients received cyclophosphamide alone every 3 weeks, escalating from 500 mg/m^2 to 1100 mg/m^2 until relapse or a total of 12 months after second-look surgery.
- If residual cancer after second-look surgery, patients went off treatment and were followed for survival.

Dose Reductions
- Grade 3 granulocyte or platelet toxicity with recovery by next cycle: dose reduced to 75% for doxorubicin and cyclophosphamide (not reduced for cisplatin).

- Grade 4 granulocyte or platelet toxicity with recovery to next cycle: dose reduced to 50% for doxorubicin and cyclophosphamide and cisplatin reduced to 25%.
- Dose could be escalated by 25% increments for each subsequent course until the full dose was reached if there was no further toxicity.

Doxorubicin
- Stopped if congestive heart failure or any other life-threatening cardiac toxicities.
- Total cumulative dose not to exceed 400 mg/m^2.

Cisplatin
- Held if blood urea nitrogen (BUN) >30 mg/dL or creatinine >2 mg/dL.
- Restarted only after BUN <25 mg/dL and creatinine <1.5 mg/dL.

ASSESSMENTS

Evaluation of Response
- Complete response (CR): disappearance of all gross disease for at least 1 month.
- Partial response (PR): 50% or greater reduction in product of each lesion size in 2 perpendicular diameters for at least 1 month.

ENDPOINTS
- Response rate (primary endpoint).

STATISTICAL CONSIDERATIONS
- Sample size projections were based on complete response rate of 35% for CA and an increase of 15% for CAP.

CONCLUSION OF TRIAL
- The addition of cisplatin to cyclophosphamide and doxorubicin (CAP) improves response rate, response duration, survival in patients with measurable disease, and progression-free interval in all patients (measurable and nonmeasurable) compared to CA alone. The addition of cisplatin is a significant step forward in the management of ovarian cancer.
- The value of maintenance therapy with cyclophosphamide is unclear. The benefit on continued treatment needs to be balanced against the risk of leukemogenesis from prolonged treatment with an alkylating agent.

Table 2.1 Results of GOG 47

Treatment arm	Cyclophosphamide + doxorubicin (CA) N = 215 evaluable	CA + cisplatin (CAP) N = 225 evaluable	Statistics
Patient characteristics			
Median age (range)	56 (25-70)	57 (23-70)	
Grade 3	38%	40%	
Stage III	65%	66%	
Stage IV	32%	30%	
Recurrent	3%	4%	
Serous	52%	54%	
Endometrioid	14%	11%	
Unspecified	19%	15%	
Mucinous	3%	5%	
Clear cell	4%	3%	
Other	7%	11%	
Treatment delivery	No details	No details	
Efficacy			
CR	25%	51%	$P<.0001$
PR	22%	24%	
Stable disease	43%	19%	
Progressive disease	9%	5%	
Response duration	8.8 months	14.6 months	$P=.02$
Progression-free interval	7.7 months	13.1 months	$P<.0001$
Survival (measurable disease)	15.7 months	19.7 months	$P<.03$
Survival (nonmeasurable disease)	18.7 months	18.9 months	NS
Toxicity			
G3/4 WBC	80/189 (42%)	116/195 (59%)	
G3/4 platelet	2/189 (1%)	17/195 (9%)	
G3/4 GI	14/194 (7%)	31/198 (16%)	

CR, complete response; GI, gastrointestinal; NS, not significant; PR, partial response; WBC, white blood cells.

- No survival advantage was seen for CAP in nonmeasurable cases. These cases ranged from minimally bulky to massive but clinically nonmeasurable disease. Most women treated with CA ended up receiving cisplatin as secondary therapy, and this may have influenced the measurement of postprotocol survival. However, this would be relevant to both measurable and nonmeasurable cases and does not necessarily account for the lack of survival difference with nonmeasurable cases.

COMMENTS

- Cisplatin was commercially available when this trial was conducted, so crossover to cisplatin use after completion of the trial may have blunted survival differences.

GOG 52 (Omura, JCO 1989)

REFERENCE

- Omura GA, et al. Randomized trial of cyclophosphamide plus cisplatin with or without doxorubicin in ovarian carcinoma: a Gynecologic Oncology Group Study. *J Clin Oncol*. 1989;7(4):457-465. PMID: 2926470. (Omura et al. 1989)

TRIAL SPONSOR

- Gynecologic Oncology Group (GOG)

RATIONALE FOR TRIAL

- GOG 47 demonstrated cyclophosphamide, doxorubicin, and cisplatin (CAP) to be superior to cyclophosphamide and doxorubicin (CA). CAP improved complete response rate, response duration, and progression-free interval. CAP improved survival only in patients with measurable disease (Omura et al. 1986).
- Prior studies suggest that doxorubicin does not confer a treatment advantage.
- This study was designed to compare CP (omitting doxorubicin) with CAP in patients with optimal cytoreduction.

PATIENT POPULATION

- N=349 evaluable patients.
- Enrolled from April 1981 to July 1985.
- Small-volume stage III ovarian cancer (<1 cm, therefore no clinically measurable lesions to follow).
- Ineligible: prior cancer, prior irradiation or chemotherapy, major organ dysfunction, history of congestive heart failure, complete disability, borderline cancers.

TREATMENT DETAILS

Arm 1: CP (cyclophosphamide + Cisplatin).
- Cyclophosphamide 1000 mg/m^2.
- Cisplatin 50 mg/m^2.
- Administered every 3 weeks for 8 cycles.

Arm 2: CAP (Cyclophosphamide + Adriamycin + Cisplatin)
- Cyclophosphamide 500 mg/m^2.
- Adriamycin (doxorubicin) 50 mg/m^2.
- Cisplatin 50 mg/m^2.
- Administered every 3 weeks for 8 cycles.
- Dosing schedules were chosen to anticipation of comparable hematologic toxicities.

Second-Look Laparotomy
- Patients without progression underwent second-look laparotomy at 6 months.
  - Negative second look—followed without additional treatment.
  - Positive second look—went off treatment part of study.

Dose Reductions
- Grade 3 granulocyte or platelet toxicity with recovery by next cycle: cyclophosphamide and doxorubicin doses were reduced to 75%; cisplatin was not decreased.
- Grade 4 granulocyte or platelet toxicity with recovery by next cycle: cyclophosphamide and doxorubicin doses were reduced to 50%; cisplatin was reduced to 75%.
- Doses could be escalated by 25% for each subsequent course until 100% if no further severe myelosuppression was noted.

Doxorubicin
- Stopped if congestive heart failure or any other life-threatening cardiac condition.
- Total cumulative dose was not to exceed 400 mg/m^2.

Cisplatin
- Held if BUN >30 mg/dL or creatinine >2 mg/dL.
- Restarted only after BUN and creatinine returned to acceptable levels.

ASSESSMENTS
- Radiographs and scans every 3 months.

Table 2.2 Results of GOG 52

Treatment arm	Cyclophosphamide + cisplatin (CP) N = 176	CP + doxorubicin (CAP) N = 173	Statistics
Patient characteristics			
Median age	56 (19-80)	53 (23-80)	
Residual disease	72%	71%	
Grade 3	33%	36%	
Stage III, optimal	100%	100%	
Serous	53%	58%	
Endometrioid	15%	12%	
Mucinous	2%	1%	
Clear cell	6%	11%	
Other	23%	18%	
Treatment delivery			
Cyclophosphamide	24% decrease in dose	21% decrease in dose	
Cisplatin	7% decrease in dose	10% decrease in dose	
Doxorubicin		22% decrease in dose	
Average cycle time	25.8 days	26.1 days	
Efficacy			
Progression-free interval	22.7 months	24.6 months	NS
Overall survival	31.2 months	38.9 months	NS
Negative second look	30.2%	32.8%	NS
Toxicity			
G3/4 leukocyte	55%	57%	NS
G3/4 thrombocytopenia	1%	2%	
G3 nausea/vomiting	3.6%	9.3%	

NS, not significant.

ENDPOINTS

- Progression-free interval (PFI) (primary endpoint).
- Frequency of negative second-look laparotomy.
- Survival.

STATISTICAL CONSIDERATIONS

Sample Size

- Study designed assuming a median PFI of 2 years for CP with a 1-tail test at the .05 level. Statistical power is 97% and 76% for a 15% and 10% increase in the 2-year PFI rate.

Statistical Tests

- Mantel-Haenszel χ^2 test to compare frequency of negative second-look laparotomy.
- Cox proportional hazards model, likelihood ratio test to compare survival.

CONCLUSION OF TRIAL

- Doxorubicin does not improve outcomes in optimal stage III ovarian cancer.

COMMENTS

- Second-look surgery does not influence survival outcomes as better options for "salvage" therapy are needed.
- Residual disease status had a large impact on progression-free interval. However, once a negative second look was documented, residual disease status no longer had an impact.
- Low grade and younger age were also favorable factors for outcome.
- Timing of chemotherapy initiation did not have an impact on survival.
- Clear cell carcinoma had the worst progression-free interval and survival.
- Cyclophosphamide dose was lower in CAP (500) vs CP (1000).

GOG 97 (McGuire, JCO 1995)

REFERENCE

- McGuire WP, et al. Assessment of dose-intensive therapy in suboptimally debulked ovarian cancer: a Gynecologic Oncology Group study. *J Clin Oncol.* 1995;13(7):1589-1599. PMID: 7602348. (McGuire et al. 1995)

TRIAL SPONSOR

- Gynecologic Oncology Group (GOG)

RATIONALE FOR TRIAL

- The current standard therapy at the time of this trial was the 2-drug regimen of cyclophosphamide and cisplatin.
- The 2-drug regimen had been shown to be as efficacious as and less toxic than a 4-drug regimen (Neijt et al. 1991).
- This trial was designed to evaluate chemotherapy dose intensity on ovarian cancer survival and response in patients with bulky residual disease.

PATIENT POPULATION
- N = 458 eligible.
- Enrolled between January 1987 and April 1990.

Inclusion Criteria
- Stage III epithelial ovarian cancer with >1 cm residual disease after surgical cytoreduction or stage IV disease.
- Patients were allowed to have clinically measurable or nonmeasurable (assessable) disease.
- GOG performance status of 0, 1, or 2.
- Adequate bone marrow (white blood cells [WBC] $>3 \times 10^9$/L, platelets $>100 \times 10^9$/L), renal (serum creatinine <2 mg/dL) and hepatic function (serum bilirubin and aspartate aminotransferase [AST] <2 times the upper limit of institutional norm)
- Study entry within 6 weeks of the surgical procedure.

Exclusion Criteria
- Borderline tumors, prior therapy, any other malignant disease other than nonmelanoma skin cancer.

TREATMENT DETAILS

Arm 1: Standard Therapy
- Cyclophosphamide 500 mg/m^2 (166 mg/m^2/wk).
- Cisplatin 50 mg/m^2 (16.6 mg/m^2/wk).
- Treatment every 3 weeks for 8 courses.

Arm 2: Intensive Therapy
- Cyclophosphamide 1000 mg/m^2 (333 mg/m^2/wk).
- Cisplatin 100 mg/m^2 (33.3 mg/m^2/wk).
- Treatment every 3 weeks for 4 courses.
- Patients in the intensive therapy group received the same total dose of chemotherapy but at 1.97 times greater dose intensity than the standard therapy group.

Management of Toxicities
- To maintain dose intensity, patients were not allowed to undergo dose reductions.
- Hematologic toxicity was managed with treatment delays. If delay was greater than 3 weeks, the patient was taken off study and monitored for survival.

- No delay was allowed for any grade gastrointestinal toxicity, G1 or G2 peripheral neurotoxicity, mild renal toxicity (creatinine ≤2 mg/dL or creatinine clearance ≥50 mL/min), or mild ototoxicity (<–10 dB reduction in high-frequency discrimination).
- Persistent and more severe neurologic, otic, or renal toxicity required removal of the patient from the study.
- If a patient developed hemorrhagic cystitis, an equitoxic dose of chlorambucil was substituted for cyclophosphamide.

ASSESSMENTS

- Baseline history and physical examination, laboratory procedures, imaging studies to assess disease measurements.
- Functional Living Index–Cancer (FLIC) given before chemotherapy, after each course of treatment, and 6 weeks after last course of treatment.
- Tumor measurements after each 2 courses of therapy.
- Second-look laparotomy performed after completing therapy on patients without measurable disease or patients who achieved a complete clinical response to determine the pathologic response rate. Failure to undergo surgery was considered a major protocol violation.
- Cancer antigen 125 (CA125) was monitored but never used as an indicator of disease status.

ENDPOINTS

- Overall survival (OS).
- Progression-free survival (PFS).
- Response.

STATISTICAL CONSIDERATIONS

- Kaplan-Meier used to estimate survival (Kaplan and Meier 1958).
- Log-rank test used to assess the independence of PFS, OS, and randomized treatment (Mantel 1966).
- Linear proportional hazards model was used to estimate the treatment effects while adjusted for other pretreatment factors (Cox 1972).
- A proportional hazards model with an interaction term was used to determine the homogeneity of the treatment effect for those with and without measurable disease.

Table 2.3 Results of GOG 97

Treatment arm	Standard-intensity CP N=235	Dose-intense CP N=223	Statistics
Patient characteristics			
Median age (range)	60 (22-80)	60 (20-83)	
Measurable disease	38%	36%	
Stage III, <2 cm	5%	9%	
Stage III, ≥2 cm	63%	57%	
Stage IV, <2 cm	8%	16%	
Stage IV, ≥2 cm	24%	19%	
Serous	70%	66%	
Endometrioid	11%	18%	
Mucinous	3%	3%	
Clear cell	4%	2%	
Other	13%	12%	
Treatment delivery			
Days between courses	21-25	22-28	
Median total dose			
Cisplatin	391 mg/m^2	394 mg/m^2	NS
Cyclophosphamide	3906 mg/m^2	3943 mg/m^2	NS
Efficacy			
Complete response	36%	30%	NS
Partial response	24%	25%	
Stable disease	32%	28%	
Progression	1%	11%	
Death before evaluation	5%	6%	
Negative SL, measurable	10%	10%	NS
Negative SL, nonmeasurable	16%	19%	
Median PFS	12.1 months	14.3 months	NS
Median OS	19.5 months	21.3 months	NS
Toxicity			
G3/4 WBC	39%	82%	<.005
G3/4 platelet	<1%	22%	<.005
G3/4 anemia	<3%	9%	<.005
G3/4 GI/vomiting	3%	16%	<.005
G3/4 renal	<1%	5%	<.005
G3/4 febrile neutropenia	0%	2%	<.005
G3/4 sepsis/infection	<2%	5%	<.05
Removed due to toxicity	7%	17%	
Death attributed to treatment	N=1	N=2	
Progression or death before completing therapy	23.8%	7.6%	

CP, cyclophosphamide+cisplatin; GI, gastrointestinal; NS, not significant; OS, overall survival; PFS, progression-free survival; SL, second look; WBC, white blood cells.

- The Kruskal-Wallis rank test adjusted for tied ranks was used to test the independence of dose intensity, total dose delivered, and severity of toxicity relative to the assigned treatment (Kruskal and Wallis 1952).
- The Mantel-Haenszel χ^2 test was used to determine the independence of treatment and response and was stratified by disease measurability (Mantel and Haenszel 1959).

CONCLUSIONS OF TRIAL

- Clinical and pathologic response rates, response duration, and survival were similar between treatment arms, but adverse events (hematologic, gastrointestinal, febrile episodes, sepsis, and renal toxicities) were more common and severe in the dose-intensive therapy group.
- This study provides no evidence to support the hypothesis that modest increases in dose intensity (without increasing total dose) have an impact on outcome.

COMMENTS

- Dose modification was rigorously controlled in this trial to maintain dose intensity.
- Neither high-dose chemotherapy (with or without autologous bone marrow rescue) nor modest dose intensification (as studied in this trial) overcame the development of chemoresistance.

GOG 111 (McGuire, NEJM 1996)

REFERENCE

- McGuire WP, et al. Cyclophosphamide and cisplatin compared with paclitaxel and cisplatin in patients with stage III and stage IV ovarian cancer. *N Engl J Med.* 1996;334(1):1-6. PMID: 7494563. (McGuire et al. 1996)

TRIAL SPONSOR

- Gynecologic Oncology Group (GOG)

RATIONALE FOR TRIAL

- At the time of trial design, the standard of care for advanced epithelial ovarian cancer in the United States was a combination of an alkylating agent and cisplatin, specifically cyclophosphamide and cisplatin. However, long-term disease control with this regimen was less than 10% in

women with incompletely resected stage III and less than 5% in women with stage IV disease.
- In 1989, a phase II trial reported that paclitaxel produced a 24% response rate in patients with platinum-resistant ovarian cancer (McGuire et al. 1989). Another phase II trial reported a 37% response rate in 1994 (Thigpen et al. 1994). This made paclitaxel the most active single-agent drug ever evaluated by the GOG in a phase II study in ovarian cancer.
- A phase I trial of paclitaxel and cisplatin demonstrated the safety of the combination when paclitaxel was given first as a 24-hour infusion (Rowinsky et al. 1991a).
- Based on the activity of paclitaxel in the salvage setting, the safety of the combination of paclitaxel and cisplatin, and the need for better treatment alternatives than the current standard of care, the GOG conducted this phase III study to evaluate the efficacy of the paclitaxel+cisplatin combination as standard first-line therapy in patients with incompletely resected stage III or any stage IV ovarian cancer.

PATIENT POPULATION
- N=386.
- Accrual began in April 1990 and completed its goal within 2 years.

Inclusion Criteria
- Stage IV or suboptimal stage III (defined as residual disease >1 cm) epithelial ovarian cancer.
- Having undergone surgical debulking; having received no prior chemotherapy or radiation; having a GOG performance status of 0 to 2 and having adequate hematologic (WBC ≥3000/mm^3, platelet count >100,000/mm^3), renal (serum creatinine <2.0 mg/dL), and liver (serum bilirubin and serum AST <2 times the upper limit of normal for the institution) function.
- Entry within 6 weeks of the debulking procedure.

Exclusion Criteria
- Borderline tumors, taking antiarrhythmic medication, any prior cancer other than nonmelanoma skin cancer.

TREATMENT DETAILS

Arm 1: Standard Therapy Group—Cyclophosphamide+Cisplatin
- Cyclophosphamide 750 mg/m^2 intravenous (IV)
- Cisplatin 75 mg/m^2 IV at rate of 1 mg/min.
- Treatment every 3 weeks for 6 courses.

Arm 2: Experimental Therapy Group—Paclitaxel and Cisplatin
- Paclitaxel 135 mg/m² IV as a 24-hour continuous infusion.
- Cisplatin 75 mg/m² IV at a rate of 1 mg/min.
- Treatment every 3 weeks for 6 courses.
- Pretreatments.
  - Dexamethasone 20 mg orally or IV 14 and 7 hours before infusion.
  - Diphenhydramine 50 mg IV 30 minutes before infusion.
  - Any histamine H_2 antagonist IV 30 minutes before infusion.

Treatment Delays
- Delayed week by week until WBC >3000/mm³ and platelet count >100,000/mm³.
- No delay allowed for any gastrointestinal toxicity, grade 1 or 2 peripheral neurotoxicity, mild renal toxicity (creatinine ≤2 mg/dL or creatinine clearance of ≥50 mL/min), or mild ototoxicity (reduction of ≤10 dB in high-frequency discrimination).

Treatment Withdrawal
- For treatment delays exceeding 3 weeks due to hematologic toxicity.
- For more severe neurologic, renal, or otic toxicity that had not resolved by the time of the next scheduled dose.
- For cardiac toxic effects (other than asymptomatic sinus bradycardia).
- For severe allergic reaction (bronchospasm, hypotension, diffuse urticaria) during the paclitaxel infusion.

Dose Modifications—Cyclophosphamide
- Reduction to 500 mg/m² for grade 4 hematologic toxicity (WBC ≤1000/mm³, absolute neutrophil count (ANC) ≤500/mm³, platelet count <25,000/mm³).
- Reescalation in subsequent dose if nadir counts not grade 4.

Dose Modifications—Paclitaxel
- Reduction to 110 mg/m² for grade 4 hematologic toxicity (WBC ≤1000/mm³, ANC ≤500/mm³, platelet count <25,000/mm³).
- Reescalation in subsequent dose if nadir counts not grade 4.

Dose Modifications—Cisplatin
- Not allowed.

ASSESSMENTS
- Imaging studies before and after every other course of therapy.
- Adverse events graded by toxicity criteria of the GOG.

- Reassessment laparotomy to determine pathologic response required for those without measurable disease and those with measureable disease and complete clinical response.

ENDPOINTS

- Progression-free survival (primary endpoint).
- Overall survival.

STATISTICAL CONSIDERATIONS

- Kaplan-Meier to estimate the cumulative proportion surviving.
- Two-tailed log-rank test to assess the independence of PFS, OS, and randomized treatment assessment.
- Linear proportional hazards analysis to estimate relative risk adjusted for pretreatment factors.
- Proportional hazards with an interaction term to assess the homogeneity of the treatment effect across prognostic groups.
- Kruskal-Wallis rank test adjusted for tiered ranks to test the independence of the severity of toxicity with the assigned treatment.
- Pearson's χ^2 test to test the independence of response and treatment.

CONCLUSION OF TRIAL

- Incorporation of paclitaxel into first-line chemotherapy for patients with incompletely resected stage III and IV epithelial ovarian cancer improves both progression-free and overall survival. Paclitaxel and cisplatin are associated with an estimated 40% reduction in the risk of death compared to cyclophosphamide and cisplatin.

COMMENTS

- At the start of the study, all women receiving paclitaxel underwent cardiac monitoring as patients receiving paclitaxel therapy had previously been reported to experience bradyarrhythmias with atrioventricular block and ventricular irritability (Rowinsky et al. 1991b). Only 7 women had grade 2 or higher cardiac episodes (first-degree heart block, ischemic events without infarction), so the requirement for cardiac monitoring was removed toward the end of the study.
- The benefit of paclitaxel did not appear to be due to a poorer than anticipated outcome among the patients receiving standard therapy.
- The benefit of paclitaxel did not appear to be limited to the subpopulations with measurable disease or stage III disease.

Table 2.4 Results of GOG 111

Treatment arm	Cisplatin + cyclophosphamide N=202	Cisplatin + paclitaxel N=184	Statistics
Patient characteristics			
Median age (range)	60 (27-80)	59 (20-84)	
Measurable disease	57%	54%	
Stage III	64%	67%	
Stage IV	36%	33%	
Serous	64%	76%	
Endometrioid	13%	8%	
Mucinous	5%	2%	
Clear cell	2%	2%	
Other	15%	12%	
Grade 1	7%	4%	
Grade 2	41%	45%	
Grade 3	52%	51%	
Treatment delivery			
Interval between cycles	21-28 days	21 days	
Completed 6 cycles	78%	87%	
Discontinuation due to			
Progression or death	11%	5%	
Toxicity or declined	10%	8%	
Efficacy			
Overall response rate	60%	73%	
Complete response (CR)	31%	51%	$P=.01$
Partial response (PR)	29%	22%	
Pathologic CR	20%	26%	NS
PFS	13 months	18 months	RR 0.7, $P<.001$
OS	24 months	38 months	RR 0.6, $P<.001$
Toxicity			
G3/4 neutropenia	83%	92%	<.05
G3/4 thrombocytopenia	3%	3%	
G3/4 anemia	8%	9%	
G3/4 gastrointestinal	11%	15%	
Fever	11%	20%	<.05
Alopecia	37%	63%	<.05
G3/4 renal	<2%	<1%	
Any neurologic	21%	28%	
Allergic reaction	0%	4%	<.05
Death due to treatment	N=6	N=4	

NS, not significant; OS, overall survival; PFS, progression-free survival; RR, relative risk.

- Paclitaxel was in limited use when this trial was conducted. Therefore, crossover occurred to a lesser degree after the conclusion of the trial and there was likely to be less blunting of the survival outcomes.

GOG 104 (Alberts, NEJM 1996)

REFERENCE

- Alberts DS, et al. Intraperitoneal cisplatin plus intravenous cyclophosphamide versus intravenous cisplatin plus intravenous cyclophosphamide for stage III ovarian cancer. *N Engl J Med.* 1996;335(26):1950-1955. PMID: 8960474. (Alberts et al. 1996)

TRIAL SPONSOR

- Gynecologic Oncology Group (GOG)

RATIONALE FOR TRIAL

- In an attempt to maximize the activity of cisplatin against ovarian cancer, trials have investigated its delivery directly into the peritoneal cavity. This results in intraperitoneal cisplatin concentrations that are 12 to 15 times greater than the concentration in plasma (Howell et al. 1982; Goel et al. 1989).
- Survival may be improved with salvage intraperitoneal chemotherapy in patients with small (<1 cm) residual masses after upfront chemotherapy and second-look surgery (Howell et al. 1987; Kirmani et al. 1991).
- This trial was conducted to compare intraperitoneal and intravenous cisplatin administration in the upfront adjuvant treatment of patients with stage III ovarian cancer and residual masses less than 2 cm in size.

PATIENT POPULATION

- N=654 enrolled, 546 eligible.
- Enrollment between June 1986 and July 1992.
- Stage III epithelial ovarian cancer with less than 2 cm residual disease.
- Surgery that included exploratory laparotomy with at least total abdominal hysterectomy, bilateral salpingo-oophorectomy, omentectomy, and debulking to optimal (<2 cm size) status.
- Enrollment within 4 weeks of surgery.
- Performance status of 0 to 2; adequate blood counts, renal function (serum creatinine ≤1.5 mg/dL or creatinine clearance ≥40 mL/min).

TREATMENT DETAILS

Arm 1: Intravenous Cyclophosphamide + Intravenous Cisplatin

- Cyclophosphamide 600 mg/m^2 in 150 mL of diluent over 60 to 90 minutes IV.
- Cisplatin 100 mg/m^2 in 500 to 1000 mL of normal saline at a rate of 1 mg/min.
- IV hydration with at least 1 L of normal saline with 3 g of magnesium sulfate and 40 g of mannitol over a period of 1 to 2 hours.
- Treatment every 3 weeks for 6 cycles.

Arm 2: Intravenous Cyclophosphamide + Intraperitoneal Cisplatin

- Cyclophosphamide 600 mg/m^2 in 150 mL of diluent over 60 to 90 minutes IV.
- Cisplatin 100 mg/m^2 in 2 L of normal saline warmed to body temperature and instilled into the peritoneal cavity as fast as possible.
- IV hydration with at least 1 L of normal saline with 3 g of magnesium sulfate and 40 g of mannitol over a period of 1 to 2 hours.
- Treatment every 3 weeks for 6 cycles.

Treatment Delays

- Delay for a maximum of 2 weeks to allow for resolution of toxic effects.

Treatment Discontinuation

- Cisplatin discontinued and cyclophosphamide increased to 1000 mg/m^2.
  - For grade 2 or higher peripheral neuropathy.
  - For serum creatinine >1.9 mg/dL.
- Treatment discontinued permanently.
  - For serum creatinine >1.9 mg/dL for 8 weeks.

ASSESSMENTS

- Serum CA125 before each cycle.
- Second-look laparotomy at completion of therapy if no clinical evidence of disease.

ENDPOINTS

- Survival.
- Pathologic complete response rate.

STATISTICAL CONSIDERATIONS

Sample Size

- Initial trial design had a power of 93% to detect a difference in the hazard ratio for death of 0.67 with a 2-sided P value of .05 and 215 patients per treatment arm.
- With a Pearson χ^2 approximation and 2-sided P value of .05, there was 85% power to detect a difference of pathologic response rate of 55% vs 40%.
- Accrual was extended for another year in January 1991 to achieve a large enough sample size to do a separate analysis of data from patients with residual tumors <0.5 cm. With the plan to accrue 560 patients (390 with tumors <0.5 cm), the power to detect a hazard ratio of 0.67 was 88%.

Statistical Tests

- Cox regression analyses.
- Two-sided Fisher's exact tests to compare toxicities.

CONCLUSION OF TRIAL

- Intraperitoneal cisplatin was associated with a 20% improvement in survival and a 24% reduction in the risk of death compared to intravenous cisplatin.
- Pathologic complete response rates are greater in the subset of patients with ≤0.5-cm residual tumor masses, supporting the observation that the penetration of intraperitoneal cisplatin is limited to a depth of 0.1 to 1 mm from the surface of the tumor (Los et al. 1989).

COMMENTS

- There was a higher rate of pathologic complete response (pCR) among patients receiving intraperitoneal compared to intravenous cisplatin. However, among the 400 patients eligible for second-look surgery (no clinical evidence of disease at completion of therapy), 103 did not undergo surgery or they had inadequate surgery, creating bias. Because of this bias, the pCR data are reported without statistical comparisons.
- Covariates associated with improved survival included (and thus included in the final Cox model).
   - No gross residual disease ($P<.001$).
   - Younger age ($P<.001$).
   - Non–clear cell and nonmucinous histology ($P<.001$).
   - Enrollment after surgery ($P<.001$).

Table 2.5 Results of GOG 104

Treatment arm	Intravenous group N=279	Intraperitoneal group N=267	Statistics
Patient characteristics			
Median age (range)	56 (21-85)	59 (24-84)	
Minimal residual <0.5 cm	72%	73%	
No gross residual	26%	25%	
Stage III	100%	100%	
Serous	66%	67%	
Endometrioid	9%	10%	
Mucinous	3%	1%	
Clear cell	2%	2%	
Other	20%	20%	
Grade 1	13%	11%	
Grade 2	30%	31%	
Grade 3	57%	58%	
Treatment delivery			
Completed 6 cycles	58%	58%	
Cisplatin discontinued for toxicity (+ increase cyclophosphamide)	40%	22%	
Efficacy			
Complete PR (second look)	36%	47%	
OS	41 months	49 months	HR 0.76, $P=.02$
OS, <0.5 cm residual	46 months	51 months	HR 0.8, $P=.10$
Toxicity			
Treatment-related death	N=0	N=2	
>G3 anemia	25%	26%	NS
>G3 granulocytopenia	69%	56%	.0002
>G3 leukopenia	50%	40%	.04
>G3 thrombocytopenia	9%	8%	NS
≥G2 abdominal pain	2%	18%	<.001
≥G2 tinnitus	14%	7%	.01
≥G2 hearing loss	15%	5%	<.001
≥G2 neuromuscular	25%	15%	.02
≥G2 pulmonary effects	0.4%	3%	.002

HR, hazard ratio; OS, overall survival; PR, pathologic response.

- Neutropenia, tinnitus, and hearing loss were experienced more frequently in the intravenous arm. Abdominal pain was experienced more frequently in the intraperitoneal arm, but pain usually resolved within 24 hours and was generally manageable with weak opioid or nonopioid drugs. Dyspnea occurred more frequently with intraperitoneal administration, likely due to compression of the base of the lungs.
- This trial was published shortly after GOG 111 (McGuire et al. 1996), which demonstrated the superiority of paclitaxel+cisplatin over cyclophosphamide+cisplatin. Ongoing studies will plan to evaluate the efficacy of intraperitoneal cisplatin with paclitaxel.

ICON2 (Lancet 1998)

REFERENCE

- ICON2: randomised trial of single-agent carboplatin against three-drug combination of CAP (cyclophosphamide, doxorubicin, and cisplatin) in women with ovarian cancer. ICON Collaborators. International Collaborative Ovarian Neoplasm Study. *Lancet.* 1998;352(9140):1571-1576. PMID: 9843101. (International Collaborative Ovarian Neoplasm Group 1998)

TRIAL SPONSORS

- International Collaborative Ovarian Neoplasm Study
  - Instituto Mario Negri in Milan, Italy
  - Swiss Institute for Cancer Research (SIAK) in Bern, Switzerland
  - Medical Research Council's Cancer Trials Office in Cambridge, United Kingdom

RATIONALE FOR TRIAL

- Five meta-analyses representing data from 45 randomized controlled trials suggest that immediate platinum-based treatment is better than non-platinum-based treatment, combination therapy is better than single-agent platinum, and there is no difference between carboplatin and cisplatin either as single agents or within combination regimens (Chemotherapy in advanced ovarian cancer . . . 1991).
- Two meta-analyses focusing on the role of doxorubicin suggest that the combination of cyclophosphamide, doxorubicin, and cisplatin (CAP)

is better than cyclophosphamide and cisplatin (CP) (Cyclophosphamide plus cisplatin . . . 1991; A'Hern and Gore 1995). The 3-drug regimen is associated with a marginal improvement in 5-year survival from 20% to 26%.
- While many believed CAP to be the most effective drug regimen for advanced ovarian cancer at this time, there was an open question as to whether single-agent platinum (the most active agent in the combination) administered at full dose would provide equivalent or better survival outcomes compared to CAP.
- Carboplatin was chosen as the single-agent platinum in this study because it is less toxic than cisplatin at optimally tolerated doses and has similar efficacy. Single-agent carboplatin was the most widely used regimen in the United Kingdom, and CAP was the most widely used regimen in Italy at this time.

PATIENT POPULATION
- N = 1526.
- Patients entered between January 1991 and July 1996.
- ICON2 was run as 3 parallel trials through (1) the Instituto Mario Negri in Milan, Italy; (2) the Swiss Institute for Cancer Research (SIAK) in Bern, Switzerland; (3) and the Medical Research Council's Cancer Trials Office in Cambridge, United Kingdom.
- Patients were recruited from 132 centers in 9 countries.
- Histologically confirmed invasive epithelial ovarian cancer; fit to receive chemotherapy; no prior chemotherapy or radiation therapy; no previous malignancy (excluding nonmelanoma skin cancer); adequate renal function.
- No restrictions on extent of surgery, but total abdominal hysterectomy, bilateral salpingo-oophorectomy, and thorough staging were recommended as the minimum procedures.
- Eligibility criteria were intentionally left wide to promote recruitment.

TREATMENT DETAILS

Arm 1: CAP (Cyclophosphamide, Adriamycin, Cisplatin)
- Cyclophosphamide 500 mg/m^2.
- Adriamycin (doxorubicin) 50 mg/m^2.
- Cisplatin 50 mg/m^2.
- One cycle every 3 weeks for 6 cycles.

Arm 2: Carboplatin
- Carboplatin area under the curve (AUC) 5.
- Dose determined by AUC method of Calvert (Calvert et al. 1989). Glomerular filtration rate (GFR) was determined by radioisotope method or the Cockcroft formula. If GFR was determined by creatinine clearance, carboplatin dose was recommended to be reduced by 10%.
- One cycle every 3 weeks for 6 cycles.

ASSESSMENTS
- Pretreatment data were collected at the time of randomization.
- Treatment and initial follow-up data were collected 6 months later.
- Further follow-data were collected 12 months after randomization and every year thereafter.

ENDPOINTS
- Five-year survival.
- OS.
- PFS.

STATISTICAL CONSIDERATIONS
Sample Size
- Five-year survival estimated to be 20% in the carboplatin group. To detect an improvement in survival with CAP to 26% with 90% power and to 25% with 85% power at a significance level of 5%, the maximum accrual target was set to 2000 patients.

Statistical Tests
- Kaplan-Meier curves, Mantel-Cox version of log-rank test.
- Stratified log-rank test to allow for differences across 3 centers.
- Cox proportional hazards model to account for imbalances in pretreatment characteristics.

CONCLUSION OF TRIAL
- There was no difference in PFS or OS between CAP and single-agent carboplatin.
- Neither treatment was more effective in any subgroup analyses, suggesting that the results of ICON2 are applicable to a broad range of patients.

Table 2.6 Results of ICON2

Treatment arm	CAP N=766	Carboplatin N=760	Statistics
Patient characteristics			
Italy	64%	64%	
United Kingdom	20%	20%	
Switzerland	7%	7%	
Other	7%	10%	
Age <55	38%	35%	
Age 55-65	31%	33%	
Age >65	31%	33%	
No residual	31%	31%	
≤2 cm residual	25%	24%	
>2 cm residual	45%	45%	
Stage I	11%	13%	
Stage II	12%	11%	
Stage III	63%	62%	
Stage IV	14%	15%	
Serous	52%	52%	
Endometrioid	13%	13%	
Mucinous	10%	9%	
Clear cell	5%	5%	
Other	21%	20%	
Grade 1	13%	11%	
Grade 2	32%	31%	
Grade 3	46%	50%	
Unknown grade	9%	10%	
Treatment delivery			
Received 6 cycles	80%	81%	
Received 0 cycles	N=34	N=14	
Efficacy			
1-year PFS	63%	60%	HR 0.92, $P=.20$
Median PFS	17 months	15.5 months	favoring CAP
2-year OS	60%	60%	HR 1, $P=.98$
Median OS	33 months	33 months	
Toxicity (collected in Italy only)			
Alopecia	70%	4%	
G 3/4 leucopenia	36%	10%	
G 3/4 Nausea, vomiting	20%	9%	
G 3/4 thrombocytopenia	6%	16%	

CAP, cyclophosphamide+Adriamycin/doxorubicin+cisplatin; HR, hazard ratio; PFS, progression-free survival; OS, overall survival.

- CAP was more toxic than carboplatin, causing more alopecia, leucopenia, nausea, and vomiting. Carboplatin caused more thrombocytopenia.
- Single-agent carboplatin is a safe and effective standard treatment option for patients with advanced ovarian cancer.

COMMENTS

- Recruitment to ICON2 was stopped in July 1996 before the planned 2000 patients had been enrolled due to an interest in testing paclitaxel-containing regimens in the context of data from GOG 111 (McGuire et al. 1996). ICON3 began recruitment in February 1995 comparing the combination of paclitaxel + carboplatin with single-agent carboplatin or CAP (International Collaborative Ovarian Neoplasm Group 2002).

GOG 132 (Muggia, JCO 2000)

REFERENCE

- Muggia FM, et al. Phase III randomized study of cisplatin versus paclitaxel versus cisplatin and paclitaxel in patients with suboptimal stage III or IV ovarian cancer: a Gynecologic Oncology Group study. *J Clin Oncol.* 2000;18(1):106-115. PMID: 10623700. (Muggia et al. 2000)

TRIAL SPONSOR

- Gynecologic Oncology Group (GOG)

RATIONALE FOR TRIAL

- Despite the activity of cisplatin in advanced ovarian cancer, the long-term survival of suboptimally cytoreduced patients remains poor.
- Paclitaxel has been established as a salvage treatment of patients with platinum-sensitive and platinum-resistant ovarian cancer (McGuire et al. 1989; Thigpen et al. 1994).
- Because the possibility existed that paclitaxel may be more active than cisplatin, this trial was designed to compare the activity of single-agent cisplatin vs single-agent paclitaxel vs combination cisplatin and paclitaxel.

PATIENT POPULATION

- N = 648 registered, 614 eligible.
- Accrual between March 1992 and May 1994.

- Histologically confirmed epithelial ovarian cancer; stage III disease with at least 1 mass >1 cm residual or any stage IV disease; no prior anticancer medications or radiation; normal marrow (granulocytes >1500/μL; platelets >100,000/μL); normal renal function (serum creatinine <1.5 mg/dL); normal liver function (alanine aminotransferase [ALT], AST <2 times normal; bilirubin <1.5 mg/dL); GOG performance score of 0, 1, or 2.
- Ineligible: borderline tumors; any other prior malignancy other than basal cell carcinoma or in situ of the cervix; primary peritoneal tumor or lack of tumor in the ovaries.
- Registration within 6 weeks of staging surgery.

TREATMENT DETAILS

- Higher single-agent doses were selected because studying lower doses might have led to less definitive conclusions.

Arm 1: Single-Agent Cisplatin
- Cisplatin 100 mg/m^2 IV.
- Repeated every 3 weeks for 6 courses.
- Dose adjustment of cisplatin by 50% for grade 2 or higher thrombocytopenia or any other grade 2 nonhematologic toxicity (with the exception of nausea and vomiting); any grade tinnitus.
- Dose held for cisplatin for any grade 3 or 4 nephropathy or neuropathy until toxicity completely resolved.

Arm 2: Single-Agent Paclitaxel
- Paclitaxel 200 mg/m^2 IV over 24 hours.
- Repeated every 3 weeks for 6 courses.
- Dose adjustment of paclitaxel to 150 mg/m^2 for any grade 4 neutropenia or grade 3 neutropenia requiring hospitalization.

Arm 3: Combination Cisplatin+Paclitaxel (Same Regimen as GOG 111) (McGuire et al. 1996)
- Paclitaxel 135 mg/m^2 IV over 24 hours.
- Cisplatin 75 mg/m^2 IV.
- Repeated every 3 weeks for 6 courses.
- Dose adjustment of paclitaxel to 110 mg/m^2 for any grade 4 neutropenia or grade 3 neutropenia requiring hospitalization.
- Dose adjustment of cisplatin by 50% for grade 2 or higher thrombocytopenia or any other grade 2 nonhematologic toxicity (with the exception of nausea and vomiting); any grade tinnitus.

- Dose held for cisplatin for any grade 3 or 4 nephropathy or neuropathy until toxicity completely resolved.

Treatment Delays
- Delay until platelet count >100,000/µL and ANC >1500/µL.
- Granulocyte colony-stimulating factors (G-CSFs) were permitted if ANC failed to recover to >1500/µL within 21 days of the last treatment despite 1 dose-level reduction or if neutropenia-related complications occurred at the reduced dose level.

ASSESSMENTS
- Baseline computed tomography (CT) scan (within 3 weeks), CA125, blood work, and exam.

ENDPOINTS
- PFS.
- OS.
- Response rate.

STATISTICAL CONSIDERATIONS

Sample Size
- Sample size provides 80% chance of detecting a true 29% decrease in the hazard ratio (40% increase in PFS) with a type I error limited to .05.

CONCLUSION OF TRIAL
- Response rates were significantly lower and progression-free survival was shorter with paclitaxel monotherapy compared to the cisplatin-containing regimens.
- There was no difference in overall survival between the 3 treatment arms.
- Combination therapy had a better toxicity profile than the high-dose monotherapy regimens.

COMMENTS
- Cisplatin and paclitaxel monotherapies were discontinued more frequently than the combination regimen due to toxicity or patient refusal (cisplatin only) or due to early progression (paclitaxel only).
- Toxicities.
  - Paclitaxel associated with more severe neutropenia, fever, and alopecia.

Table 2.7 Results of GOG 132

Treatment arm	Cisplatin N=200	Paclitaxel N=213	Cisplatin+paclitaxel N=201
Patient characteristics			
Age <50	23%	23%	22%
Age 50-69	59%	59%	61%
Age ≥70	18%	18%	16%
Measurable disease	61%	61%	62%
Stage III	65%	72%	73%
Stage IV	35%	28%	27%
Serous	71%	74%	65%
Endometrioid	7%	7%	10%
Mucinous	2%	3%	2%
Clear cell	1%	1%	4%
Other	19%	15%	16%
Grade 1	8%	9%	6%
Grade 2	41%	39%	37%
Grade 3	51%	52%	57%
Treatment delivery			
Completed 6 courses	69%	71%	81%
Discontinuation due to			
Toxicity or refusal	17%	4%	7%
Early progression	7%	20%	6%
Efficacy			
CR	42%	21%	43%
PR	25%	21%	23%
No response	33%	57%	33%
Pathologic CR	Not assessed	6%	24% ($P<.03$)
Median PFS	16.4 months	10.8 months	14.1 months
Median OS	30.2 months	25.9 months	26.3 months
Toxicity			
G3/4 granulocytopenia	48%	96%	94%
G3/4 thrombocytopenia	4%	3%	3%
G3/4 anemia	11%	6%	8%
G3/4 GI toxicity	33%	10%	18%
G3/4 renal toxicity	4%	0%	<1%
G3/4 neurologic toxicity	11%	1%	5%

CR, complete response; GI, gastrointestinal; OS, overall survival; PFS, progression-free survival; PR, partial response.

- ○ Cisplatin associated with more severe anemia, thrombocytopenia, neurotoxicity, nephrotoxicity, and gastrointestinal toxicity.
- Salvage therapy was initiated before clinical progression in all 3 treatment arms.
  - ○ Among patients receiving cisplatin only, 52% received paclitaxel as next nonprotocol regimen.
  - ○ Among patients receiving paclitaxel only, 69% received a regimen containing cisplatin or carboplatin as next nonprotocol regimen.
  - ○ Among patients receiving combination cisplatin and paclitaxel, 39% received further cisplatin or carboplatin and 40% received a regimen containing neither platinum nor paclitaxel as next nonprotocol regimen.
- GOG initiated this trial before the results of GOG 111 were available (McGuire et al. 1996).
- This trial needs to be considered in the context of GOG 111 (McGuire et al. 1996) and OV-10 (Piccart et al. 2000), 2 trials that both demonstrated the superiority of cisplatin+paclitaxel over cisplatin+cyclophosphamide. In contrast, GOG 132 demonstrates no difference between cisplatin+paclitaxel vs cisplatin alone (Muggia et al. 2000).
  - ○ Both paclitaxel and cisplatin were commercially available at the time of GOG 132, and many patients crossed over early (before disease progression) after participating in the trial. While this may be responsible for blunting of a survival difference, if one exists, this trial was not designed to evaluate differences between concurrent and sequential treatment strategies, and one cannot conclude that these are equivalent strategies from these data. However, these data are provocative and suggest that sequential therapy may be an acceptable treatment strategy for future studies.
  - ○ During GOG 111, paclitaxel was not commercially available. During the European-Canadian OV-10 trial, paclitaxel was available, but it was not generally used until demonstrated progression. Based on the OV-10 study, the withholding of paclitaxel until clinical progression is not an acceptable treatment strategy.
  - ○ The divergent results between GOG 132 and GOG 111/OV-10 might be explained by the higher dose of cisplatin (100 mg/m^2) in the GOG 132 regimen. This might also be explained by a possible antagonistic effect of cyclophosphamide when combined with cisplatin. However, when considered in the context of the available literature, there is no direct evidence to suggest this to be the case.

Danish Netherlands Trial (Neijt, JCO 2000)

REFERENCE

- Neijt JP, et al. Exploratory phase III study of paclitaxel and cisplatin versus paclitaxel and carboplatin in advanced ovarian cancer. *J Clin Oncol.* 2000;18(17):3084-3092. PMID: 10963636. (Neijt et al. 2000)

TRIAL SPONSOR

- Supported by grants from Bristol-Meyers Squibb.

RATIONALE FOR TRIAL

- Cisplatin + paclitaxel was recommended as the current standard of care. However, paclitaxel was infused over 24 hours and administration required hospitalization for at least 48 hours. Administration of paclitaxel over 3 hours at a higher dose resulted in a different toxicity profile (Eisenhauer et al. 1994; Connelly et al. 1996).
- The substitution of carboplatin for cisplatin results in an improved toxicity profile with less nephrotoxicity, ototoxicity, and neurotoxicity but more myelotoxicity when used as a single agent. However, carboplatin was found to be less effective than cisplatin in a number of solid tumors, and its use was not recommended in the initial treatment of ovarian cancer where the goal of treatment was long-term survival and cure (Vermorken et al. 1993; Lokich and Anderson 1998).
- This exploratory trial was conducted to evaluate the combination of paclitaxel (3-hour infusion) with cisplatin or carboplatin to address the following questions:
  - How many cycles are safe and feasible when administered to outpatients?
  - Is neurotoxicity less with carboplatin compared to cisplatin?
  - Are the regimens equal in efficacy?
  - Is there enough activity to justify the costs of a larger randomized study?

PATIENT POPULATION

- N = 213; 208 eligible.
- Accrual between March 1994 and March 1997.
- Epithelial ovarian cancer, International Federation of Gynecology and Obstetrics (FIGO) stages IIB to IV.
- Adequate bone marrow function (WBC $>3 \times 10^9$/L; platelet count $>100 \times 10^9$/L); adequate renal function (serum creatinine >120 µmol/L;

creatinine clearance >60 mL/min/1.73 m^2); adequate liver function (bilirubin level >25 µmol/L).
- Exclusion criteria: World Health Organization (WHO) performance status of 4; age >75 years or <18 years; complete bowel obstruction; symptomatic brain metastases; prior chemotherapy or radiation therapy; history of ventricular arrhythmia; history of congestive heart failure; myocardial infarction within 6 months of randomization; borderline tumors; second malignant disease; active infection; other serious medical conditions; prior allergic reactions to Cremophor EL.

TREATMENT DETAILS

Arm 1: Paclitaxel + Cisplatin (Administered as Inpatient)
- Paclitaxel 175 mg/m^2 IV over 3 hours.
- Cisplatin 75 mg/m^2 IV.
- Treatment every 3 weeks for 6 cycles.

Arm 2: Paclitaxel + Carboplatin (Administered as Outpatient)
- Paclitaxel 175 mg/m^2 IV over 3 hours.
- Carboplatin AUC 5 IV. GFR based on creatinine clearance, EDTA (ethylenediaminetetraacetic acid) clearance, or the Cockcroft-Gault formula (Cockroft and Gault 1976). Dose (mg) = 5 × (GFR + 25) (Calvert et al. 1989).
- Treatment every 3 weeks for 6 cycles

Standard Premedications
- Dexamethasone 20 mg orally 12 and 6 hours prior to chemotherapy.
- Diphenhydramine 50 mg IV.
- Cimetidine 300 mg IV (or ranitidine 50 mg IV).
- Antiemetics at investigators discretion.

Dose Reductions
- According to nadirs and nadir duration (Neijt et al. 1997).

Treatment Continuations
- Six cycles of treatment unless progressive disease or unacceptable toxicity.
- If assessable disease and no change in disease status after 6 cycles, then 2 additional courses and additional treatment at the discretion of the investigator.
- If partial response, treatment continuation until progression or toxicity.

- If complete response, then 3 additional courses after date of documented response.
- If nonassessable disease, then treatment with 6 cycles until progression or toxicity with subsequent treatment at the discretion of the investigator.

Surgery
- Initial cytoreductive surgery.
- If unresectable disease at time of initial surgery, then maximum cytoreductive surgery recommended as soon at tumor masses were deemed resectable.
- Second-look laparotomy was not recommended.

ASSESSMENTS
- Baseline CA125, CT scan, labs.
- Blood counts weekly.
- CA125 with each cycle of treatment, 1 month after completing therapy and every 3 months thereafter.
- Pelvic examination after 3 and 6 cycles.
- Scans performed at the time CA125 started to increase or when progressive disease suspected on exam. Scans repeated after 3 courses if normal CA125 level at study entry or if CA125 values had not decreased to normal values after 3 courses.

ENDPOINTS
- PFS.

STATISTICAL CONSIDERATIONS

Sample Size
- With a PFS estimate of 20 months for cisplatin+paclitaxel, the study was designed with α of .05 and power of 80% to detect a hazard ratio of 1.67 (PFS as low as 12 months for carboplatin+paclitaxel). Assuming an accrual over 3 years, a total number of 196 patients were needed with 140 events.
- PFS and OS analyzed with Kaplan-Meier survival curves with P values calculated by the log-rank and Breslow tests for significance.

Statistical Tests
- Neurotoxicity-free period assessed by Kaplan-Meier.
- Cox proportional hazards model used for effects of treatment, age, WHO performance status, residual tumor size, FIGO stage, grade,

Table 2.8 Results of the Danish Netherlands Trial

Treatment arm	Paclitaxel + cisplatin N = 108	Paclitaxel + carboplatin N = 100	Statistics
Patient characteristics			
Median age	56 years	56 years	
Residual disease ≤1 cm	44%	41%	
Residual disease >1 cm	56%	59%	
Stage II	10%	11%	
Stage III	69%	70%	
Stage IV	20%	19%	
Serous	60%	55%	
Endometrioid	14%	5%	
Mucinous	5%	6%	
Clear cell	1%	6%	
Other	20%	28%	
Grade 1	5%	11%	
Grade 2	33%	20%	
Grade 3	39%	47%	
Unknown grade	23%	22%	
Treatment delivery			
6 cycles (at least)	79%	89%	
12 cycles	3%	4%	
Discontinued for toxicity	17%	5%	
Efficacy			
Overall response	62%	66%	
Clinical complete	35%	40%	
Partial	26%	25%	
No change	19%	16%	
Progression	11%	13%	
Median PFS			HR 1.07 (95% CI, 0.78-1.48)
Median OS	30 months	32 months	HR 0.85 (95% CI, 0.59-1.24)
Toxicity (6 cycles)			
G3/4 hemoglobin	1%	6%	NS
G3/4 granulocytes	50%	70%	<.01
G3/4 platelets	1%	6%	<.01
G2/3 fever	8%	11%	NS
G3 nausea	17%	14%	<.01
G3 neurotoxicity	6%	2%	NS

CI, confidence interval; HR, hazard ratio; NS, not significant; PFS, progression-free survival; OS, overall survival.

histology, body weight, body surface, and baseline laboratory values on PFS.

CONCLUSION OF TRIAL

- The paclitaxel+carboplatin combination is safe and easy to administer to outpatients and is less toxic than paclitaxel+cisplatin. Due to the small number of patients and the wide confidence intervals around survival outcomes, conclusions about efficacy cannot be made with this study.

COMMENTS

- Toxicities.
  - No difference in hair loss, fever, mucositis, diarrhea, allergic reactions, pulmonary toxicity, cutaneous complications, cardiac events, arthralgia, myalgia, constipation, or renal toxicities.
  - Neurotoxicity (greater than grade 1) occurred earlier with paclitaxel+cisplatin.
  - Neurotoxicity occurred in the paclitaxel+carboplatin arm, but it was less frequent, was less severe, and occurred later compared to the neurotoxicity occurring in the cisplatin-containing arm.
- CA125 assessments were performed and elevations were the first sign of progressive disease in 70% of patients who had an elevated level at study entry.
- Because this study determined treatment duration differently from other studies, many patients received more than 6 cycles of treatment. Likely due to the better tolerability of the carboplatin-containing regimen, more women on this arm received prolonged treatment. It is not clear whether this resulted in an impact on PFS.
- Univariate analysis found the following factors to predict worse PFS: residual disease, stage, low hemoglobin levels, high platelet counts, and high number of granulocytes. These findings may implicate interleukin 6 (IL-6) and C-reactive protein in poor outcome. The prognostic impact of hemoglobin, platelets, and granulocytes disappears in a multivariate analysis that included tumor mass, suggesting that IL-6 cytokine release may be related to tumor size.

OV-10 (Piccart, JNCI 2000)

REFERENCE

- Piccart MJ, et al. Randomized intergroup trial of cisplatin-paclitaxel versus cisplatin-cyclophosphamide in women with advanced epithelial ovarian cancer: three-year results. *J Natl Cancer Inst.* 2000;92(9): 699-708. PMID: 10793106. (Piccart et al. 2000)

TRIAL SPONSORS

- EORTC (European Organization for Research and Treatment of Cancer)
- NOCOVA (Nordic Gynecological Cancer Study Group)
- NCI-C-CTG (National Cancer Institute of Canada Clinical Trials Group)
- Scottish Group

RATIONALE FOR TRIAL

- GOG 111 was conducted in the United States and reported better outcome with paclitaxel-cisplatin than cyclophosphamide-cisplatin in suboptimally debulked stage III/IV ovarian cancer patients (abstract at ASCO in 1993, published in 1996) (McGuire et al. 1996).
- This was a confirmatory trial conducted in Europe and Canada.
- In contrast to the administration of Taxol over 24 hours in GOG 111, Taxol was given as a 3-hour infusion in this trial. A prior European-Canadian collaborative trial found a PFS advantage for Taxol 175 mg/m^2 administration over 3 hours in a 2 × 2 factorial design evaluating paclitaxel dose (135 or 175 mg/m^2) and infusion time (3 hours or 24 hours) in patients with recurrent ovarian cancer (Eisenhauer et al. 1994).

PATIENT POPULATION

- N = 680 recruited.
- Trial organized in April 1994, accrual completed in August 1995.

Inclusion Criteria

- Histologically confirmed epithelial ovarian cancer, stage IIB, IIC, III, or IV.
- Initial surgery within 8 weeks.
- Optimal (≤1 cm residual) or suboptimal (>1 cm residual) cytoreduction.

Exclusion Criteria
- WHO performance status of 4.
- Inadequate bone marrow function (neutrophil count <1.5 × 10^9/L; platelet count <100 × 10^9/L).
- Inadequate liver function (bilirubin >25 μmol/L).
- Inadequate renal function.
- Prior chemotherapy or radiotherapy.
- Complete bowel obstruction.
- Brain metastases.
- Borderline histology.
- Carcinoma of unknown origin.
- Atrial or ventricular arrhythmias.
- Congestive heart failure.
- Myocardial infarction within 6 months.
- Second malignant disease excluding basal cell carcinoma of the skin or in situ carcinoma of the cervix.
- Inability to follow up.
- Active infection.
- Other serious underlying medical conditions.

TREATMENT DETAILS

Arm 1: Cyclophosphamide + Cisplatin (CP)
- Cyclophosphamide 750 mg/m^2 IV rapid injection.
- Cisplatin 75 mg/m^2 IV over 1 hour.
- Administered every 3 weeks.
- Premedications with antiemetics.
- Hydration: 1-L prehydration over 3 hours + posthydration of 1 L over 3 hours (outpatient) or 2 to 3 L over 15 hours (inpatient).

Arm 2: Taxol + Cisplatin (TP)
- Paclitaxel 175 mg/m^2 IV over 3 hours. Dose was escalated to 200 mg/m^2 IV in the second cycle if no febrile neutropenia.
- Cisplatin 75 mg/m^2 IV over 1 hour.
- Premedications.
  - Dexamethasone 20 mg orally 12 hours and 6 hours before paclitaxel.
  - Diphenhydramine 50 mg IV 30 minutes before paclitaxel.
  - Ranitidine 50 mg IV 30 minutes before paclitaxel.
  - Antiemetics.

- Hydration: 1-L prehydration over 3 hours + posthydration of 1 L over 3 hours (outpatient) or 2 to 3 L over 15 hours (inpatients).

Dose Modifications and Drug Substitutions
- For febrile neutropenia or prolonged myelosuppression (G4 neutropenia and/or thrombocytopenia for 2 successive weekly counts):
  - Paclitaxel reduced 20%.
  - Cyclophosphamide reduced 20%.
  - Cisplatin dose not reduced.
  - G-CSF used only if toxic effects occurred despite dose reduction.
- Substitution of carboplatin for cisplatin.
  - Severe renal toxicity (creatinine clearance <45 mL/min per 1.73 m^2).
  - Substantial hearing loss.
  - WHO grade 3 or 4 neurotoxicity.
- Discontinuation of paclitaxel.
  - WHO grade 3 or 4 neurotoxicity.
  - Severe hypersensitivity reactions.
  - Severe cardiac arrhythmias.

Other Treatment Details
- Interval cytoreduction and second-look surgeries allowed.
- Patients who had progressed were allowed to receive any secondary treatment at the investigator's discretion, including taxanes.
- Patients without disease progression after 6 cycles could receive another 3 cycles of optional protocol treatment.
- Cyclophosphamide + cisplatin—options for 3 additional cycles.
  - Cyclophosphamide + cisplatin.
  - Cyclophosphamide + carboplatin.
  - Cyclophosphamide.
  - Cisplatin.
  - Carboplatin.
- Paclitaxel + cisplatin—options for 3 additional cycles.
  - Paclitaxel + cisplatin.
  - Paclitaxel + carboplatin.
  - Paclitaxel.
  - Cisplatin.
  - Carboplatin.
  - Cyclophosphamide + carboplatin.

ASSESSMENTS

- Clinical and radiologic assessment after 3 cycles of therapy.
- Final response status was assigned after 6 cycles of therapy by clinical and radiologic assessment or by second-look surgery.
- CA125 measurements were not used to assess response, except for normalization required for complete response status.
- CT scans were performed at baseline and after 3 cycles, 6 cycles, and 9 cycles.
- Once off protocol therapy, patients were monitored with exam and CA125 assessment every 3 months for 2 years and every 6 months thereafter. CT scans were not performed routinely but were ordered in the setting of symptoms or CA125 elevation.

ENDPOINTS

- PFS (defined as date of randomization to date of progression, death, or start of new therapy).
- Clinical response rate.
- Overall survival (defined as date of randomization to date of death).
- Quality of life.
- Cost-effectiveness.
- Potential use of CA125 as a surrogate for patient outcome.

STATISTICAL CONSIDERATIONS

Sample Size

- Target accrual of 600 patients to have an 80% probability of detecting an increase in the median PFS by 33% with a 2-sided significance level of 5%. Calculations were based on an accrual time of 18 months.

Statistical Tests

- Kaplan-Meier curves with 2-sided unstratified log-rank test.
- Cox proportional hazards regression model.
- Two-sided χ^2 test or 2-sided Fisher's exact test.
- Two-sided Kruskal-Wallis test.

CONCLUSION OF TRIAL

- This trial confirms the conclusions of GOG 111, which demonstrated the superiority of paclitaxel+cisplatin over cyclophosphamide+cisplatin.

Table 2.9 Results of OV-10

Treatment arm	Cyclophosphamide + cisplatin (CP) N=338	Paclitaxel + cisplatin (TP) N=342	Statistics
Patient characteristics			
Median age (range)	58 (22-85)	58 (23-79)	
No residual	15.7%	17.5%	
Residual disease ≤1 cm	18.6%	21.1%	
Residual disease >1 cm	65.4%	61.1%	
Stage II	6.8%	6.4%	
Stage III	72.5%	74.9%	
Stage IV	20.7%	18.7%	
Serous	62.7%	68.7%	
Endometrioid	13.6%	9.1%	
Mucinous	5.3%	3.5%	
Clear cell	5.3%	4.4%	
Other	13.0%	14.3%	
Grade 1	8.6%	8.2%	
Grade 2	25.4%	26.9%	
Grade 3	56.8%	57.6%	
Unknown grade	9.2%	7.3%	
Treatment delivery			
Median cycles (range)	6 (0-10)	6 (0-10)	
>6 cycles	26.2%	33.3%	
Switch to carboplatin	8.9%	11.8%	
Cisplatin dose reduction	21.4%	30.1%	$P<.001$
Cisplatin dose delay	59.8%	36.3%	
Paclitaxel dose increase		71.1%	
D/C for toxicity	4.5%	6.5%	
Crossover to paclitaxel	48%		
Efficacy			
Pathologic CR	25%	42.5%	
Microscopic residual	20.5%	23%	
Overall response	44.7%	58.6%	$P=.01$
Complete response	27.3%	40.7%	$P=.01$
Partial response	17.4%	17.9%	
Stable disease	15.5%	11.7%	
Progressive disease	13.0%	4.9%	
Median PFS	11.5 months	15.5 months	HR 0.74, $P=.0005$
Median OS	25.8 months	35.6 months	HR 0.73, $P=.0016$
Toxicity (first 6 cycles)			
G3/4 neutropenia	71%	64%	
Febrile neutropenia	3%	2%	

Table 2.9 Results of OV-10 *(continued)*

Treatment arm	Cyclophosphamide+ cisplatin (CP) N=338	Paclitaxel+ cisplatin (TP) N=342	Statistics
G3/4 thrombocytopenia	5%	2%	
G3/4 nausea	19%	13.3%	
G3/4 vomiting	17%	10%	
G3 stomatitis	0%	0.6%	
G3 alopecia	20%	50%	
G3 arthralgia	0.6%	3%	
G3 myalgia	0%	6%	
G3/4 neurosensory	0.6%	14.3%	
G3 neuromotor	0.3%	3%	
G3 ototoxicity	4%	2%	
Severe hypersensitivity	1%	4%	

CR, complete response; D/C, discontinued; HR, hazard ratio; OS, overall survival; PFS, progression-free survival.

COMMENTS

- Accrual completed in 1995, 4 months before GOG 111 was published (McGuire et al. 1996).
- A total of 680 patients were accrued in only 15 months and marked a turning point in the ability to conduct intergroup trials.
- PFS was selected as the primary endpoint as more crossover to paclitaxel was anticipated. Despite the 48% crossover rate, this study found PFS and OS differences in favor of the paclitaxel-containing regimen (vs 8% crossover rate in GOG 111).
- Differences between OV-10 and GOG 111.
  - OV-10 had broader inclusion criteria with inclusion of stage II patients, inclusion of patients with suboptimal cytoreduction, ability of patients to undergo secondary cytoreduction, and interval debulking surgery.
  - OV-10 allowed up to 9 cycles of chemotherapy, administered paclitaxel over 3 hours rather than 24 hours, mandated dose escalation of paclitaxel, and allowed substitution of carboplatin for cisplatin in the setting of toxicity.
- The rate of neurotoxicity of 14% in OV-10 was higher than the 4% rate reported in GOG 111.
  - This may be attributed to the paclitaxel dose escalation (built into the protocol due to the uncertainties of optimal dosing schedule) and the option to give 9 cycles of treatment (built into the protocol to

account for the possibility that prior evidence supporting 6 cycles did not apply to this new regimen).
- This trial provides strong level I evidence to support paclitaxel+cisplatin as the new standard of care, and it refutes the claim that paclitaxel administration should be delayed until relapse.

GOG 114 (Markman, JCO 2001)

REFERENCE

- Markman M, et al. Phase III trial of standard-dose intravenous cisplatin plus paclitaxel versus moderately high-dose carboplatin followed by intravenous paclitaxel and intraperitoneal cisplatin in small-volume stage III ovarian carcinoma: an intergroup study of the Gynecologic Oncology Group, Southwestern Oncology Group, and Eastern Cooperative Oncology Group. *J Clin Oncol.* 2001;19(4):1001-1007. PMID: 11181662. (Markman et al. 2001)

TRIAL SPONSORS

- Gynecologic Oncology Group (GOG)
- Southwest Oncology Group (SWOG)
- Eastern Cooperative Oncology Group (ECOG)

RATIONALE FOR TRIAL

- Current standard of care is platinum+paclitaxel, but the majority of patients still die of ovarian cancer.
- Studies suggest the utility of giving cisplatin by the intraperitoneal (IP) route (Alberts et al. 1996; Markman 1998).
- This trial also employed the concept of administering systemic chemotherapy to chemically debulk residual tumors by giving 2 cycles of moderately high-intensity carboplatin (AUC 9) before administering IP chemotherapy (Shapiro et al. 1997).

PATIENT POPULATION

- N=523 patients entered, 462 eligible.
- Enrollment from August 1992 to April 1995.

Inclusion Criteria
- Stage III epithelial ovarian cancer.
- Tumor debulking to optimal residual (<1 cm).

- Entry within 6 weeks of surgery.
- Adequate bone marrow (WBC ≥3000 cells/mm^3; platelets ≥100,000/mm^3); adequate renal function (creatinine clearance ≥50 mL/min); adequate hepatic function (bilirubin ≤1.5 times normal; serum ALT ≤3 times normal function); GOG performance status of 0, 1, or 2.

Exclusion Criteria
- Borderline tumors.
- Suboptimal residual disease.
- Stage IV disease.
- Prior chemotherapy or radiotherapy.
- Septicemia, severe infection acute hepatitis, or severe bleeding.
- GOG performance status of 3 or 4.
- Other malignancy excluding nonmelanoma skin cancer.
- Congestive heart failure, unstable angina, or myocardial infarction within 6 months.
- Not expected to tolerate the hemodynamic effects of sinus bradycardia.
- Abnormal cardiac conduction.
- Taking medications known to affect cardiac conduction.

TREATMENT DETAILS
- Originally designed as a 3-arm trial with 1 arm receiving cisplatin+cyclophosphamide. When the results of GOG 111 showed inferiority of this regimen to paclitaxel+cisplatin (McGuire et al. 1996), this arm was discontinued and the 66 patients enrolled to this arm were not analyzed.

Arm 1: Paclitaxel IV + Cisplatin IV
- Paclitaxel 135 mg/m^2 IV over 24 hours.
- Cisplatin 75 mg/m^2 IV on day 2.
- Administered every 21 days for 6 cycles.

Arm 2: High-Dose Carboplatin Followed by Paclitaxel IV + Cisplatin IP
- Carboplatin AUC 9 IV for 2 courses every 28 days. Dose calculated by Calvert formula (Calvert et al. 1989) with glomerular filtration rate being considered equivalent to the creatinine clearance, which was calculated by the Jelliffe method (Jelliffe 1973).
- Paclitaxel 135 mg/m^2 IV over 24 hours on day 1.

- Cisplatin 100 mg/m² IP on day 2. Administered in 2 L of normal saline through an implantable peritoneal dialysis catheter (ie, Tenckhoff catheter).
- Paclitaxel and cisplatin administered every 21 days for 6 cycles.

Premedications
- Standard prophylaxis to prevent paclitaxel hypersensitivity (dexamethasone, diphenhydramine, either cimetidine or ranitidine).
- Antiemetics and hydration programs were left to the discretion of the investigator.

Treatment Modifications
- To maintain dose intensity, dose reductions were not allowed.
- Treatments were delayed until WBC ≥3000 cells/mm³ and platelets ≥100,000/mm³.
- Grade 3 or 4 peripheral neuropathy resulted in treatment interruption until resolution to a maximum of grade 1.

ASSESSMENTS
- Second-look surgery performed within 8 weeks for all patients without evidence of progressive disease.
- Frequency of CT scans not stated in manuscript.

ENDPOINTS
- PFS (defined as date from entry onto the protocol to the date of appearance of disease as determined clinically or radiographically—not surgically).
- OS (defined as date from entry onto the protocol to the date of death).

STATISTICAL CONSIDERATIONS

Sample Size
- Accrual goal of 440 patients and follow-up until 150 deaths had occurred to provide 80% power to detect a 33% decrease in the hazard ratio at the .05 level (1-sided).

Statistical Tests
- Kaplan-Meier survival analyses, log-rank test.
- Cox model.
- Pearson's χ^2 test significance level of .20.
- Mann-Whitney U test.

Table 2.10 Results of GOG 114

Treatment arm	IV paclitaxel+ IV cisplatin N=227	Carboplatin+ IV paclitaxel+ IP cisplatin N=235	Statistics
Patient characteristics			
Age <51	37%	33%	
Age 51-70	51%	58%	
Age >70	12%	9%	
No residual	36%	35%	
Residual disease ≤1 cm	64%	65%	
Stage III	100%	100%	
Serous	70%	63%	
Endometrioid	10%	14%	
Mixed	9%	9%	
Other	11%	14%	
Grade 1	14%	11%	
Grade 2	40%	39%	
Grade 3	46%	50%	
Treatment delivery			
Received 6 courses	86%	71%	
Refusal of second look	15.0%	22.6%	
Efficacy			
Median PFS	22.2 months	27.9 months	HR 0.78, $P=.01$
Median OS	52.2 months	63.2 months	HR 0.81, $P=.05$
Toxicity			
G3/4 WBC	62%	77%	Significant
G3/4 platelets	3%	49%	Significant
G3/4 hematologic	88%	92%	
G3/4 gastrointestinal	17%	37%	Significant
G3/4 cardiovascular	3%	4%	
G3/4 neurologic	9%	12%	
G3/4 infection	2%	5%	
G3/4 metabolic	1%	10%	Significant
Deaths	N=2	N=2	

HR, hazard ratio; IP, intraperitoneal; IV, intravenous; OS, overall survival; PFS, progression-free survival; WBC, white blood cells.

CONCLUSIONS OF TRIAL

- Because the improvement in survival was of borderline significance and at the expense of greater toxicity, the experimental arm in this trial is not recommended for use.
- This study confirms the relative safety as well as the survival advantage of administering IP cisplatin compared to IV cisplatin (as seen in GOG 104) (Alberts et al. 1996).
- Given the superior outcomes with paclitaxel plus cisplatin over cyclophosphamide and cisplatin (as seen in GOG 111 and OV-10) (McGuire et al. 1996; Piccart et al. 2000), it is important to study the impact of IP cisplatin when combined with paclitaxel (design of GOG 172) (Armstrong et al. 2006).

COMMENTS

- This study was designed recognizing that the results would not give a clear answer regarding the separate effects of high-dose IV carboplatin or IP cisplatin. Because the increases in survival with the experimental arm were marginal and at the expense of greater toxicity, the question of future directions from this study are raised.
- Due to the imbalance and higher than expected refusals of second-look procedures, the endpoint of pathologic response was thought to be likely biased and was not reported.

ICON3 (Lancet 2002)

REFERENCE

- International Collaborative Ovarian Neoplasm Group. Paclitaxel plus carboplatin versus standard chemotherapy with either single-agent carboplatin or cyclophosphamide, doxorubicin, and cisplatin in women with ovarian cancer: the ICON3 randomised trial. *Lancet.* 2002;360 (9332):505-515. PMID: 12241653. (International Collaborative Ovarian Neoplasm Group 2002)

TRIAL SPONSORS

- Istituto Mario Negri in Milan, Italy
- Swiss Group for Cancer Research (SAKK) in Bern, Switzerland
- Nordic Society for Gynecologic Oncology (NSGO) in Odense, Denmark

ICON3

- Medical Research Council (MRC) Cancer Trials Office in Cambridge, United Kingdom

RATIONALE FOR TRIAL

- The ICON2 trial compared single-agent carboplatin with the 3-drug regimen of cyclophosphamide, Adriamycin, and cisplatin (CAP) and found no difference in progression-free or overall survival between the treatment arms (International Collaborative Ovarian Neoplasm Group 1998).
- Based on GOG 111, OV-10, and GOG 132, many have suggested that paclitaxel and cisplatin should be the standard of care for advanced ovarian cancer (McGuire et al. 1996; Muggia et al. 2000; Piccart et al. 2000).
- Because of the equivalence of cisplatin and carboplatin and the concern over neurotoxicity when cisplatin and paclitaxel are administered together, others have suggested that carboplatin and paclitaxel should be given as routine treatment (GOG 158, AGO/OVAR-3, Neijt trials) (Neijt et al. 2000; du Bois et al. 2003; Ozols et al. 2003).
- ICON3 aims to compare paclitaxel+carboplatin against a non-taxane-containing platinum-based regimen. At the time of trial initiation, the results from ICON2 were not yet mature and a firm recommendation for the regimens in the control arm (carboplatin vs CAP) could not be made.

PATIENT POPULATION

- N=2074 enrolled.
- Enrollment from February 1995 to October 1998 from 130 centers in 8 countries.
- Invasive epithelial ovarian cancer; fit to receive chemotherapy; no other malignant disease; no prior chemotherapy or radiotherapy.
- Minimum recommended surgical procedure was total abdominal hysterectomy, bilateral salpingo-oophorectomy, and thorough staging.

TREATMENT DETAILS

- The treating physician could choose the control regimen (carboplatin or CAP), but this had to be specified before randomization.

Control Group—Carboplatin

- Dose determined by the AUC method of Calvert (Calvert et al. 1989) of 5 (GFR+25) mg.

Control Group—CAP
- Cyclophosphamide 500 mg/m^2 IV.
- Doxorubicin 50 mg/m^2 IV.
- Cisplatin 50 mg/m^2 IV.

Experimental Group—Paclitaxel + Carboplatin
- Paclitaxel 175 mg/m^2 IV over 3 hours.
- Carboplatin (same dosing as control arm).

ASSESSMENTS
- Data were collected pretreatment and after each cycle of treatment. During follow-up, data were collected every 3 months for the first 2 years, every 6 months for the next 3 years, and every year thereafter.

ENDPOINTS
- OS (time from randomization to death from any cause).
- PFS (time from randomization to first appearance of progressive disease or death from any cause) and toxicity.

STATISTICAL CONSIDERATIONS

Sample Size
- Power analysis based on expectation of 2-year survival of 50% in the control groups. An accrual target of 1000 patients in the control groups was selected to detect a 10% difference in 2-year survival from 50% to 60% with 85% power and 5% significance level, translating into a hazard ratio of 0.74.
- One year into the trial, the trial sample size was increased to a new target of 2000 patients to detect more a subtle difference of 7% difference from 50% to 57% 2-year survival with 85% power and 5% significance level, corresponding to a hazard ratio of 0.81.

Statistical Tests
- Kaplan-Meier survival curves for OS and PFS were compared using the Mantel-Cox version of the log-rank test. The stratified log-rank test was used to account for the 2 control groups, the differences across the 4 participating centers, and the difference in randomization ratios (1:1 at 2 centers and 2:1 at 2 centers).
- χ^2 test for interaction or χ^2 test for trend used to test of differences in the relative size of effect in different subgroup.

Table 2.11 Results of ICON3

Treatment arm	Carboplatin N=943	Paclitaxel, carboplatin N=478	CAP N=421	Paclitaxel, carboplatin N=232
Patient characteristics				
Median age	59.4	60.7	56.9	56.6
No residual	27%	28%	38%	34%
Residual disease <2 cm	26%	26%	19%	19%
Residual disease ≥2 cm	47%	46%	44%	47%
Stage I	8%	9%	10%	9%
Stage II	11%	10%	12%	13%
Stage III	65%	64%	63%	63%
Stage IV	16%	17%	15%	15%
Serous	54%	57%	51%	54%
Endometrioid	16%	14%	16%	16%
Mucinous	7%	7%	9%	7%
Clear cell	5%	6%	7%	6%
Other	18%	16%	16%	17%
Grade 1	9%	13%	12%	11%
Grade 2	35%	28%	39%	34%
Grade 3	56%	60%	49%	55%

(continued)

Table 2.11 Results of ICON3

Treatment arm	Carboplatin N=943	Paclitaxel, carboplatin N=478	CAP N=421	Paclitaxel, carboplatin N=232
Treatment delivery				
Total dose	73% Carboplatin	74% Paclitaxel 70% Carboplatin	72% Cyclophosphamide 71% Doxorubicin 75% Cisplatin	79% Paclitaxel 80% Carboplatin
Efficacy				
OS	35.4 months	36.1 months		
PFS	16.1 months	17.3 months		
Toxicity (G3/4)				
Alopecia	4%	73%	76%	80%
Nausea and vomiting	9%	9%	23%	10%
Hematologic	32%	25%	33%	29%
Fever, antibiotics	3%	10%	23%	13%
Sensory neuropathy	1%	19%	3%	18%
Motor neuropathy	<1%	3%	1%	1%

CAP, cyclophosphamide+Adriamycin/doxorubicin+Cisplatin; OS, overall survival; PFS, progression-free survival.

(continued)

CONCLUSIONS OF TRIAL
- The combination of paclitaxel + carboplatin is not superior to single-agent carboplatin or CAP.
- Paclitaxel + carboplatin is more toxic and causes more fever, alopecia, and sensory neuropathy than carboplatin alone.
- ICON3 suggests that single-agent carboplatin, CAP, and paclitaxel + carboplatin are all safe and have similar efficacy as first-line treatments for ovarian cancer.

COMMENTS
- In the context of other phase III trials, ICON3 seems to contradict the findings of GOG 111 (McGuire et al. 1996) and OV-10 (Piccart et al. 2000) but are in line with GOG 132 (Muggia et al. 2000). One explanation is that the control arm of cisplatin + cyclophosphamide (as given in GOG 111 and OV-10) is inferior to the control arm of single-agent platinum (as given in GOG 132 and ICON3).
- About one-third of patients in the ICON3 control arms went on to receive a taxane later. This raises the question of the optimum time to use paclitaxel in the treatment of advanced ovarian cancer and whether this would be at the time of progression after single-agent platinum.

GOG 158 (Ozols, JCO 2003)

REFERENCE
- Ozols RF, et al. Phase III trial of carboplatin and paclitaxel compared with cisplatin and paclitaxel in patients with optimally resected stage III ovarian cancer: a Gynecologic Oncology Group study. *J Clin Oncol.* 2003;21(17):3194-200. PMID: 12860964. (Ozols et al. 2003)

TRIAL SPONSOR
- Gynecologic Oncology Group (GOG)

RATIONALE FOR TRIAL
- The GOG 111 and OV-10 studies both demonstrated superiority of cisplatin + paclitaxel over the control treatment of cisplatin + cyclophosphamide (McGuire et al. 1996; Piccart et al. 2000).
- Carboplatin is an analogue of cisplatin with less hematologic toxicity and comparable efficacy.

- A 1993 International Ovarian Cancer Consensus Conference recommended that carboplatin should not be routinely used in the upfront treatment of patients with small-volume stage III ovarian cancer (Vermorken et al. 1993).
- A GOG pilot study found the combination of carboplatin and paclitaxel to be active with an overall response rate of 75% and a complete response rate of 67% (Bookman et al. 1996).
- GOG 158 was designed as a noninferiority study to compare the efficacy and toxicity of carboplatin+paclitaxel vs the standard regimen of cisplatin+paclitaxel.

PATIENT POPULATION
- N=840, 792 eligible.
- Stage III epithelial ovarian cancer with <1 cm residual disease.
- No prior chemotherapy; GOG performance status of 0 to 2; WBC ≥3000/µL; platelets ≥100,000/µL; serum creatinine ≤2.0 mg/dL; serum bilirubin and AST levels of no more than 2 times the institutional upper limit of normal.

TREATMENT DETAILS

Control Arm: Paclitaxel + Cisplatin
- Paclitaxel 135 mg/m^2 IV over 24 hours.
- Cisplatin 75 mg/m^2 IV at a rate of 1 mg/min.
- Treatment every 3 weeks for 6 cycles.

Experimental Arm: Paclitaxel + Carboplatin
- Paclitaxel 175 mg/m^2 IV over 3 hours.
- Carboplatin AUC 7.5 mg/mL/min. Dose based on the Calvert formula of AUC × (GFR + 25). Creatinine clearance was calculated using the Jelliffe formula (Jelliffe 1973).

Premedications Before Paclitaxel
- Dexamethasone 20 mg orally 12 and 6 hours before treatment.
- Diphenhydramine 50 mg IV 30 minutes before treatment.
- Cimetidine 300 mg IV 30 minutes before treatment.

Treatment Modifications
- If ANC ≤1000/µL and/or platelets <100,000/µL, then cycle delay, dose reduction, and addition of G-CSF in this sequence.
- No dose modification for uncomplicated nadirs.

- If delay of 2 weeks or less, no dose modification and no G-CSF.
- If delay of 2 to 3 weeks, dose modification.
- If recurrent delays of more than 2 weeks or febrile neutropenia, G-CSF added at dose of 5 µg/kg/d for 14 days starting 24 hours after the completion of chemotherapy.
- No cycle delay for gastrointestinal toxicity, grade 1 to 2 peripheral neuropathy, or mild renal toxicity (serum creatinine ≤2 mg/dL or creatinine clearance ≥50 mL/min).
- Discontinuation of protocol therapy for more severe renal or neurologic toxicity that had not resolved before the next scheduled dose of therapy.

ASSESSMENTS

- Because eligibility included tumors <1 cm only, imaging procedures were not required until after the completion of 6 cycles of chemotherapy.
- The decision of whether to undergo second-look laparotomy was made at the time of random assignment.

ENDPOINTS

- OS and PFS (measured from the date of random assignment to treatment).

STATISTICAL CONSIDERATIONS

Sample Size
- A sample size of 720 patients was set with an estimated 3 years of follow-up to observe 382 recurrences before testing the noninferiority hypothesis. This was a 1-sided test with the probability of a type I and type II error both set at 0.1 for a hazard ratio of 1.3 (favoring cisplatin plus paclitaxel). These characteristics were chosen to detect a moderate-size loss of efficacy with the use of carboplatin plus paclitaxel.

Statistical Tests
- Cumulative proportions of survival were based on Kaplan-Meier procedures.
- Relative risk estimates of treatment effects were calculated with the Cox model adjusting for prognostic factors.
- The Kruskal-Wallis rank test adjusted for ties was used to test the independence of severity of toxicity (grade 0 to 4) to the assigned treatment.

Table 2.12 Results of GOG 158

Treatment arm	Paclitaxel and cisplatin N=400	Paclitaxel and carboplatin N=392	Statistics
Patient characteristics			
Age 21-50	33%	29%	
Age 51-70	56%	58%	
Age 71-90	11%	13%	
No residual	36%	35%	
Residual disease ≤1 cm	64%	65%	
Stage III	100%	100%	
Serous	70%	74%	
Endometrioid	11%	9%	
Mucinous	3%	2%	
Clear cell	3%	5%	
Other	14%	9%	
Grade 1	11%	9%	
Grade 2	35%	36%	
Grade 3	54%	55%	
Optional second look	50%	49%	
Treatment delivery			
Received 6 cycles	85%	87%	
Efficacy			
Median PFS	19.4 months	20.7 months	RR 0.88 (0.75-1.03)
Median OS	48.7 months	57.4 months	RR 0.84 (0.70-1.02)
pCR	46%	53%	
Toxicity			
G3/4 leukopenia	63%	59%	$P<.05$
G3/4 thrombocytopenia	5%	39%	$P<.05$
G3/4 granulocytopenia	93%	89%	
G3/4 gastrointestinal	23%	10%	$P<.05$
G/34 neurologic	8%	7%	
G3/4 metabolic	8%	3%	$P<.05$
G3/4 genitourinary	3%	1%	$P<.05$
G1/2 pain	15%	26%	$P<.05$

pCR, pathologic complete response; OS, overall survival; PFS, progression-free survival; RR, relative risk.

CONCLUSION OF TRIAL
- The combination of paclitaxel plus carboplatin is not inferior to the combination of paclitaxel plus cisplatin in patients with small-volume stage III epithelial ovarian cancer.

COMMENTS
- This trial was designed as a noninferiority trial, not to determine the superiority of carboplatin over cisplatin.
    - The 16% reduced risk of death with carboplatin is suggestive of a possible increase in efficacy over cisplatin.
    - The carboplatin dose (AUC 7.5) may have resulted in more platinum exposure than the cisplatin dose (75 mg/m^2).
    - In trials combining carboplatin with cyclophosphamide, there was no benefit to increasing doses of carboplatin (Jakobsen et al. 1997; Gore et al. 1998). The pharmacodynamic interaction between carboplatin and paclitaxel may favor higher doses of carboplatin.
- Other prospective randomized trials comparing paclitaxel + carboplatin vs paclitaxel + cisplatin:
    - Danish Netherlands Trial (Neijt et al. 2000) had an insufficient number of patients to determine statistical equivalency.
    - Arbeitsgemeinschaft Gynakologische trial from Germany (du Bois et al. 2003) showed no difference in PFS or OS between treatments. Paclitaxel was administered as 185 mg/m^2 over 3 hours (vs 135 mg/m^2 over 24 hours in GOG 158) and carboplatin was dosed at AUC 6 (vs AUC 7.5 in GOG 158).
    - Both the Netherlands and German trials included patients with stage II to IV disease.
- GOG 158 fails to support the concern that a 3-hour infusion of paclitaxel is less efficacious than a 24-hour infusion.
- Different toxicity profiles.
    - Cisplatin was responsible for more gastrointestinal and metabolic toxicity.
    - There was no difference in neurotoxicity between arms. This is in contrast to the results of the 2 European trials that both showed less neurotoxicity with carboplatin. This may be because cisplatin was combined with a 3-hour infusion of paclitaxel in the control arms.
- Median survival after recurrence was 23 months without difference between treatment groups.

- While this trial demonstrates carboplatin + paclitaxel to be the treatment of choice for patients with small-volume stage III ovarian cancer, it also highlights the need for more effective therapies. More than 70% of patients experienced recurrence with the majority occurring in the first 2 years following therapy.
- GOG 182 was designed subsequently to test the addition of a third drug to the carboplatin and paclitaxel base.

AGO/OVAR-3 (du Bois, JNCI 2003)

REFERENCE

- du Bois A, et al. A randomized clinical trial of cisplatin/paclitaxel versus carboplatin/paclitaxel as first-line treatment of ovarian cancer. *J Natl Cancer Inst.* 2003;95(17):1320-9. PMID: 12953086. (du Bois et al. 2003)

TRIAL SPONSOR

- Arbeitsgemeinschaft Gynakologische Onkologie (AGO) Ovarian Cancer Study Group

RATIONALE FOR TRIAL

- In the 1980s, 2 trials demonstrated improved survival when cisplatin was added to doxorubicin and cyclophosphamide (Neijt et al. 1984; Omura et al. 1986). Subsequent studies showed no difference between 2-drug and 3-drug regimens (Bertelsen et al. 1987; Omura et al. 1989), resulting in the combination of cisplatin and cyclophosphamide being considered the standard of care for about a decade.
- In the 1990s, paclitaxel replaced cyclophosphamide in the first-line treatment of advanced ovarian cancer (McGuire et al. 1996; Piccart et al. 2000). Paclitaxel plus cisplatin was considered the new standard of care, but this was challenged by the results of the ICON3 trial (International Collaborative Ovarian Neoplasm Group 2002).
- Despite these advances, more than 50% of patients with advanced ovarian cancer die within 5 years of original diagnosis. This makes tolerability of treatment and quality-of-life important considerations in ongoing research. Carboplatin is better tolerated than cisplatin when combined with cyclophosphamide with no loss in efficacy (Alberts et al. 1992; Swenerton et al. 1992).
- Several phase I/II studies tested the feasibility of combining carboplatin with paclitaxel (du Bois et al. 1997). The maximum tolerated dose

of paclitaxel ranged from 175 to 275 mg/m² and the maximum tolerated dose of carboplatin ranged from 300 to 550 mg/m² or AUC 5 to AUC 7.5.
- This trial and GOG 158 were both designed as noninferiority studies to test the efficacy and toxicity of carboplatin vs cisplatin when combined with paclitaxel.

PATIENT POPULATION
- N = 883 screened, 798 eligible.
- Enrollment between November 1995 and November 1997.

Inclusion Criteria
- Histologically confirmed FIGO stage IIB to IV epithelial ovarian cancer.
- Radical debulking surgery within 6 weeks or random assignment.
- Adequate hematologic, renal, and hepatic function: ANC >1.5 × 10⁹ cells/L, platelet count >100 × 10⁹ cells/L, serum creatinine and bilirubin <1.25 times upper normal limit.

Exclusion Criteria
- Low malignant potential tumors.
- ECOG performance status >2 or Karnofsky index <60%.
- Estimated GFR <60 mL/min.
- Other malignancies.
- Previous chemotherapy, immunotherapy, or radiotherapy for ovarian cancer.
- Severe neuropathy.
- Cardiac arrhythmias.
- Congestive heart failure.

TREATMENT DETAILS

Arm 1: Paclitaxel Plus Cisplatin (PT)
- Paclitaxel 185 mg/m² IV over 3 hours (dose capped at 400 mg).
- Cisplatin 75 mg/m² IV over 30 minutes (dose capped at 165 mg).

Arm 2: Paclitaxel Plus Carboplatin (TC)
- Paclitaxel 185 mg/m² IV over 3 hours (dose capped at 400 mg).
- Carboplatin AUC 6 IV over 30 to 60 minutes (dose capped at 880 mg). Calculated by the method of Calvert (Calvert et al. 1989) of AUC × (GRF +25). GFR estimated by the Jelliffe formula (Jelliffe 1973).

- This dose was the maximum tolerated dose (MTD) in a preceding phase I/II trial (du Bois et al. 1997).

Dose Reductions Allowed for Toxicity
- Level 1.
  - Carboplatin AUC 5.
  - Cisplatin 60 mg/m^2.
  - Paclitaxel 160 mg/m^2.
- Level 2.
  - Carboplatin AUC 4.
  - Cisplatin 50 mg/m^2.
  - Paclitaxel 135 mg/m^2.
- Treatment delayed for ANC <1.5 × 10^9 cells/L or platelet count <100 × 10^9 cells/L.
- Prophylaxis with G-CSF was not allowed, but supportive use could be initiated if ANC recovery took more than 36 days.

Premedications
- Dexamethasone 20 mg single dose before paclitaxel.
- Clemastine 2 mg IV 30 minutes before paclitaxel.
- Cimetidine 300 mg IV 30 minutes before paclitaxel.
- Antiemetics: serotonin type 3 receptor antagonists and corticosteroids.
- Hydration with cisplatin: pre- and postchemotherapy hydration to avoid nephrotoxicity.

Treatment Discontinuation
- For disease progression during therapy.

Treatment Continuation
- Patients with partial remission and residual tumor after 6 cycles could receive additional treatment cycles.

ASSESSMENTS
- Chemistries before each treatment cycle.
- Hematologic parameters measured weekly.
- Quality of life measured by the EORTC quality-of-life questionnaire (QLQ)–C30, version 2.0 (Aaronson et al. 1993) after each treatment cycle and 3 and 6 months after completion of treatment.
- Tumor measurement was recorded before each treatment cycle by physical examination and before each third treatment cycle by imaging in patients with measurable or evaluable disease. Imaging consisted

of ultrasound, x-ray, computed tomography, or magnetic resonance imaging (MRI), and a consistent modality was used at baseline and follow-up.
- Second-look surgery was not recommended.
- Follow-up visits were schedule every 3 months for the first 2 years and every 6 months thereafter until 5 years after treatment cessation.

ENDPOINTS

- Proportion of patients without progression at 2 years (primary endpoint).
- Toxicity.
- Response to treatment.
- Quality of life.
- Overall survival (measured from time of randomization).
- Progression-free survival time (measured from time of randomization).

STATISTICAL CONSIDERATIONS

Stratification
- Patients were stratified based on residual tumor size and FIGO stage.
  - Stratum 1: patients with residual tumor ≤1 cm and FIGO stage IIB, IIC, or III.
  - Stratum 2: residual tumor >1 cm or FIGO stage IV.

Sample Size
- This was a noninferiority trial with a sample size of 692 patients to exclude a difference between the proportion of patients without progression at 2 years of more than 8% between arms with 80% power and α of 5%. This calculation was based on the assumption of an equal number of patients per stratum and a dropout rate of 10%. During the trial, the sample size was increased to 798 patients to account for more patients in stratum 1.

CONCLUSION OF TRIAL

- Because carboplatin is more tolerable than cisplatin with equal treatment efficacy, the combination of carboplatin with paclitaxel may be in the best interest of patients with advanced ovarian cancer.

COMMENTS

- There was greater toxicity and worse quality of life with cisplatin compared to carboplatin.

Table 2.13 Results of AGO/OVAR-3

Treatment arm	Paclitaxel+ cisplatin N=386	Paclitaxel+ carboplatin N=397	Statistics
Patient characteristics			
Median age (range)	57.7 years	56.7 years	
Stratum 1 (≤1 cm, II, III)	59.3%	52.9%	
Stratum 2 (>1 cm, IV)	40.7%	47.1%	
Residual ≤1 cm	65.9%	59.5%	
Residual >1 cm	34.1%	40.5%	
Stage II	7.5%	9.3%	
Stage III	76.4%	72.5%	
Stage IV	16.1%	18.1%	
Serous	69.9%	70.8%	
Other	30.1%	29.2%	
Grade 1	6.7%	9.5%	
Grade 2	37.3%	38.5%	
Grade 3	56.0%	52.0%	
Treatment delivery			
Received 6 cycles	84.0%	87.7%	
Treatment delay >7 days	10.3%	14.0%	
Dose reductions	10.5%	11.2%	
Efficacy			
Complete response	43.3%	36.5%	
Partial response	33.3%	41.9%	
Stable disease	10.0%	10.8%	
Progressive disease	13.3%	10.8%	
No progression at 2 years	40.0%	37.5%	NS
Median PFS	19.1 months	17.2 months	HR 1.095 (95% CI, 0.89-1.23)
Strata 1	24.2 months	26.0 months	HR 0.91 (95% CI, 0.72-1.15)
Strata 2	14.3 months	13.4 months	HR 1.14 (95% CI, 0.91-1.43)
Median OS	44.1 months	43.3 months	HR 1.05 (95% CI, 0.87-1.26)
Strata 1	55.4 months	59.4 months	HR 0.92 (95% CI, 0.70-1.22)
Strata 2	30.7 months	31.4 months	HR 1.08 (95% CI, 0.85-1.38)
Toxicity			
G3/4 platelets	1%	12.9%	
G3/4 anemia	3.9%	5.9%	
G3/4 leukopenia	10.8%	31.9%	
G3/4 neutropenia	22.0%	37.0%	
Febrile neutropenia	3.6%	8.0%	
G3/4 infections	22.6%	35.6%	
G3 nausea	13.8%	5.4%	
G3 vomiting	9.1%	2.3%	
Any ototoxicity	16.9%	8.8%	
Any renal toxicity	19.9%	5.4%	
G3/4 sensory neuropathy	13.5%	7.2%	

CI, confidence interval; HR, hazard ratio; NS, not significant; PFS, progression-free survival; OS, overall survival.

- Response rates were higher with cisplatin than carboplatin, but this did not translate into improved survival.
- Patients receiving carboplatin had greater myelosuppression, but this rarely led to symptoms such as febrile neutropenia or nonneutropenic infections.
- This trial supports the findings from other trials of platinum plus paclitaxel chemotherapy (McGuire et al. 1996; Neijt et al. 2000; Piccart et al. 2000).
  - Direct comparisons of toxicities are difficult due to the different grading systems used.
  - Gastrointestinal and neurologic toxicities are less with carboplatin.
  - The median OS time with paclitaxel+cisplatin is higher in this trial than others (44.1 months vs 38 months [McGuire et al. 1996], 35.6 months [Piccart et al. 2000], and 30 months [Neijt et al. 2000]), which likely reflects a patient population with more favorable tumor characteristics.

SCOTROC—Scottish Randomised Trial in Ovarian Cancer (Vasey, JNCI 2004)

REFERENCE

- Vasey PA, et al. Phase III randomized trial of docetaxel-carboplatin versus paclitaxel-carboplatin as first-line chemotherapy for ovarian carcinoma. *J Natl Cancer Inst.* 2004;96(22):1682-1691. PMID: 15547181. (Vasey et al. 2004)

TRIAL SPONSOR

- Scottish Gynaecological Cancer Trials Group
- Supported by grants from Aventis Pharmaceuticals

RATIONALE FOR TRIAL

- Docetaxel is a semisynthetic taxane with superior activity to anthracyclines and paclitaxel in metastatic breast cancer.
- Phase II trials of docetaxel in ovarian cancer demonstrate activity comparable to paclitaxel.
- The combination of docetaxel and carboplatin was found to be feasible.

PATIENT POPULATION
- N = 1077.
- Recruited from 83 international centers between October 1988 and May 2000.
- Women 18 years and older.
- Histologically confirmed epithelial ovarian cancer, stages IC to IV.
- ECOG performance status of 0 to 2.
- No prior chemotherapy or radiotherapy.
- Adequate bone marrow, hepatic, and renal function.
- Excluded if peripheral neuropathy more than grade 2.
- Randomization within 6 weeks of surgery.
- First treatment cycle within 2 weeks of randomization.

TREATMENT DETAILS

Arm 1: Paclitaxel + Carboplatin
- Paclitaxel 175 mg/m^2 IV over 3 hours.
- Carboplatin AUC 5 IV over 1 hour.

Arm 2: Docetaxel + Carboplatin
- Docetaxel 75 mg/m^2 IV over 1 hour.
- Carboplatin AUC 5 over 1 hour.

Paclitaxel Treatment Details
- Dexamethasone 20 mg 12 and 6 hours prior to chemotherapy.
- Chlorpheniramine 10 mg or diphenhydramine 50 mg 1 hour prior to chemotherapy.
- Ranitidine 50 mg or cimetidine 300 mg 1 hour prior to chemotherapy.
- Starting dose 175 mg/m^2 over 3 hours.
- Dose reduction to 135 mg/m^2 over 3 hours for complicated grade 4 neutropenia.
- Discontinued for deterioration of liver function or neurotoxicity grade 3 or more.
- Hypersensitivity reactions—infusion stopped, symptoms treated, paclitaxel reinfused within 3 hours if appropriate.

Docetaxel Treatment Details
- Dexamethasone 8 mg twice a day for 3 days starting on day prior to chemotherapy.
- Starting dose 75 mg/m^2 over 1 hour.
- Dose reduction to 60 mg/m^2 over 1 hour for complicated grade 4 neutropenia.

- Discontinued for deterioration of liver function or neurotoxicity grade 3 or more.
- Hypersensitivity reactions—infusion stopped, symptoms treated, docetaxel reinfused within 3 hours if appropriate.

Carboplatin Treatment Details
- Carboplatin dose calculated by Calvert formula with edetic acid to measure GFR.
- Starting dose AUC 5 in both treatment arms.
- Dose reduction to AUC 4 for complicated grade 4 thrombocytopenia.

Antiemetics
- Granisetron 3 mg.
- Ondansetron 8 mg.

Treatment Delays
- Allowed for up to 2 weeks for:
  - ANC <1500/µL.
  - Platelets <100,000 /µL.
  - Mucositis grade 3 or more.
  - Skin toxicity grade 2 or more.

Dose Reductions
- Complicated grade 4 neutropenia.
  - G-CSF 300 mg/d added for persistent neutropenia despite dose reduction of paclitaxel or docetaxel.
  - Prophylactic antibiotics added for all subsequent cycles.

Interval Cytoreduction
- Allowed between cycles 3 and 4.

Treatment Continuation
- If partial response or complete response with elevated CA125, 3 cycles of carboplatin AUC 7 allowed for up to 3 additional cycles.

ASSESSMENTS
- CT scan at baseline and after cycles 3 and 6—classified according to Response Evaluation Criteria in Solid Tumors (RECIST).
- CA125 at baseline and before each cycle—classified according to method of Rustin.
- Toxicity assessed by NCI-CTC, version 2.0.
- Quality of life assessed before each cycle and at 6 months and then every 4 months for up to 2 years using EORTC QLQ-C30 (version 3.0) and EORTC QLQ-OV28 (version 1).

Table 2.14 Results of SCOTROC

Treatment arm	Paclitaxel-carboplatin N=538	Docetaxel-carboplatin N=539	Statistics
Patient characteristics			
Median age (range)	59 years (19-84)	59 years (21-85)	
Stage IC-II	20%	19%	
Stage III-IV	80%	81%	
No residual	33%	33%	
≤2 cm residual	30%	30%	
>2 cm residual	37%	37%	
Serous	44%	44%	
Endometrioid	10%	12%	
Clear cell	4%	5%	
Mucinous	2%	4%	
Other	38%	34%	
Grade 3	54%	54%	
Treatment delivery			
Withdrawal from protocol	21%	15%	
Additional carboplatin AUC 7	13%	11%	
Efficacy			
Median PFS (95% CI)	14.8 months (13.5-16.1)	15 months (13.3-16.6)	HR 0.97, P=NS
2-year survival	68.9%	64.2%	HR 1.13, P=NS
Complete response	28%	28%	P=NS
Toxicity			
G3-4 neutropenia	84%	94%	$P<.001$
G4 neutropenia+fever	2%	11%	$P<.001$
G4 neutropenia >7 days	3%	14%	$P<.001$
G3-4 thrombocytopenia	10%	9%	P=NS
G3-4 anemia	8%	11%	P=NS
Deaths	N=1	N=2	
G2-4 neurosensory	30%	11%	$P<.001$
G2-4 neuromotor	7%	3%	$P<.001$
Other toxicities	More arthralgia, myalgia, alopecia, abdominal pain	More gastrointestinal toxicity, peripheral edema, allergic reactions, nail changes	

AUC, area under the curve; CI, confidence interval; HR, hazard ratio; NS, not significant; PFS, progression-free survival.

- Neurotoxicity assessment at some centers with 12 questions and 5 neurologic tests to report NScore at baseline, after cycles 3 and 6, at 6 months and every 4 months for up to 2 years.
- Follow-up every 2 months with exam and CA125. CT scans for rising CA125.

ENDPOINTS

- Progression-free survival (primary endpoint).
- Overall survival.
- Quality of life.

STATISTICAL CONSIDERATIONS

Sample Size
- Study designed with 80% power to detect a difference of 25% increase in median PFS from 17 to 21.25 months. Required 1050 patients with minimum follow-up of 1 year.

CONCLUSIONS OF TRIAL

- Similar efficacy between arms and acceptable toxicities in both arms.
- Compared to paclitaxel-carboplatin, docetaxel-carboplatin resulted in greater myelosuppression but less neurotoxicity during therapy and follow-up.
- Docetaxel-carboplatin is an alternative to treatment with paclitaxel-carboplatin in the upfront treatment of patients with stage IC to IV ovarian cancer.

COMMENTS

- This trial has shorter survival times compared to other trials. Authors state this may be due to different patient populations (more residual disease) or the broad definition of progressive disease used in this trial.
- According to the authors, the higher rate of neurotoxicity of 30% reported in the paclitaxel-carboplatin arm may be due to the more comprehensive approach to neurotoxicity monitoring in this trial.

GOG 172 (Armstrong, NEJM 2006)

REFERENCE

- Armstrong DK, et al. Intraperitoneal cisplatin and paclitaxel in ovarian cancer. *N Engl J Med*. 2006;354(1):34-43. PMID: 16394300. (Armstrong et al. 2006)

TRIAL SPONSOR

- Gynecologic Oncology Group (GOG)

RATIONALE FOR TRIAL

- Most patients with advanced ovarian cancer attain clinical remission, but the majority eventually relapse and die of disease.
- The intensity of intravenous therapy is limited by myelotoxicity. However, several drugs can be administered directly into the peritoneal cavity. Intraperitoneal administration of chemotherapy allows for tumor to receive sustained exposure to high concentrations of drug while bone marrow and other normal tissues are relatively spared.
- Two prior GOG trials (GOG 104 and GOG 114) evaluated intraperitoneal administration of cisplatin in patients with low-volume ovarian cancer. GOG 104 demonstrated a survival advantage with intraperitoneal cisplatin, but paclitaxel was not administered in the regimen (Alberts et al. 1996). GOG 114 demonstrated a PFS advantage and only borderline OS advantage with intraperitoneal cisplatin, but the interpretation of the trial was complicated by the use of 2 cycles of moderately intensive carboplatin, which added to the toxicity of the treatment (Markman et al. 2001).
- Intraperitoneal chemotherapy had not been widely accepted and used based on high cost, high toxicity, and lack of familiarity with intraperitoneal administration and catheter-placement techniques.

PATIENT POPULATION

- N=429 enrolled, 415 eligible.
- Enrollment between March 1998 and January 2001.
- Stage III epithelial ovarian cancer with <1 cm residual mass after surgery.
- GOG performance status of 0 to 2.
- Normal blood counts, adequate renal and hepatic function.
- Ineligibility criteria: prior chemotherapy or radiation; second primary cancer; low malignant potential tumors.

TREATMENT DETAILS

Arm 1: Intravenous Therapy
- Paclitaxel 135 mg/m^2 IV over 24 hours on day 1.
- Cisplatin 75 mg/m^2 IV on day 2.
- Treatment given every 3 weeks for 6 cycles.

Arm 2: Intravenous/Intraperitoneal Therapy
- Paclitaxel 135 mg/m^2 IV over 24 hours on day 1.
- Cisplatin 100 mg/m^2 IP on day 2.
- Paclitaxel 60 mg/m^2 IP on day 8.
- Intraperitoneal chemotherapy was reconstituted in 2 L of warmed normal saline and infused as rapidly as possible.
- Treatment given every 3 weeks for 6 cycles.

Premedications
- Standard premedications to prevent paclitaxel hypersensitivity.
- Hydration and antiemetics given before cisplatin.

Treatment Delays
- If ANC <1500 cells/mm^3, platelets <100,000/mm^3, or serum creatinine >2 mg/dL, then treatment delay, dose reduction, then addition of G-CSF (in this sequence)
- If grade 3 or 4 peripheral neuropathy, creatinine >2 mg/mL or creatinine clearance <50 mL/min, then treatment was postponed.
- If treatment was delayed for more than 3 weeks, patients were removed from study.
- In the intraperitoneal therapy group:
   - For grade 2 abdominal pain, the dose of intraperitoneal drug was reduced.
   - For grade 3 abdominal pain, recurrent grade 2 abdominal pain after dose reduction, or intraperitoneal catheter complications, dosing was changed to intravenous.
- For grade 2 peripheral neuropathy, the dose of cisplatin was reduced.
- For cisplatin-related toxic effects requiring discontinuation of protocol therapy, carboplatin was substituted for cisplatin.

ASSESSMENTS
- At registration, patients decided whether they would undergo second-look laparotomy.
- Physical exam, history, complete blood count (CBC), chemistries, and CA125 were measured at baseline, at the completion of therapy, every 3 months for 24 months, then after 6 months thereafter.
- Quality-of-life assessment with the Functional Assessment of Cancer Therapy—Ovarian (FACT-O) instrument (Basen-Engquist et al. 2001) at registration, before cycle 4, 3 to 6 weeks after cycle 6 and 12 months after the completion of therapy.

ENDPOINTS

- PFS (measured from date of randomization).
- OS (measured from date of randomization).
- Quality of life.

STATISTICAL CONSIDERATIONS

Stratification Factors

- Patients were randomized with stratification according to residual disease and decision of whether to undergo second-look surgery.

Sample Size

- A sample size of 384 patients with follow-up to observe 208 recurrences and 208 deaths allowed testing for a hazard ratio of 1.5 (favoring intraperitoneal administration) for recurrence and survival using a 1-sided log-rank test with 90% power and an α level of .05.

Statistical Tests

- Kaplan-Meier to estimate the cumulative proportions of survival (Kaplan and Meier 1958).
- Cox model to estimate the relative risk and confidence intervals for treatment effects on progression and death (Cox 1972).
- Adjusted estimates were based on covariates of age and histology.
- Wilcoxon rank-sum test to test the independence of the risk of severe and life-threatening toxic effects from treatment.
- Quality-of-life assessments were analyzed with linear models with an unstructured covariance matrix. Covariance parameters were estimated with the restricted maximum likelihood.

CONCLUSION OF TRIAL

- Intravenous/intraperitoneal chemotherapy improves survival at the expense of greater toxicity in patients with optimally debulked stage III ovarian cancer.

COMMENTS

- Intraperitoneal therapy was associated with significantly worse fatigue, pain, and hematologic, gastrointestinal, neurologic, and metabolic toxicities.
  - The increased toxicity with intraperitoneal therapy might be attributed to the higher dose of cisplatin. The rationale for the higher dose

Table 2.15 Results of GOG 172

Treatment arm	Intravenous N=210	Intraperitoneal N=205	Statistics
Patient characteristics			
Age 21-50	27%	31%	
Age 51-70	62%	56%	
Age 71-80+	10%	13%	
No residual	36%	38%	
Residual disease ≤1 cm	64%	62%	
Stage III	100%	100%	
Serous	81%	77%	
Endometrioid	6%	8%	
Clear cell	4%	5%	
Other	9%	9%	
Grade 1	9%	12%	
Grade 2	40%	35%	
Grade 3	50%	52%	
Elected second look	49%	49%	
Treatment delivery			
Completed 6 cycles	83%	42%	
Efficacy			
Pathologic CR	41%	57%	
Median PFS	18.3 months	23.8 months	RR 0.80, $P=.05$
With gross residual	15.4 months	18.3 months	RR 0.81, NS
With no visible residual	35.2 months	37.6 months	RR 0.80, NS
Median OS	49.7 months	65.6 months	RR 0.75, $P=.03$
With gross residual	39.1 months	52.6 months	RR 0.44, NS
With no visible residual	78.2 months	Not yet reached	RR 0.69, NS
Toxicity			
Treatment-related death	N=4	N=5	
G3/4 leukopenia	64%	76%	$P<.001$
G3/4 thrombocytopenia	4%	12%	$P=.002$
G3/4 gastrointestinal	24%	46%	$P<.001$
G3/4 renal	2%	7%	$P=.03$
G3/4 cardiovascular	5%	9%	$P=.06$
G3/4 neurologic	9%	19%	$P=.001$
G3/4 fever	4%	9%	$P=.02$
G3/4 infection	6%	16%	$P=.001$
G3/4 fatigue	4%	18%	$P<.001$
G3/4 metabolic	7%	27%	$P<.001$
G3/4 pain	1%	11%	$P<.001$
G3/4 hepatic	<1%	3%	$P=.05$

CR, complete response; NS, not significant; PFS, progression-free survival; OS, overall survival; RR, relative risk.

is that capillary uptake of cisplatin from the intraperitoneal surfaces is slow and incomplete. This results in prolonged but lower systemic exposure compared to intravenous administration (Schneider 1994).
    ○ The increased toxicity with intraperitoneal therapy might be attributed to the use of intraperitoneal paclitaxel. Paclitaxel has very slow intraperitoneal clearance and remains in the peritoneal cavity for 1 week after administration (Francis et al. 1995). The peritoneal clearance could be altered by administration after intraperitoneal cisplatin.
    ○ It is not known whether altering the treatment regimen to reduce toxicity will compromise its efficacy.
- Quality of life was worse with intraperitoneal therapy at cycle 4 and 3 to 6 weeks after treatment. However, there was no difference in quality of life between groups at 1 year after treatment.
- Patients who had a left colonic or rectosigmoid resection were less likely to receive all 6 cycles of intraperitoneal therapy.
- The single-lumen venous-access catheter attached to an implantable subcutaneous port is associated with minimal fibrous sheath formation and less risk of bowel obstruction or perforation compared to the fenestrated intraperitoneal catheter (Alberts et al. 2002).
- The median OS time of 65.6 months in the patients receiving intraperitoneal therapy is the longest survival reported in a GOG phase 3 trial.

GOG 182/ICON5 (Bookman, JCO 2009)

REFERENCE

- Bookman MA, et al. Evaluation of new platinum-based treatment regimens in advanced-stage ovarian cancer: a Phase III Trial of the Gynecologic Cancer Intergroup. *J Clin Oncol*. 2009;27(9):1419-1425. PMID: 19224846. (Bookman et al. 2009)

TRIAL SPONSORS

- Gynecologic Oncology Group (GOG)
- Medical Research Council in the United Kingdom (MRC-UK) representing the International Collaborative Ovarian Neoplasm (ICON) group
- Australia and New Zealand Gynecologic Oncology Group (ANZGOG; Camperdown, Australia)

- Istituto Mario Negri (Milan, Italy)
- Southwest Oncology Group
- Five other groups managed by the National Cancer Institute (NCI)

RATIONALE FOR TRIAL

- Despite response rates of greater than 80%, long-term survival of ovarian cancer remains poor as a result of recurrence and drug resistance.
- While platinum and taxanes are the core of primary treatment, other drugs have demonstrated activity in the recurrent setting, including topotecan, gemcitabine, and pegylated liposomal doxorubicin (Gordon et al. 2004; ten Bokkel Huinink et al. 2004; Pfisterer et al. 2006a).
- A multiarm, multistage study was designed to compare 4 different treatment arms against a single reference arm of carboplatin and paclitaxel.
- This collaborative trial with a target accrual of 4000 patients would report clinical outcomes but also provide an international database, including outcomes in patients with uncommon histologies and genetic mutations associated with cancer risk.

PATIENT POPULATION

- N=4312 enrolled.
- Patients enrolled between February 2001 and September 2004.
- Stage III or IV epithelial ovarian cancer, either optimal (≤1 cm) or suboptimal residual disease.
- GOG performance status of 0, 1, or 2.
- Labs: ANC ≥1500/μL, platelets ≥100,000/μL, creatinine ≤1.5 times upper limit of normal, bilirubin ≤1.5 times upper limit of normal, AST and alkaline phosphatase ≤2.5 times upper limit of normal.
- Baseline sensory or motor neuropathy of grade 1 or lower by the NCI Common Toxicity Criteria version 2.
- Breast cancer: eligible if disease free for at least 3 years.
- Early-stage synchronous endometrial cancer: eligible if minimal invasion and no high-grade features.
- Ineligible: low malignant potential tumors, carcinosarcoma, nonepithelial histology.

TREATMENT DETAILS

- Dose and schedule were designed to maximize delivery of newer agents, preserve exposure to paclitaxel and carboplatin, and equilibrate the risk of hematologic toxicity.

Arm 1: CP (Carboplatin Paclitaxel)
- Cycles 1 to 8.
  - Carboplatin AUC 6 IV on day 1.
  - Paclitaxel 175 mg/m^2 IV over 3 hours on day 1.

Arm 2: CPG (Carboplatin Paclitaxel + Gemcitabine)
- Cycles 1 to 4.
  - Carboplatin AUC 5 IV on day 1.
  - Paclitaxel 175 mg/m^2 IV over 3 hours on day 1.
  - Gemcitabine 800 mg/m^2 IV over 30 minutes on day 1 and day 8.
- Cycles 5 to 8.
  - Carboplatin AUC 5 IV on day 1.
  - Paclitaxel 175 mg/m^2 IV over 3 hours on day 1.

Arm 3: CPD (Carboplatin Paclitaxel + Pegylated Liposomal Doxorubicin)
- Cycles 1 to 8.
  - Carboplatin AUC 5 IV on day 1.
  - Paclitaxel 175 mg/m^2 IV over 3 hours on day 1.
- Cycles 1, 3, 5, and 7.
  - Pegylated liposomal doxorubicin (PLD) 30 mg/m^2 IV on day 1 (dosing of PLD every 3 weeks was associated with unacceptable risk of mucosal, skin, and/or hematologic toxicity due to prolonged clearance, and tolerability is improved with use in alternating cycles).

Arm 4: CT → CP (Carboplatin Topotecan → Carboplatin Paclitaxel)
- Cycles 1 to 4.
  - Topotecan 1.25 mg/m^2/d IV on days 1, 2, and 3.
  - Carboplatin AUC 5 IV on day 3 (delay to day 3 based on evidence of sequence-specific hematologic toxicity in phase I trials).
- Cycles 5 to 8.
  - Carboplatin AUC 6 IV on day 1.
  - Paclitaxel 175 mg/m^2 IV over 3 hours on day 1.

Arm 5: CG → CP (Carboplatin Gemcitabine → Carboplatin Paclitaxel)
- Cycles 1 to 4.
  - Gemcitabine 1000 mg/m^2 IV on day 1 and day 8.
  - Carboplatin AUC 6 IV on day 8 (delay to day 8 based on evidence of sequence-dependent hematologic toxicity in patients with lung cancer).

- Cycles 5 to 8.
  - Carboplatin AUC 6 IV on day 1.
  - Paclitaxel 175 mg/m² IV over 3 hours on day 1.

Supportive Measures
- Prophylactic hematopoietic growth factors were not required but could be added after cycle delay and/or dose reduction for recurrent toxicity.

Surgery
- Interval cytoreduction allowed between the fourth and fifth cycles for patients with suboptimal residual disease if the intent was declared at registration.
- Reassessment second-look surgery was not allowed as this approach provides no clinical benefit and surgical assessment of small-volume disease could interfere with determination of PFS (Greer et al. 2005).

ASSESSMENTS
- Not stated in manuscript.
- International criteria were adopted to permit use of CA125 to identify progression after completion of primary therapy (Rustin et al. 2006).

ENDPOINTS
- OS.
- PFS.
- Toxicities.
- Complications.
- Dose intensity.
- Cumulative dose delivery.

STATISTICAL CONSIDERATIONS

Sample Size
- In patients receiving the control CP regimen, the estimated median PFS and OS were 15 months and 36 months, respectively.
- An event-triggered interim analysis was scheduled to occur after 240 PFS events in the control CP arm to eliminate regimens that demonstrated insufficient activity. A regimen was continued if the relative PFS event rate was at least 7% lower than the reference arm by pairwise PFS comparisons using a stratified log-rank test (Peto and Peto 1972).
- The sample size provided 90% power to declare a regimen superior if it reduced the risk of death by 25% compared to the reference arm with α limited to 0.125 (0.05/4; 2-tail test) for each pairwise comparison

Table 2.16 Results of GOG 182/ICON5

Treatment arm	CP N = 864	CPG N = 864	CPD N = 862	CT → CP N = 861	CG → CP N = 861
Patient characteristics					
Median age	57.5 years	59.1 years	59.5 years	58.5 years	59.3 years
Microscopic	About 25%	About 25%	About 25%	About 25%	About 25%
≤1 cm residual	About 45%	About 45%	About 45%	About 45%	About 45%
>1 cm residual	About 30%	About 30%	About 30%	About 30%	About 30%
Stage III	83.8%	86.7%	86.2%	86.4%	83.7%
Stage IV	16.2%	13.3%	13.8%	13.7%	16.3%
Serous	About 80%	About 80%	About 80%	About 80%	About 80%
Endometrioid	About 10%	About 10%	About 10%	About 10%	About 10%
Mucinous	About 1%	About 1%	About 1%	About 1%	About 1%
Clear cell	About 1%	About 1%	About 1%	About 1%	About 1%
Other	About 5%	About 5%	About 5%	About 5%	About 5%
Treatment delivery					
Overall, 79% completed 8 cycles					
Efficacy					
Median PFS, 16 mo	HR 1.00 (ref)	HR 1.028, NS	HR 0.984, NS	HR 1.066, NS	HR 1.037, NS
Median OS, 44.1 mo	HR 1.00 (ref)	HR 1.006, NS	HR 0.952, NS	HR 1.051, NS	HR 1.114, NS
Toxicity					
≥G4 ANC	About 60%	About 75%	About 70%	About 58%	About 58%
≥G3 PLT	About 25%	About 60%	About 40%	About 29%	About 58%
≥G3 Hgb	About 15%	About 20%	About 17%	About 18%	About 21%
≥G3 fever	About 10%	About 16%	About 16%	About 10%	About 10%
≥G2 hepatic	About 5%	About 11%	About 5%	About 5%	About 9%
≥G2 neuropathy	About 25%	About 27%	About 25%	About 15%	About 16%
≥G2 pulmonary	About 11%	About 13%	About 12%	About 11%	About 16%
≥G3 GI	About 10%	About 15%	About 14%	About 13%	About 10%

ANC, absolute neutrophil count; CG, carboplatin+gemcitabine; CP, carboplatin+paclitaxel; CPD, carboplatin+paclitaxel+pegylated liposomal doxorubicin; CPG, carboplatin+paclitaxel+gemcitabine; CT, carboplatin+topotecan; GI, gastrointestinal; Hgb, hemoglobin; HR, hazard ratio; NS, not significant; PFS, progression-free survival; OS, overall survival; PLT, platelets.

(Schoenfeld 1981). This effect size was comparable to an increase in the 3-year surviving proportion from 50% to 59.3%.

CONCLUSION OF TRIAL

- The addition of a third cytotoxic agent to paclitaxel and carboplatin provided a benefit in PFS or OS after optimal or suboptimal cytoreduction for ovarian cancer.

COMMENTS

- At the time of the interim analysis, none of the experimental regimens reduced the PFS event rate by at least 7% compared to the control arm, so the study was closed in September 2004 to further accrual.
- Extent of cytoreductive surgery was an important prognostic factor for OS (second only to stage).
  - Suboptimal (>1 cm): PFS 13 months, OS 33 months.
  - Gross optimal (≤1 cm): PFS 16 months, OS 40 months.
  - Microscopic residual: PFS 29 months, OS 68 months.
- This trial accrued approximately 1200 patients per year, representing about 6.25% of all women with newly diagnosed ovarian cancer in the United States during this period.

JGOG 3016 (Katsumata, Lancet 2009; Katsumata, Lancet Oncol 2013)

REFERENCES

- Katsumata N, et al. Dose-dense paclitaxel once a week in combination with carboplatin every 3 weeks for advanced ovarian cancer: a phase 3, open-label, randomised controlled trial. *Lancet*. 2009;374(9698):1331-1338. PMID: 19767092. (Katsumata et al. 2009)
- Katsumata N, et al. Long-term results of dose-dense paclitaxel and carboplatin versus conventional paclitaxel and carboplatin for treatment of advanced epithelial ovarian, fallopian tube, or primary peritoneal cancer (JGOG 3016): a randomised, controlled, open-label trial. *Lancet Oncol*. 2013;14(10):1020-6. PMID: 23948349. (Katsumata et al. 2013)

TRIAL SPONSOR

- Japanese Gynecologic Oncology Group (JGOG)

RATIONALE FOR TRIAL

- Standard first-line chemotherapy for advanced ovarian cancer consists of paclitaxel and carboplatin given every 3 weeks. The 3rd International Gynecologic Cancer Consensus Conference in 2004 recommended paclitaxel 175 mg/m^2 over 3 hours plus carboplatin AUC 5 to 7.5 mg/mL per minute over 30 to 60 minutes every 3 weeks for 6 cycles as first-line chemotherapy (du Bois et al. 2005b).

- The addition of another drug to paclitaxel and carboplatin given either concurrently or sequentially has not improved outcomes (du Bois et al. 2006b; Bookman et al. 2009; Hoskins et al. 2010).
- Dose-dense weekly administration of paclitaxel may be a strategy to improve survival as the duration of exposure, even at low concentrations, can result in adequate cytotoxicity (Lopes et al. 1993; Jordan et al. 1996). Phase 2 trials combining dose-dense paclitaxel with carboplatin have demonstrated feasibility and efficacy (Rose et al. 2005; Sehouli et al. 2008).
- This trial was conducted to compare standard paclitaxel and carboplatin dosing against a regimen containing dose-dense weekly paclitaxel with carboplatin.

PATIENT POPULATION

- N = 637 enrolled, 631 eligible.
- Recruited from 85 centers in Japan from April 2003 to December 2005.
- Stage II to IV epithelial ovarian cancer, fallopian tube cancer, peritoneal cancer.
- Patient with a cytological diagnosis only had to meet the following criteria:
  - Cytological diagnosis of adenocarcinoma.
  - An abdominal mass of at least 2 cm in diameter on abdominal images.
  - A CA125/carcinoembryonic antigen (CEA) ratio >25 (Yedema et al. 1992) or no evidence of gastrointestinal cancer if CA125/CEA ratio ≤25.
- ECOG performance status of 0 to 3.
- Adequate organ function: ANC >1500 cells per µL; platelet count >100,000 cells per µL; serum bilirubin <25.7 µmol/L; serum AST <100 IU/L; serum creatinine <132.6 µmol/L.
- Exclusions: prior chemotherapy; low malignant potential tumor; synchronous or metachronous malignant disease within 5 years other than carcinoma in situ.

TREATMENT DETAILS

Arm 1: Conventional Paclitaxel + Carboplatin
- Paclitaxel 180 mg/m^2 IV over 3 hours on day 1.
- Carboplatin AUC 6 mg/mL per minute IV over 1 hour on day 1; dose calculated with formula of Calvert (Calvert et al. 1989) using creati-

nine clearance calculated by method of Jelliffe (Jelliffe 1973), not glomerular filtration rate.
- Standard premedications prior to paclitaxel to prevent hypersensitivity.
- Treatment every 3 weeks for 6 cycles.
- Hematologic parameters to treat—day 1: ANC >1000 cells/μL, platelets >75,000 cells/μL.
- Treatment was delayed for a maximum of 3 weeks.

Arm 2: Dose-Dense Paclitaxel + Carboplatin
- Paclitaxel 80 mg/m² IV over 1 hour on days 1, 8, and 15.
- Carboplatin AUC 6 mg/mL per minute IV over 1 hour on day 1; dose calculated with formula of Calvert (Calvert et al. 1989) using creatinine clearance calculated by method of Jelliffe (Jelliffe 1973), not glomerular filtration rate.
- Standard premedications prior to paclitaxel to prevent hypersensitivity.
- Treatment every 3 weeks for 6 cycles.
- Hematologic parameters to treat—day 1: ANC >1000 cells/μL, platelets >75,000 cells/μL.
- Hematologic parameters to treat—days 8 and 15: ANC >500 cells/μL, platelets >50,000 cells/μL.
- Treatment was delayed for a maximum of 3 weeks.

Dose Modifications
- Carboplatin reduced for hematologic toxicity, including febrile neutropenia, ANC <500 cells/μL persisting for ≥7 days, platelets <10,000 cells/μL, platelets 10,000 to 50,000 cells/μL with bleeding tendencies, or treatment delayed for more than 1 week for hematologic toxicity.
  ○ Level 1 reduction to AUC 5 mg/mL per minute.
  ○ Level 2 reduction to AUC 4 mg/mL per minute.
- Paclitaxel reduced for nonhematologic toxicity, including grade 2 or higher peripheral neuropathy.
  ○ Conventional dose level 1 reduction to 135 mg/m².
  ○ Conventional dose level 2 reduction to 110 mg/m².
  ○ Dose-dense dose level 1 reduction to 70 mg/m².
  ○ Dose-dense dose level 2 reduction to 60 mg/m².

Supportive Measures
- Patients did not receive G-CSF unless they had treatment delays or neutropenic complications.

Treatment Continuation
- Patients with partial or complete responses received an additional 3 cycles of chemotherapy.

Surgery
- Interval debulking surgery after 2 to 4 cycles of chemotherapy was allowed.
- Secondary debulking surgery or second-look surgery after 6 cycles of chemotherapy was allowed.

ASSESSMENTS
- Radiological studies at baseline and after 2, 4, and 6 cycles of chemotherapy. After discontinuation of protocol therapy, patients had follow-up every 3 months for the first 2 years and every 6 months thereafter with exam and CA125. CT scans were performed for symptoms or elevated CA125 levels.
- CA125 criteria for disease progression (Oken et al. 1982).
  - Patients with raised CA125 before treatment with return to normal after treatment needed to show reelevation of CA125 to 2 times the upper limit of normal.
  - Patients with raised CA125 before treatment that did not return to normal need to show evidence of CA125 ≥2 times the nadir level.
  - Patients with CA125 in the normal range before treatment needed to show evidence of CA125 ≥2 times the upper limit of normal with at least 2 values recorded at least 1 week apart.
- In patients with measurable disease, clinical and radiographic measurements had priority over CA125 levels and progression during treatment could not be based on CA125 measurements alone.
- Assessment of response had to be confirmed on 2 occasions at least 4 weeks apart.

ENDPOINTS
- PFS (measured from date of randomization) (primary endpoint).
- OS.
- Response rates.
- Adverse events.

STATISTICAL CONSIDERATIONS

Sample Size
- Hypothesis was that the dose-dense regimen would prolong PFS by 37.5% (from 16 months with conventional therapy to 22 months with dose-dense therapy). In April 2003, a sample size of 380 patients was planned to detect this difference with 80% power, 2-sided log-rank test, and α of .05.
- In January 2005, the sample size was increased to 600 to detect a smaller prolongation of PFS of 31.3% (from 16 to 21 months) with 80% power, 2-sided log-rank test, α of 0.05, accrual of 3 years, and a follow-up of 1.5 years.

Statistical Tests
- Cumulative survival curve and median PFS time were estimated by the Kaplan-Meier method.
- Two-sided χ^2 tests or 2-sided Fisher's exact tests were used to compare proportions of adverse events between groups.
- Fisher's exact test was used to compare responses.

CONCLUSIONS OF TRIAL

- Dose-dense paclitaxel with carboplatin improves survival compared to the conventional 3-week regimen with a 29% lower risk of disease progression and a 25% lower risk of death.
- With long-term follow-up, dose-dense treatment improves survival compared to conventional treatment and may be considered a new standard of care for first-line treatment of ovarian cancer.

COMMENTS FROM 2009 PUBLICATION

- With a Cox proportional hazards model, PFS was longer in the dose-dense treatment group across all subgroups except for in patients with clear-cell or mucinous tumors.
- The concept of dose density is based on the hypothesis that shorter intervals between chemotherapy exposures would be more effective than dose escalation in reducing tumor burden (Norton 2001).
- Dose-dense administration was associated with more hematologic toxicity and more dose delays and modifications.
- Despite improving PFS and OS, the response rate did not differ. A lower dose of paclitaxel has antiangiogenic activity (Klauber et al. 1997), and

Table 2.17 Results of JGOG 3016

Treatment arm	Conventional regimen N=319	Dose-dense regimen N=312	Statistics
Patient characteristics			
Median age (range)	57 (25-84)	57 (25-87)	
Residual disease ≤1 cm	45%	46%	
Residual disease >1 cm	55%	54%	
Cytology only	11%	11%	
Primary debulking	89%	89%	
Interval debulking	9%	11%	
Second-look surgery	18%	12%	
Stage II	17%	20%	
Stage III	67%	65%	
Stage IV	16%	15%	
Serous	57%	55%	
Endometrioid	12%	12%	
Mucinous	3%	7%	
Clear cell	12%	10%	
Other	16%	15%	
Grade 1	13%	13%	
Grade 2	22%	19%	
Grade 3	23%	25%	
Unknown grade	43%	42%	
Treatment delivery			
Completed 6+ cycles	73%	62%	
Treatment delays	67%	76%	$P=.02$
Dose reductions	35%	48%	$P=.001$
Efficacy			
In 2009 publication			
Median PFS	17.2 months	28.0 months	HR 0.71, $P=.0015$
OS at 3 years	65.1%	72.1%	HR 0.75, $P=.03$
Overall response	53%	56%	$P=$ NS
In 2013 publication			
Median PFS	17.5 months	28.2 months	HR 0.76, $P=.0037$
Median OS	62.2 months	100.5 months	HR 0.79, $P=.039$
OS at 5 years	51.1%	58.7%	
PFS, residual >1 cm	12.1 months	17.6 months	HR 0.71, $P=.0029$
PFS, residual ≤1 cm	60.9 months	Median not reached	HR 0.74, $P=.08$
OS, residual >1 cm	33.5 months	51.2 months	HR 0.75, $P=.0027$
OS, residual ≤1 cm	Median not reached	Median not reached	HR 0.76, $P=.23$
PFS, serous/other	17.5 months	28.7 months	HR 0.70, $P=.0007$

Table 2.17 Results of JGOG 3016 *(continued)*

Treatment arm	Conventional regimen N=319	Dose-dense regimen N=312	Statistics
PFS, clear cell/mucinous	16.7 months	18.7 months	HR 1.06, $P=.84$
OS, serous/other	61.2 months	100.5 months	HR 0.76, $P=.0252$
OS, clear cell/mucinous	62.2 months	Median not reached	HR 0.92, $P=.776$
Toxicity			
Higher with dose-dense			
G3/4 anemia	44%	69%	$P=.0001$
No difference			
G3/4 neutropenia	88%	92%	$P=$NS
G3/4 thrombocytopenia	38%	44%	$P=$NS
G3/4 motor neuropathy	4%	5%	$P=$NS
G3/4 sensory neuropathy	6%	7%	$P=$NS
G3/4 hypersensitivity	1.6%	1.9%	$P=$NS

HR, hazard ratio; NS, not significant; PFS, progression-free survival; OS, overall survival.

antiangiogenic agents might promote tumor dormancy by maintaining tumor size and prevention outgrowth (Folkman 1971).
- Frequency of neurotoxicity was similar between the groups. This may be due to the fact that patients receiving dose-dense therapy discontinued treatment more frequently.

COMMENTS FROM 2013 PUBLICATION

- The median OS in patients with optimally resected disease (<1 cm residual) who received conventional treatment (62.2 months) was better than in other trials conducted in Europe and the United States, demonstrating that Asian patients with ovarian cancer have better survival than non-Asian patients. This may be due to biological differences, environmental factors, socioeconomic differences, and/or response to treatment.
- In the subgroup analyses, the greatest benefit of the dose-dense regimen was in patients with optimally cytoreduced (<1 cm) non–clear cell and nonmucinous histologies (ie, serous or other). Other treatment strategies are needed for clear cell and mucinous tumors.
- Carboplatin was dosed with the formulas of Calvert and Jelliffe without adjustment of serum creatinine concentrations. Glomerular filtration rate was estimated using the enzymatic peroxidase-antiperoxidase method, which can result in excessive dosing and more myelosuppression. Other methods to calculate the GFR have been proposed (Ando et al. 2000; Levey et al. 2006; Matsuo et al. 2009), but no consensus

exists. Based on an analysis demonstrating no association between relative dose intensity of carboplatin and PFS or OS, possible excessive doses of carboplatin are not thought to have contributed to the survival differences seen in this trial.
- Dose-dense regimens are also being evaluated in MITO-7, ICON8, and GOG 262. The best dosing schedule has yet to be established.

MITO-2 (Pignata, Oncology 2009; Pignata, JCO 2011)

REFERENCES

- Pignata S, et al. Carboplatin and pegylated liposomal doxorubicin for advanced ovarian cancer: preliminary activity results of the MITO-2 phase III trial. *Oncology.* 2009;76(1):49-54. PMID: 19039248. (Pignata et al. 2009)
- Pignata S, et al. Carboplatin plus paclitaxel versus carboplatin plus pegylated liposomal doxorubicin as first-line treatment for patients with ovarian cancer: the MITO-2 randomized phase III trial. *J Clin Oncol.* 2011;29(27):3628-3635. PMID: 21844495. (Pignata et al. 2011)

TRIAL SPONSOR

- Multicentre Italian Trials in Ovarian Cancer (MITO)
- Integrated Therapeutics Group (ITG)—no role in trial design and data interpretation
- Schering-Plough Italy provided experimental drug—no role in trial design and data interpretation
- Nonprofit Italian Association for Cancer Research

RATIONALE FOR TRIAL

- After treatment for ovarian cancer, the risk of recurrence and death remains high.
- Standard treatment affects quality of life due to toxicities that include alopecia, neurotoxicity, and fatigue.
- Anthracyclines were used in first-line treatment of ovarian cancer before the introduction of taxanes and a meta-analysis demonstrated the addition of doxorubicin improved survival (Cyclophosphamide plus cisplatin . . . 1991; Fanning et al. 1992; A'Hern and Gore 1995; Muggia et al. 1997; West and Zweig 1997). However, safety concerns with

anthracyclines include dose-limiting acute toxicity of myelosuppression and gastrointestinal toxicities and chronic cumulative cardiotoxicity and alopecia.
- PLD is doxorubicin encapsulated in liposomes coated with methoxypolyethylene glycol, which prolongs the circulation of the drug and its concentration in the tumor. This formulation results in a different pharmacokinetic and toxicity profile (Theodoulou and Hudis 2004). Compared to anthracyclines, PLD has less myelotoxicity, alopecia, nausea, vomiting, and cardiomyopathy but has more skin and mucosal toxicity, including palmar-plantar erythrodysesthesia (PPE) and stomatitis (Muggia et al. 1997; O'Brien et al. 2004).
- In second-line treatment for platinum-sensitive ovarian cancer, a randomized trial demonstrated PLD treatment to have better survival than topotecan treatment as well as a favorable toxicity profile (Gordon et al. 2004).
- A phase II study by the Group d'Investigateurs Nationaux pour l'Etude des Cancers Ovariens treated patients with platinum-sensitive relapsed ovarian cancer with carboplatin AUC 5 and PLD 30 mg/m^2 every 4 weeks and demonstrated a 63% response rate, median PFS of 9.4 months, and median OS of 32 months. Toxicities included severe neutropenia (about 50%), fever (3%), PPE (32%), and neuropathy (28%) but was well tolerated overall (Ferrero et al. 2007).
- Several phase I and II studies combine PLD and carboplatin in relapsed ovarian cancer (Goncalves et al. 2003; du Bois et al. 2006a; du Bois et al. 2007; Ferrero et al. 2007; Alberts et al. 2008a).
- This trial was designed to evaluate whether carboplatin/PLD has superior PFS to carboplatin/paclitaxel in first-line treatment of advanced ovarian cancer. To provide the same dose intensity of carboplatin in both arms, the carboplatin/PLD was dosed on an every 3-week schedule.

PATIENT POPULATION

- N = 820 enrolled.
- Enrolled between January 2003 and November 2007.
- Cytologic or histologic diagnosis of epithelial ovarian cancer, stages IC to IV.
- Age less than 75 years.
- ECOG performance status of 0, 1, or 2.
- Life expectancy ≥3 months.

- Adequate bone marrow, kidney, and liver function.
- Exclusions: prior chemotherapy; clinically relevant heart disease; other concomitant diseases representing contraindications to treatment drugs; prior or concomitant other malignancy except nonmelanoma skin cancer or carcinoma in situ of the uterine cervix.

TREATMENT DETAILS

Arm 1: Standard Arm: Paclitaxel + Carboplatin
- Paclitaxel 175 mg/m^2 IV on day 1 every 3 weeks. Paclitaxel was diluted in 250 mL of normal saline and infused over 3 hours.
- Carboplatin AUC 5 IV on day 1 every 3 weeks. Doses were calculated according to the Calvert formula with creatinine clearance estimated by the Cockcroft formula. Carboplatin was diluted in 250 mL of 5% dextrose in water (D5W) and infused over 30 minutes.
- Treatment for 3 cycles with assessment and a further 3 cycles if stable or responding disease.

Arm 2: Experimental Arm: Carboplatin + PLD
- Carboplatin AUC 5 IV on day 1 every 3 weeks.
- PLD 30 mg/m^2 IV on day 1 every 3 weeks. PLD was diluted in 250 mL of D5W and infused over 60 minutes after carboplatin infusion.
- Treatment for 3 cycles with assessment and a further 3 cycles if stable or responding disease.

Conditions for Retreatment
- Leukocytes >3000/μL, neutrophils >1500/μL, platelets ≥100,000/μL, absence of grade 2 or more organ toxicity (excluding alopecia).

Dose Modifications
- Twenty percent dose reduction for all drugs if ANC <500/μL or platelets <50,000/μL for more than 7 days.
- Twenty percent reduction of carboplatin and paclitaxel for neuropathy.
- Carboplatin reduced to AUC 4 for creatinine clearance <60 mL.
- For grade 2 or more skin toxicity, PLD was delayed for up to 2 weeks or until toxicity resolved to grade 1 or less; otherwise, PLD was interrupted; 25% subsequent dose reduction if grade 3 or 4 skin toxicity cleared within 2 weeks.

Treatment Discontinuation
- For treatment delays of ≥2 weeks.

ASSESSMENTS

- CT or MRI of the abdomen and pelvis at baseline and after 3 and 6 cycles of chemotherapy.
- Quality of life was assessed with the EORTC QLQ-C30 (Aaronson et al. 1993).
- Toxicity graded according to the National Institute Common Toxicity Criteria (version 2.0).
- RECIST version 1.0 used for evaluation of response (Therasse et al. 2000).
  - Progression defined as 20% increase in the sum of the largest diameters of known lesions; appearance of new lesions; increase in CA125 level of more than 25%; death from any cause.

ENDPOINTS

- PFS (primary endpoint).
- OS.
- Treatment activity.
- Toxicity.
- Quality of life.

STATISTICAL CONSIDERATIONS

Sample Size

- In total, 820 patients and 632 progression events were needed for 80% power of detecting a 0.80 hazard ratio of progression with a 2-tailed α of 0.05. This represented an improvement in PFS from 18 to 22.5 months. No interim analyses were planned.
- At the time of analysis, only 556 events had occurred due to a relatively good prognosis population (>50% optimal debulking, one-third with no residual disease, high proportion of early-stage patients). This number of events allowed for detection of a hazard ratio (HR) of 0.79 with 80% power.

Stratification Factors

- Stratification variables included center, residual disease (absent, ≤1 cm, >1 cm, no primary surgery), stage (IC, II, III, IV), and ECOG performance status (0, 1, 2).

Statistical Tests

- Inverted Kaplan-Meier method (Schemper and Smith 1996) to calculate median follow-up and Kaplan-Meier product-limit method to

Table 2.18 Results of MITO-2

Treatment arm	Standard (PC) N=410	Experimental (C-PLD) N=410	Statistics
Patient characteristics			
Median age (range)	57 (21-77)	57 (25-77)	
No residual	36.1%	36.6%	
Residual disease ≤1 cm	17.1%	19.3%	
Residual disease >1 cm	28.3%	27.1%	
No surgery	18.5%	17.1%	
Stage IC	9.0%	9.0%	
Stage II	9.8%	9.5%	
Stage III	59.8%	60.5%	
Stage IV	21.5%	21.0%	
Serous	63%	66%	
Endometrioid	12%	12%	
Mucinous	2.9%	3.2%	
Clear cell	3.7%	2.9%	
Other	18.1%	16.1%	
Grade	Not reported	Not reported	
Treatment delivery			
No treatment	1.0% (N=4)	1.5% (N=6)	
Received 6 cycles	86.5%	81.1%	
Cycles delayed for toxicity	11.5%	34.5%	
Discontinuation			
Progression/death	5.6%	7.2%	
Toxicity/refusal	5.1%	9.4%	
Violation/other	2.0%	1.5%	
Efficacy			
Median PFS	16.8 months	19.0 months	HR 0.95, P=NS
Median OS	53.2 months	61.6 months	HR 0.89, P=NS
ORR	59%	57%	P=NS
Toxicity			
Deaths	N=4	N=2	
Worse with PC			
Alopecia	63%	14%	$P<.001$
Any diarrhea	13%	6%	$P<.001$
≥G3 neuropathy	3%	<1%	$P=.003$
Worse with C-PLD			
≥G3 thrombocytopenia	2%	16%	$P<.001$
≥G3 anemia	4%	10%	$P<.001$
Skin toxicities	6%	21%	$P<.001$
Stomatitis	<10%	19%	$P<.001$

Table 2.18 Results of MITO-2 *(continued)*

Treatment arm	Standard (PC) N=410	Experimental (C-PLD) N=410	Statistics
No difference			
≥G3 leukopenia	19%	15%	NS
≥G3 neutropenia	50%	43%	NS
Febrile neutropenia	2%	<2%	NS
Infections	<4%	<3%	NS
Bleeding	<1%	<1%	NS

C-PLD, carboplatin+pegylated liposomal doxorubicin; HR, hazard ratio; NS, not significant; PFS, progression-free survival; ORR, overall response rate; OS, overall survival; PC, paclitaxel+carboplatin.

estimate PFS and OS curves (Kaplan and Meier 1958). Curves compared with the log-rank test (Mantel 1966).
- Cox proportional hazards model used to assess treatment effect adjusted by baseline prognostic variables.
- χ^2 used to compared the difference in overall response rates.
- Exact linear rank test used to compare patters of toxicity, considering all grades.
- χ^2 and Fisher's exact tests used to compare rates of severe toxicity.
- Quality-of-life analyses were performed according to the EORTC manual (Fayers 2001).

CONCLUSION OF TRIAL

- Carboplatin and PLD does not improve survival compared to carboplatin and paclitaxel but can be considered as an alternative front-line therapy for ovarian cancer due to its different toxicity profile. This might be a particular consideration for patients at high risk of neurotoxicity or those wishing to avoid alopecia.

COMMENTS

- Residual disease and stage were independent predictors of PFS. There was no heterogeneity of treatment effect.
- There were no reported differences in quality of life except for more loss of appetite with the experimental arm and more diarrhea in the standard arm.
- Toxicity profiles were dramatically different. Carboplatin/PLD was associated with less hair loss and less neurotoxicity but with more skin toxicity and stomatitis. Carboplatin and PLD also caused

worse hematologic toxicity but within acceptable limits for clinical practice.
- These authors previously demonstrated that residual neurotoxicity occurs frequently after carboplatin and paclitaxel treatment and 14% have persistent symptoms even after 1 year (Pignata et al. 2006). Residual neurotoxicity may affect later treatment choices.
- The MITO-2 study adds to the data regarding the role of anthracyclines in ovarian cancer treatment with prior data suggesting the addition of doxorubicin to improve survival outcomes (A'Hern and Gore 1995).
- The final MITO-2 analysis was done with fewer events than planned (556 instead of 632 events) due to the favorable prognostic factors of enrolled patients. A much longer follow-up time would have been required, and this may have resulted in dilution of PFS differences.

AGO-OVAR9 (du Bois, JCO 2010)

REFERENCE
- du Bois A, et al. Phase III trial of carboplatin plus paclitaxel with or without gemcitabine in first-line treatment of epithelial ovarian cancer. *J Clin Oncol.* 2010;28(27):4162-4169. PMID: 20733132. (du Bois et al. 2010)

TRIAL SPONSORS
- Gynecologic Cancer Intergroup
- Arbeitsgemeinschaft Gynaekologische Onkologie Studiengruppe Ovarialkarzinom (AGO-OVAR)
- Groupe d'Investigateurs Nationaux pour l'Etude des Cancers Ovariens (GINECO)
- Nordic Society of Gynecologic Oncology (NSGO)

RATIONALE FOR TRIAL
- A possible method for improving survival in advanced ovarian cancer is to add a non-cross-resistant drug to platinum and paclitaxel.
- Gemcitabine was thought be a good candidate based on:
  - It has single-agent activity in relapsed ovarian cancer comparable to standard liposomal doxorubicin in randomized trials (Mutch et al. 2007; Ferrandina et al. 2008).

- It can be combined with platinum in platinum-sensitive ovarian cancer (du Bois et al. 2001; Brewer et al. 2006).
  - The combination has been shown to have higher efficacy than carboplatin alone in this population (Pfisterer et al. 2006a).
  - It can be added as a third drug to platinum and taxane, which would allow assessment of a triplet regimen without compromising therapy by withholding a standard drug (Gupta et al. 2005; Hensley et al. 2006; Friedlander et al. 2007).
- This trial was designed to compare paclitaxel/carboplatin/gemcitabine (du Bois et al. 2005a) to paclitaxel/carboplatin in advanced ovarian cancer.

PATIENT POPULATION

- N = 1784 screened, 1742 eligible.
- Between 2002 and 2004, 1742 patients were enrolled (175 in stratum 1, 891 in stratum 2, and 676 in stratum 3).
- FIGO stages I to IV ovarian cancer with upfront debulking surgery within 6 weeks before random assignment.
- Adequate hematologic, renal, and hepatic function defined as ANC ≥ 1500 cells/µL, platelets $\geq 100,000$ cells/µL, and serum creatinine and bilirubin ≤ 1.25 times upper normal limit.
- Exclusions: low malignant potential tumors; ECOG performance status >2; an estimated glomerular filtration rate of <50 mL/min; other malignancies; pervious chemotherapy, immunotherapy, or radiotherapy; severe neuropathy; cardiac arrhythmias; or congestive heart failure.

TREATMENT DETAILS

Arm 1: Paclitaxel, Carboplatin (TC)

- Paclitaxel 175 mg/m^2 IV over 3 hours on day 1 every 3 weeks.
- Carboplatin AUC 5 IV over 30 to 60 minutes on day 1 every 3 weeks.

Arm 2: Paclitaxel, Carboplatin, Gemcitabine (TCG)

- Paclitaxel 175 mg/m^2 IV over 3 hours on day 1 every 3 weeks.
- Carboplatin AUC 5 IV over 30 to 60 minutes on day 1 every 3 weeks.
- Gemcitabine 800 mg/m^2 IV over 30 to 60 minutes on days 1 and 8 every 3 weeks.

Dosing Details and Supportive Measures

- Paclitaxel maximum dose of 385 mg. Dose reduction to 150 mg/m^2 (level 1) or 135 mg/m^2 (level 2).

- Carboplatin—dose calculated according to formula of Calvert (Calvert et al. 1989). GFR estimated using Jelliffe formula (Jelliffe 1973). Maximum dose of 800 mg. Dose reduction to AUC 4 (level 1/level 2).
- Gemcitabine—maximum dose of 1600 mg. Dose reduction by omission of day 8 dose (level 1).
- Dose reductions allowed for hematologic and nonhematologic toxicity.
- Treatment cycles were delayed for ANC <1500 cells/μL or platelet count <100,000 cells/μL.
- Primary prophylaxis with granulocyte colony-stimulating factor (G-CSF) or granulocyte macrophage colony-stimulating factor (GM-CSF) was not allowed.
- Supportive G-CSF/GM-CSF could be initiated at the discretion of the investigator.
- All patients received antiallergic and antiemetic premedications.
- Treatment was discontinued for disease progression.
- Patients with partial remission after 6 cycles of treatment could receive additional cycles.

ASSESSMENTS

- Tumor measurements were made before each cycle by exam, before every third cycle by imaging (in patients with measurable or evaluable disease), and after the last cycle. Tumor response was graded by RECIST (Therasse et al. 2000).
- Adverse events and toxicities were graded according to the National Cancer Institute Common Toxicity Criteria (NCI-CTC). Toxicities were evaluated per course and per patient to capture the worst score over all courses.
- Quality of life was evaluated by using global health status/quality-of-life score of the EORTC QLQ-C30, version 3.0 (Aaronson et al. 1993) and the OV-28 module specific for ovarian cancer, version 1.0 (Greimel et al. 2003). Quality of life was assessed at baseline, after the third and last treatment cycles, and 3 months after completion of treatment, and responses were evaluated according to the EORTC guidelines.
- Follow-up visits were scheduled every 3 months in the first 2 years and every 6 months thereafter for a total of 5 years.

ENDPOINTS

- OS (defined as time from random assignment to death from any cause) (primary endpoint).

- PFS.
- Response to treatment.
- Toxicity.
- Quality of life.

STATISTICAL CONSIDERATIONS

Stratification Factors
- Patients were stratified according to residual tumor size and FIGO stage.
  - Stratum 1: FIGO I to IIA disease.
  - Stratum 2: FIGO IIB to IIIC and residual <1 cm.
  - Stratum 3: Residual tumor ≥1 cm or FIGO stage IV.

Sample Size
- To detect a clinically meaningful HR of 0.818, which corresponds to an increased median survival of 8 months, and to compensate for a 10% loss to follow-up rate, recruitment of 1716 patients was planned.

Statistical Tests
- Kaplan-Meier method used to analyze time-to-event data.
- Log-rank test used to compare survival distributions between groups.
- Cox proportional hazards model used to estimate hazard ratios.
- Method of Blyth-Still-Casella used to estimate response rates.
- Exact methods for stratified testing including the Zelens exact test were used to compare response rates.
- Wilcoxon-Mann-Whitney test was used to compare global health score and its difference from baseline (reflecting summary quality-of-life measures).

CONCLUSION OF TRIAL
- The addition of gemcitabine to the paclitaxel and carboplatin backbone increased treatment burden, increased toxicities, and reduced PFS in patients with advanced epithelial ovarian cancer.

COMMENTS
- Exploratory analysis of different prognostic subgroups demonstrated no evidence of benefit from addition of gemcitabine to treatment of any subgroup.

Table 2.19 Results of AGO-OVAR9

Treatment arm	TC N=882	TCG N=860	Statistics
Patient characteristics			
Median age (range)	60 (23-82)	59 (20-80)	
Residual disease ≤1 cm	70.9%	69.2%	
Residual disease >1 cm	29.1%	30.8%	
Stage I	8.6%	8.2%	
Stage II	9.4%	10.1%	
Stage III	65.8%	65.3%	
Stage IV	16.2%	16.3%	
Serous	73.7%	75.1%	
Mucinous/clear cell	4.5%	4.7%	
Other	21.8%	20.2%	
Grade 1	10.7%	6.9%	
Grade 2	29.1%	33.7%	
Grade 3	60.2%	59.4%	
Treatment delivery			
Received at least 6 cycles	87.2%	86.2%	
Received >6 cycles	15.8%	15.8%	
Treatment delay >7 days	7.5%	11.6%	$P<.001$
At least 1 dose reduction	8.7%	15.1%	$P<.001$
Efficacy			
Objective response rate	77.5%	86.2%	$P=.0303$
Median PFS	19.3 months	17.8 months	$P<.01$
Median OS	51.5 months	49.5 months	$P=NS$
Toxicity			
Worse with TCG			
G3/4 hemoglobin	4.3%	17.8%	$P<.001$
G3/4 leukocytes	28.1%	70.2%	$P<.001$
G3/4 neutrophils	62.1%	81.5%	$P<.001$
G3/4 platelets	4.7%	35.8%	$P<.001$
Febrile neutropenia	2.3%	6.6%	$P<.001$
Transfusion blood	10.0%	32.5%	$P<.001$
Supportive care EPO	11.6%	26.7%	$P<.001$
Supportive care G-CSF	12.8%	28.0%	$P<.001$
Supportive care antibiotic	14.1%	21.6%	$P<.001$

EPO, epogen; G-CSF, granulocyte colony-stimulating factor; NS, not significant; PFS, progression-free survival; OS, overall survival; TC, taxol+carboplatin; TCG, taxol+carboplatin+gemcitabine.

- The addition of gemcitabine resulted in a disadvantage to survival in early ovarian cancer patients and a disadvantage to PFS in advanced disease, and it added to hematologic toxicity and fatigue.
- The addition of a third drug may have a detrimental effect by affecting immune suppression (Zhang et al. 2003; Alberts et al. 2008).
- More than 10,000 patients have been enrolled in intergroup trials that have evaluated the addition of anthracyclines, topotecan, and gemcitabine to standard therapy (du Bois et al. 2006b; Pfisterer et al. 2006b; Bookman et al. 2009). These trials consistently show no added benefit but increased toxicities with the addition of the third drug.
- Despite this evidence, the next generation of trials in the GCIG network is using the same design of addition of a third drug sequentially or concurrently to TC, but these new trials are using targeted therapies (bevacizumab, erlotonib, pazopanib, vargatef). This strategy is based on the assumption that the model did not fail, but the wrong drugs were selected for use (Hoskins 2009).
- Promising results from phase II studies do not always translate into success in phase III (Zia et al. 2005). Most phase II studies choose a primary endpoint of response rate, but this is a surrogate endpoint that does not necessarily correlate with survival. Response is only measured in the subgroup of patients with bulky disease, and the addition of a third drug may speed the disappearance of these masses. Survival is more dependent on the regrowth of chemoresistant tumor masses, which are not reduced by the addition of the third agent.
- The selection of drugs for phase III evaluation might be improved by the use of different endpoints that are more reflective of chemoresistant disease. This includes time to treatment failure in relation to prior recurrence-free survival (Harrison et al. 2007). Another approach may be the use of tumor kinetics seen in phase II studies to predict the survival gain achievable in phase III (Claret et al. 2009).

OV16 (Hoskins, JNCI 2010)

REFERENCE
- Hoskins P, et al. Advanced ovarian cancer: phase III randomized study of sequential cisplatin-topotecan and carboplatin-paclitaxel vs carboplatin-paclitaxel. *J Natl Cancer Inst.* 2010;102(20):1547-1556. PMID: 20937992. (Hoskins et al. 2010)

TRIAL SPONSOR

- Gynecologic Cancer Intergroup
  - NCIC Clinical Trials Group (NCIC CTG)
  - European Organization for Research and Treatment of Cancer–Gynecologic Cancer Group (EORTC-GCG)
  - Grupo de Investigacion de Cancer de Ovario (GEICO)

RATIONALE FOR TRIAL

- A potential strategy to improve the efficacy of treatment of advanced ovarian cancer is to add a third cytotoxic agent to the backbone of standard paclitaxel and carboplatin.
- Topotecan is a camptothecin analogue that has single-agent activity in recurrent ovarian cancer, including platinum-resistant disease (Creemers et al. 1996; Kudelka et al. 1996; ten Bokkel Huinink et al. 1997; Bookman et al. 1998; Hoskins et al. 1998).
- To address the issue the issue of myelosuppression with paclitaxel + carboplatin + topotecan triple therapy, the NCIC Clinical Trials Groups (NCIC-CTG) tested a regimen that consisted of sequential doublets of cisplatin + topotecan followed by carboplatin + paclitaxel and found sufficient phase II activity to warrant a phase III study (Hoskins et al. 2000).
- This trial was designed to evaluate the efficacy of topotecan when combined with standard front-line chemotherapy for advanced ovarian cancer.

PATIENT POPULATION

- N = 819 enrolled.
- Enrollment between August 2001 and June 2005.
- Newly diagnosed stage IIB to IV epithelial ovarian, fallopian tube, or primary peritoneal cancer and completed all planned primary surgery.
- Diagnosis based on:
  - Histologic findings, or
  - Cytology if the patient had a pelvic mass with an abdominal metastasis ≥2 cm in diameter, a normal mammogram within the preceding 6 weeks, and CA125 to CEA ratio ≥25. If CA125 to CEA ratio <25, patients were eligible if colonoscopy/barium enema and gastroscopy/barium meal were negative.
- No prior chemotherapy.

- ECOG performance status of 0 or 1.
- Adequate hematologic reserve and liver function.
  - Granulocytes ≥2000/µL.
  - Platelets ≥150,000/µL.
  - Creatinine less than or equal to upper normal limit.
- Exclusions: borderline ovarian tumors, prior nonsurgical therapy for ovarian cancer, other malignancy other than nonmelanoma skin cancer, in situ carcinoma of the cervix, or a solid tumor treated with curative intent and no evidence of disease for ≥5 years; myocardial infarction within 6 months; second- or third-degree heart block unless a pacemaker had been implanted; contraindication to high-volume saline diuresis; preexisting hearing loss; neuropathy greater than grade 1.

TREATMENT DETAILS

Arm 1: Standard Treatment
- Eight cycles every 3 weeks.
  - Paclitaxel 175 mg/m^2 IV over 3 hours on day 1.
  - Carboplatin AUC 5 IV over 30 minutes on day 1.

Arm 2: Experimental Treatment
- Four cycles every 3 weeks.
  - Cisplatin 50 mg/m^2 IV over 60 minutes on day 1.
  - Topotecan 0.75 mg/m^2 IV over 30 minutes on days 1 through 5.
- Four cycles every 3 weeks.
  - Paclitaxel 175 mg/m^2 IV over 3 hours on day 1.
  - Carboplatin AUC 5 over 30 minutes (or per institutional standard) IV on day 1.

Administration Details
- Carboplatin dosed using either the measured glomerular filtration rate by nuclear renogram or a calculated GFR using the Cockcroft formula.
- All drugs were administered in solution as per the product monograph.
- Hydration and premedications were administered per local institutional standards and were not specified by protocol.

Treatment Delays
- Until granulocytes ≥1500/µL and platelets >100,000/µL.

Dose Reductions and Discontinuations
- Granulocytes ≤500/µL for >7 days; platelets <25,000/µL; febrile neutropenia; grade 3 or more infection.

- Topotecan decreased by 25% in the next cycle (no change in cisplatin dosing).
- Paclitaxel deceased by 25 mg/m^2 and carboplatin decreased by 1 AUC.
• Arthralgia or myalgia.
- Grade 3: paclitaxel decreased by 25 mg/m^2.
- Grade 4: paclitaxel discontinued.
• Grade 4 anaphylaxis (life threatening).
- Protocol therapy discontinued.
• Neurotoxicity.
- Grade 2: paclitaxel decreased by 25 mg/m^2.
- Grade 3: protocol therapy discontinued.
• Mucositis.
- Grade 2 or more: paclitaxel decrease by 25 mg/m^2.
• Renal toxicity after rehydration.
- With creatinine at 1 to 1.5 × upper limit of normal: cisplatin decreased by 25%.
- With creatinine >1.5 × upper limit of normal: protocol therapy discontinued.

Surgery
• Interval debulking was allowed after 3 or 4 cycles of therapy for those not optimally debulked at the time of study entry.

ASSESSMENTS

• On day 1 of each cycle: physical exam, CBC, serum creatinine, AST or ALT, serum CA125.
• On day 15 of each cycle: CBC.
• Imaging with CT scan or MRI prior to cycle 1 to obtain baseline measures except when no debulking had been done or when optimal debulking had been achieved. Further imaging after cycle 4 (or cycle 3 if interval debulking had been planned) and after cycle 8 or earlier if progression was suspected.
• Quality of life assessed using the EORTC QLQs C30 (Aaronson et al. 1993) and OV28 (Cull et al. 2001) module at baseline and on day 1 of cycles 3, 5, and 7; at the end of the last cycle; and 3 and 6 months after completing protocol therapy.
- QLQ C30 contains 9 multi-item scales. Five functional scales measure physical, role, cognitive, emotional, and social domains. Three

symptom scales measure fatigue, pain, and nausea and vomiting. The final scale is a global health and quality-of-life scale.
- The OV28 module assess symptoms that may be specific to ovarian cancer or its treatment, including abdominal symptoms, peripheral neuropathy, hormonal symptoms, attitude to disease treatment, and sexual functioning.
• After treatment, follow-up every 3 months for the first 3 years, then every 6 months for the next 2 years, then annually thereafter. History and physical exam, CA125 assessed at each visit.
- Progression was defined by Gynecologic Cancer Intergroup definition, including objective progression using RECIST criteria (Therasse et al. 2000) or CA125 progression (Vergote et al. 2000).
- RECIST progression: either a 20% increase in the sum of diameters over the nadir or the appearance of new disease.
- CA125 progression: increase to more than twice the upper limit of normal (or of the nadir value if levels had not normalized) and confirmed at least 1 week later. CA125 values measured within 4 weeks of surgery or other abdominal procedure such as paracentesis were not considered in this evaluation.

ENDPOINTS
• PFS, defined as time from randomization to time of first observation of disease progression or death from any cause (primary endpoint).
• OS.
• Adverse effects.
• Quality of life.
• Objective response (in patients with measurable disease by RECIST).
• CA125 normalization rates 3 months after randomization.

STATISTICAL CONSIDERATIONS

Stratification Factors
• Patients were stratified based on treatment center, age (≤65 or >65), extent of surgery (no debulking, no residual, residual <1 cm, residual ≥1 cm).

Sample Size
• Assuming PFS of 16 months with standard therapy, this trial was designed to have 80% power to detect a 25% improvement in PFS from a median of 16 months to 20 months (HR, 0.8) using a 2-sided α of 5%.

At the time of final analysis, 631 progression events would be needed, requiring recruitment of 800 patients over 2 years and 29 months of follow-up.

Statistical Tests

- Stratified log-rank test used to compare PFS and OS.
- Cochran-Mantel-Haenszel test used to compare CA125 normalization rates with adjustment for stratification factors.
- Cox proportional hazards model used to assess treatment effect after adjusting for potential confounding factors and to identify factors predictive of PFS. Covariates included:
  - Treatment.
  - Stratification factors.
  - Stage (II vs III/IV).
  - Grade (1/2 vs 3/undifferentiated/unknown).
  - Histology (serous vs other).
  - Performance status (0 vs 1).
- The assumption of proportionality in the Cox model was assessed by Schoenfeld residuals.
- Fisher's exact test was used to compare the incidence of adverse events between arms.
- Wilcoxon rank-sum test was used to compare changes of quality-of-life scores from baseline between treatment arms.

CONCLUSION OF TRIAL

- The addition of topotecan to paclitaxel and carboplatin does not improve outcomes and adds to the toxicity profile in the treatment of advanced ovarian cancer.

COMMENTS

- More mature OS outcomes will be reported after continued follow-up.
- The results of this study parallel those of the GOG 182-ICON5 study, which demonstrated no improvement in survival with the addition of a third cytotoxic agent to the paclitaxel and carboplatin backbone in the treatment of advanced ovarian cancer (Bookman et al. 2009).
  - In GOG 182-ICON5, topotecan was dosed at 1.25 mg/m^2 per day for 3 days; topotecan was combined with carboplatin, which was given on day 3 rather than day 1; and the topotecan doublet was given in the last 4 cycles of therapy.

Table 2.20 Results of OV16

Treatment arm	Standard treatment N=410	Experimental sequential doublets N=409	Statistics
Patient characteristics			
Median age (range)	57 (33-75)	57 (28-78)	
No residual	22%	22%	
Residual disease <1 cm	20%	25%	
Residual disease ≥1 cm	36%	33%	
No debulking	20%	19%	
Measurable disease	47%	48%	
Stage II	8.0%	9.0%	
Stage III	64.6%	67.2%	
Stage IV	27.3%	23.7%	
Serous	68%	65%	
Endometrioid	5%	7%	
Mucinous	2%	2%	
Clear cell	5%	6%	
Other	19%	21%	
Grade	Not reported	Not reported	
Treatment delivery			
Completed 8 cycles	81%	78%	
At least 1 cycle delay	50%	85%	
Dose reductions	18%	43%	
Interval debulking	17.4%	13.5%	
Efficacy			
Objective response	77.2%	67.9%	$P=.04$
Complete response	37.3%	31.1%	Not reported
CA125 normalization	66.3%	57.5%	$P=.006$
Median PFS	16.2 months	14.6 months	HR 1.10 (95% CI, 0.94-1.28)
Median OS	42.1 months	42.3 months	NS
Toxicity			
Death	N=2	N=2	
Worse with experimental			
G4 granulocytopenia	58%	85%	$P<.001$
Febrile neutropenia	6%	22%	$P<.001$
G3/4 thrombocytopenia	9%	46%	$P<.001$
Thromboembolic events	2%	7%	$P<.001$
Nausea	77%	84%	$P=.01$

(continued)

Table 2.20 Results of OV16 *(continued)*

Treatment arm	Standard treatment N=410	Experimental sequential doublets N=409	Statistics
Vomiting	41%	57%	$P<.001$
Hospitalization	7.1%	11.3%	
Erythropoietin use	13.4%	25.8%	
G-CSF use	13.7%	34.7%	
Worse with standard			
Neurosensory	84%	74%	$P<.001$
Allergic reactions	35%	24%	$P<.001$

CA125, cancer antigen 125; CI, confidence interval; G-CSF, granulocyte colony-stimulating factor; HR, hazard ratio; NS, not significant; PFS, progression-free survival; OS, overall survival.

- In this current trial, topotecan was dosed at 0.75 mg/m² per day for 5 days, topotecan was combined with cisplatin which was given on day 1, and the topotecan doublet was given in the first 4 cycles of therapy.
- The hypothesis that the 5-day topotecan schedule with day 1 cisplatin would be synergistic was not observed to be true in this study.
- Topotecan has been tested as triplet and consolidation therapy, but no trial has demonstrated a survival benefit (De Placido et al. 2004; Pfisterer et al. 2006b; Bookman et al. 2009). The cells that are resistant to platinum and taxanes do not appear to be responsive to topotecan treatment.
- For a drug to be non-cross-resistant, it should have activity against refractory tumors (cancer that grows during treatment). In 4 single-agent studies of topotecan in the refractory setting, only 9% of patients responded to treatment (Creemers et al. 1996; ten Bokkel Huinink et al. 1997; Bookman et al. 1998; Hoskins et al. 1998). Future trials should evaluate drugs that demonstrate more efficacy against refractory cells.
- Phase III ovarian cancer trials that use the PFS endpoint (whose median is approximately 15 months for front-line trials) for early stopping often complete accrual before sufficient progression events have been seen to perform an interim analysis. This trial suggests that CA125 normalization rates at 3 months may be predictive of treatment efficacy and would provide an earlier opportunity to perform futility analyses in future phase III studies. This endpoint would require confirmatory validation as an endpoint predictive of PFS in other trials.

ICON7 (Perren, NEJM 2011; Oza, Lancet Oncol 2015)

REFERENCES

- Perren TJ, et al. A phase 3 trial of bevacizumab in ovarian cancer. *N Engl J Med*. 2011;365(26):2484-96. PMID: 22204725. (Perren et al. 2011)
- Oza AM, et al. Standard chemotherapy with or without bevacizumab for women with newly diagnosed ovarian cancer (ICON7): overall survival results of a phase 3 randomised trial. *Lancet Oncol*. 2015;16(8):928-936. PMID: 26115797. (Oza et al. 2015)

TRIAL SPONSORS

- Gynecologic Cancer InterGroup (GCIG) Internal Collaboration on Ovarian Neoplasms (ICON7)
- Led by UK Medical Research Council Clinical Trials Unit (MRC CTU)
- Participating GCIG Groups:
  - AGO-OVAR
  - ANZGOG
  - GINECO
  - GEICO
  - MRC/NCRI
  - NSGO
  - NCIC CTG

RATIONALE FOR TRIAL

- Although intraperitoneal chemotherapy administration improves survival, this is an option limited to patients with small-volume residual disease.
- Angiogenesis leads to tumor growth and metastasis and is an attractive target as ovarian cancers frequently express vascular endothelial growth factor (VEGF).
- Bevacizumab is a monoclonal antibody that binds to VEGF-A with demonstrated efficacy in colorectal, lung, renal, breast, and brain cancers (Hurwitz et al. 2004; Eskens and Sleijfer 2008). Phase 2 trials have shown efficacy in women with ovarian cancer (Burger et al. 2007; Cannistra et al. 2007; Garcia et al. 2008).
- This trial (like GOG 218) was designed to evaluate the addition of bevacizumab to standard chemotherapy in front-line treatment of ovarian cancer.

PATIENT POPULATION
- N = 1528 enrolled.
- From December 2006 to February 2009, patients were enrolled from 263 centers in the United Kingdom, Germany, France, Canada, Australia, New Zealand, Denmark, Finland, Norway, Sweden, and Spain.
- Newly diagnosed ovarian cancer that was either
  ○ High-risk, stage I or IIA clear cell, or grade 3 ovarian cancer (enrollment limited to 10% of total study population) or
  ○ Advanced stage IIB to IV epithelial ovarian, fallopian tube, or peritoneal cancer.
- ECOG performance status of 0, 1, or 2.
- Adequate coagulation values, bone marrow, liver, and renal function.
- No plans for further surgery before disease progression.
- Exclusions: other tumor types; previous systemic therapy; planned surgery; uncontrolled hypertension.
- A high-risk subgroup was defined as at risk for progression and had similar patient characteristics to those enrolled in GOG 218. This subgroup included the following:
  ○ Stage IV.
  ○ Inoperable stage III.
  ○ Suboptimally debulked stage III (>1 cm residual).

TREATMENT DETAILS

Arm 1: Standard Chemotherapy (PC)
- Paclitaxel 175 mg/m^2 IV every 3 weeks for 6 cycles.
- Carboplatin AUC 5 or 6 IV every 3 weeks for 6 cycles.

Arm 2: Standard Chemotherapy + Bevacizumab (PCB)
- Paclitaxel 175 mg/m^2 IV every 3 weeks for 6 cycles.
- Carboplatin AUC 5 or 6 IV every 3 weeks for 6 cycles.
- Bevacizumab 7.5 mg/kg IV every 3 weeks during chemotherapy until 12 additional cycles or disease progression. To prevent delayed wound healing, bevacizumab was started with cycle 1 if chemotherapy started >4 weeks after surgery and delayed until cycle 2 if chemotherapy started ≤4 weeks from surgery.

ASSESSMENTS
- Clinical assessments and CA125 were performed before each cycle of chemotherapy, every 6 weeks in year 1, every 3 months in years 2 and 3, every 6 months in years 4 and 5, and then yearly thereafter.

- After disease progression, assessments were performed every 6 months for 5 years, then yearly thereafter.
- CT or MRI was performed at baseline, after cycles 3 and 6, at 9 and 12 months after randomization, every 6 months in years 2 and 3, and then as clinically indicated until disease progression.
- Quality of life was assessed with the EORTC QLQ-C30 and QLQ-OV28 questionnaires.
- Progression was defined by RECIST criteria (Therasse et al. 2000) and did not include asymptomatic progression by CA125 levels only.
- The biologic progression-free interval as calculated from date of randomization to date of first CA-125-based progression (Rustin et al. 2004) or first RECIST-based progression.

ENDPOINTS

- PFS (calculated from date of randomization) (primary endpoint).
- OS.
- Biologic progression-free interval.
- Response to therapy.
- Toxicity.
- Quality of life.
- Laboratory results.
- Worsened ECOG performance status.
- Health economics and translational research.

STATISTICAL CONSIDERATIONS

Stratification Factors
- Patients were stratified by GCIG group, FIGO stage, and residual disease (stage I to III with ≤1 cm residual disease, stage I to III with >1 cm residual disease, stage III inoperable or stage IV), and planned interval between surgery and chemotherapy (≤4 weeks or >4 weeks).

Sample Size
- Primary analysis was carried out with an unstratified log-rank test for the difference in PFS between the 2 groups. The trial was designed to detect a 28% increase in median PFS from 18 months with standard chemotherapy to 23 months with the addition of bevacizumab (HR, 0.81) with 90% power at the 5% significance level. A sample size of 1520 women and a total of 684 events (disease progression or death) were required. After submission of the primary analysis of PFS, regulatory

authorities requested an OS analysis with at least 365 deaths (50% of the required total number of deaths).
- Study was also powered to detect a difference in OS. This analysis needed 715 deaths to detect an improvement in OS from 43 to 53 months (HR, 0.81) with 80% power at a 2-sided significance level of 5%.

Statistical Tests
- Log-rank test stratified by factors used for randomization.
- Cox regression analyses adjusted for baseline covariates when proportional hazards could be assumed.
- When nonproportional hazards, flexible parametric survival models (Royston and Parmar 2002) to smooth survival curves were used.
- Interaction analyses to evaluate differences in size of treatment effects in subgroups classified by baseline characteristics, risk of progression, and stratification factors.
- Hazard functions to analyze the magnitude and timing of treatment effect.

CONCLUSIONS OF TRIAL
- Bevacizumab improved PFS by about 2 months and increased the response rate by about 20% in patients with ovarian cancer. Survival benefits were greater among patients at high risk for progression with improved PFS of 3.6 months.
- Final overall survival results (Oza et al. 2015).
  - No difference in overall survival in the trial population as a whole.
  - OS benefit of 4 months seen in highest risk subgroup.

COMMENTS
- The benefit of bevacizumab changed over time with maximum impact at 12 months. The benefit disappeared by 24 months. The maximum treatment effect coincided with the end of bevacizumab treatment and suggest that prolonged therapy beyond 12 months may further improve outcomes.
- Because results showed evidence of nonproportional hazards, the restricted mean difference (the difference in areas under the whole length of the PFS curves) was a better estimate of treatment effect in this trial. The restricted mean difference of PFS was 20.3 months vs 21.8 months for standard therapy vs bevacizumab, for a mean difference of 1.5 months.

Table 2.21 Results of ICON7

Treatment arm	Standard chemotherapy (PC) N = 764	Bevacizumab (PCB) N = 764	Statistics
Patient characteristics			
Median age (range)	57 (18-81)	57 (24-82)	
≤1 cm residual	74%	74%	
>1 cm residual	26%	26%	
Inoperable	2%	2%	
High risk (III >1 cm/IV)	31%	30%	
Stage I/IIA	10%	9%	
Stage IIB/IIC	9%	9%	
Stage III	69%	68%	
Stage IV	12%	13%	
Serous	69%	69%	
Endometrioid	7%	8%	
Mucinous	2%	2%	
Clear cell	8%	9%	
Other	13%	12%	
Grade 1	7%	5%	
Grade 2	19%	23%	
Grade 3	74%	71%	
Treatment delivery			
Received 6 cycles	91%	94%	
Efficacy			
Reported in 2011			
Overall response rate	48%	67%	$P<.001$
Median PFS	17.4 months	19.8 months	HR 0.87, $P=.04$
High-risk group	10.5 months	16.0 months	HR 0.73, $P=.002$
Median OS	Not reached	Not reached	HR 0.85, $P=$NS
High-risk group	28.8 months	36.6 months	HR 0.64, $P=.002$
Reported in 2015			
Median OS	44.6 months	45.5 months	$P=$NS
Non-high-risk group	49.7 months	48.4 months	$P=$NS
High-risk group	34.5 months	39.3 months	HR 0.78, $P=.03$
Clear cell	48.0 months	47.6 months	$P=$NS
Low stage, high grade	56.2 months	57.5 months	$P=$NS
Low-grade serous	50.4 months	50.5 months	$P=$NS
Updated PFS analysis	17.5 months	19.9 months	$P=$NS
High-risk group	10.5 months	16.0 months	HR 0.73, $P=.001$

(continued)

Table 2.21 Results of ICON7 *(continued)*

Treatment arm	Standard chemotherapy (PC) N = 764	Bevacizumab (PCB) N = 764	Statistics
Toxicity			
Deaths	N = 1	N = 4	
Worse with bevacizumab			
Bleeding	12%	39%	
≥ G2 hypertension	2%	18%	
≥ G3 thromboembolism	3%	7%	
GI perforations	N = 3	N = 10	

GI, gastrointestinal; HR, hazard ratio; NS, not significant; PFS, progression-free survival; OS, overall survival.

- The addition of bevacizumab did not affect chemotherapy delivery but increased the range of toxic effects, including hypertension and bowel perforation.
- Differences between ICON7 and GOG 218: (1) patient population in ICON7 include patients with high-risk early-stage disease; (2) half of the dose of bevacizumab was used (7.5 mg/kg vs 15 mg/kg) for a shorter maintenance period (12 cycles vs 16 cycles).
- The bevacizumab dose used in ICON7 is one of the licensed doses for metastatic colorectal cancer but is half the dose for metastatic breast cancer.
- Final OS analysis demonstrated an association between increasing disease severity and greater benefit of bevacizumab.
- Women who might not benefit from bevacizumab in the upfront setting:
  - Early-stage I/II disease, even if high grade or clear cell histology.
  - Optimally debulked (<1 cm residual) stage III disease.
  - Low-grade serous cancer.
  - Low-stage, high-risk tumors.
- The maximum PFS benefit coincided with the duration of bevacizumab treatment. The overall survival difference outlasts the duration of exposure and suggests a durable benefit in the high-risk group. The possibility of additional benefit with extension of treatment is being evaluated in the BOOST trial (NCT01426890).
- Data from ICON7 support early use of bevacizumab based on risk and disease burden. The role of repeated administration of bevacizumab

in the recurrent setting after upfront use is being evaluated in the MITO16MANGO2b trial (NCT01802749). Benefit to this approach in colorectal and breast cancer (Bennouna et al. 2013; von Minckwitz et al. 2014).
- Trial suggests that residual tumor burden with active angiogenesis is necessary for drug activity.
- Cost-effectiveness would be improved with an effective biomarker predicting response.
  - May not work as well in immunologically active subtype.
  - May benefit mesenchymal subtype.

GOG 218 (Burger, NEJM 2011)

REFERENCE

- Burger RA, et al. Incorporation of bevacizumab in the primary treatment of ovarian cancer. *N Engl J Med*. 2011;365(26):2473-2483. PMID: 22204724. (Burger et al. 2011)

TRIAL SPONSOR

- Gynecologic Oncology Group (GOG)

RATIONALE FOR TRIAL

- VEGF and angiogenesis promote ovarian cancer progression and are inversely correlated with survival.
- Bevacizumab is a humanized anti-VEGF monoclonal antibody that inhibits tumor angiogenesis and has single-agent activity against epithelial ovarian cancer in phase II trials (Burger et al. 2007; Cannistra et al. 2007).
- This trial (like ICON7) was performed to evaluate the addition of bevacizumab to standard chemotherapy and as maintenance in the frontline treatment of ovarian cancer.

PATIENT POPULATION

- N = 1873 enrolled.
- Between October 2005 and June 2009, patients were enrolled from 336 institutions in the United States, Canada, South Korea, and Japan.
- Stage III or IV epithelial ovarian, primary peritoneal, or fallopian tube cancer.

- Standard abdominal surgery with maximal debulking effort within 12 weeks of study entry.
- GOG performance status of 0, 1, or 2.
- No history of clinically significant vascular events or intestinal obstruction.
- Patients with optimal resection (<1 cm residual lesions) were originally excluded but then later included after protocol modification in July 2007.

TREATMENT DETAILS

Arm 1: Standard Chemotherapy (PC)
- Treatment every 3 weeks for 22 cycles.
- Paclitaxel 175 mg/m^2 IV on day 1 during cycles 1 to 6.
- Carboplatin AUC 6 IV on day 1 during cycles 1 to 6.
- Placebo during cycles 2 to 22.

Arm 2: Standard Chemotherapy + Initiation Bevacizumab (PCB)
- Treatment every 3 weeks for 22 cycles.
- Paclitaxel 175 mg/m^2 IV on day 1 during cycles 1 to 6.
- Carboplatin AUC 6 IV on day 1 during cycles 1 to 6.
- Bevacizumab 15 mg/kg added during cycles 2 to 6.
- Placebo during cycles 7 to 22.

Arm 3: Standard Chemotherapy + Initiation Bevacizumab + 15 Months of Bevacizumab Maintenance (PCB + B)
- Treatment every 3 weeks for 22 cycles.
- Paclitaxel 175 mg/m^2 IV on day 1 during cycles 1 to 6.
- Carboplatin AUC 6 IV on day 1 during cycles 1 to 6.
- Bevacizumab 15 mg/kg added during cycles 2 to 22.

Treatment Discontinuation
- For disease progression, unacceptable toxic effects, completion of all 22 cycles or withdrawal.

Supportive Care Measures
- Myeloid growth factor allowed only to manage febrile neutropenia, grade 4 neutropenia (ANC <500/mm^3) for 7 days or longer or for subsequent prophylaxis

Dose Modifications
- For limiting peripheral neuropathy or hypersensitivity, paclitaxel was replaced with docetaxel 75 mg/m^2.

- For weight change >10%, bevacizumab dose was modified.
- Bevacizumab was delayed or discontinued based on duration and severity of:
  - Hypertension: systolic blood pressure >150 mm Hg or diastolic blood pressure >90 mm Hg.
  - Proteinuria: urine protein-to-creatinine ratio 3.5.
  - Wound or bowel wall disruption (any grade, cycle 2 or later).
  - Reversible posterior leukoencephalopathy syndrome.
  - Arterial thrombosis of grade 3 at any time or grade 2 during cycle 2 or later.
  - Venous thrombosis.
  - Coagulopathy.
  - Intestinal obstruction.
  - Hypersensitivity of grade 3 or greater.

ASSESSMENTS

- Before cycle 1: physical exam, CA125 level, and CT or MRI of at least abdomen and pelvis.
- For patients without progression, imaging after cycles 3, 6, 10, 14, 18, and 22.
- Serum CA125 and physical exams performed before each cycle during cycles 1 to 6, every other cycle during cycles 7 to 22, every 3 months for 2 years, every 6 months for years 3 to 5, and annually thereafter.
- Adverse events were recorded with every cycle using the National Cancer Institute Common Terminology Criteria for adverse events (Version 3) and until 30 days after last study treatment.
- Quality of life measured by the Functional Assessment of Cancer Therapy–Ovary Trial Outcome Index (FACT-O TOI) survey (Basen-Engquist et al. 2001) before cycles 1, 4, 7, 13, 22, and 6 months after completing study therapy.

ENDPOINTS

- Primary endpoint was initially OS, then changed to PFS in October 2008. This occurred when patients and investigators contested maintaining the blinding of treatment assignments after disease progression, which would be necessary to maintain the integrity of the data for an OS endpoint.
- PFS was calculated from date of enrollment to progression by RECIST (Therasse et al. 2000), increase in CA125 according to GCIG criteria

(Rustin et al. 2001) in patients who had completed chemotherapy, global deterioration of health, or death from any cause. If patients were free of progression, data were censored at the date of the last radiographic assessment.

STATISTICAL CONSIDERATIONS

Stratification Factors
- Patients were stratified by GOG performance status, cancer stage, and debulking status (stage III optimal, stage III suboptimal, stage IV).

Sample Size
- A sample size of 1800 was estimated to provide 90% power to detect a 23% reduction in the hazard of progression with either of the 2 bevacizumab-containing regimens compared to the control regimen while limiting the overall 1-sided type I error for both comparisons to 2.5%.

Statistical Tests
- Relative hazard ratios were estimated with the proportional hazards model (Cox 1972).
- Differences in FACT-O TOI scores were assessed with a linear mixed model adjusted for baseline score and age.
- Differences in adverse events were examined by Fisher's exact test (Mehta and Petal 1983).
- Hypotheses were tested at a 1.67% significance level to account for multiple comparisons.

Other Considerations
- Treatment assignments could be revealed to investigators and patients in the setting of documented disease progression.
- Database was locked on February 5, 2010.

CONCLUSION OF TRIAL
- The addition of bevacizumab during and up to 10 months after paclitaxel and carboplatin chemotherapy extends median PFS by 4 months but does not have an impact on OS in patients with advanced epithelial ovarian cancer.

Table 2.22 Results of GOG 218

Treatment arm	PC N=625	PCB N=625	PCB+B N=623
Patient characteristics			
Median age (range)	60 (25-86)	60 (24-88)	60 (22-89)
White	84.2%	83.0%	83.6%
Asian	6.6%	5.9%	6.3%
Black	4.0%	4.5%	4.3%
Hispanic	3.4%	4.5%	4.0%
Other	1.9%	2.1%	1.8%
Stage III, ≤1 cm	34.9%	32.8%	34.7%
Stage III, >1 cm	40.6%	41.0%	38.8%
Stage IV	24.5%	26.2%	26.5%
Serous	86.6%	83.0%	84.1%
Endometrioid	3.4%	2.2%	3.9%
Mucinous	1.0%	0.8%	1.3%
Clear cell	1.9%	3.7%	3.2%
Other	7.2%	10.2%	7.5%
Grade 1	5.8%	4.5%	2.9%
Grade 2	16.3%	13.8%	15.6%
Grade 3	71.2%	74.4%	73.8%
Unknown grade	6.7%	7.4%	7.7%
Treatment delivery			
Completed therapy	16%	17%	24%
Discontinuation			
Disease progression	48%	42%	26%
Adverse events	12%	15%	17%
Efficacy			
Median PFS[a]	10.3 months	11.2 months (P=NS)	14.1 months (P=.001)
Median OS[a]	39.3 months	38.7 months (P=NS)	39.7 months (P=NS)
Toxicity			
Deaths	1%	1.6%	2.3%
Worse with bevacizumab			
≥G2 hypertension[a]	7.2%	16.5% (P<.05)	22.9% (P<.05)
No difference			
GI perforation, fistula	1.2%	2.8%	2.6%
≥G3 proteinuria	0.7%	0.7%	1.6%
≥G2 pain	41.6%	41.5%	47.0%
≥G4 neutropenia	57.5%	63.3%	63.3%
Venous thrombosis	5.8%	5.3%	6.7%

(continued)

Table 2.22 Results of GOG 218 *(continued)*

Treatment arm	PC N=625	PCB N=625	PCB+B N=623
Arterial thrombosis	0.8%	0.7%	0.7%
Wound disruption	2.8%	3.6%	3.0%
CNS bleeding	0	0	0.3%
Non-CNS bleeding	0.8%	1.3%	2.1%
PRES	0	0.2%	0.2%

CNS, central nervous system; GI, gastrointestinal; NS, not significant; PFS, progression-free survival; OS, overall survival; PC, paclitaxel+carboplatin; PCB, paclitaxel+carboplatin+bevacizumab; PCB+B, paclitaxel+carboplatin+bevacizumab followed by bevacizumab maintenance; PRES, posterior reversible encephalopathy syndrome.
$^a P$ values are compared to PC control arm.

COMMENTS

- Bevacizumab (or placebo) was added in cycle 2 rather than cycle 1 to decrease the risk of wound-healing complications. The maintenance treatment time of 15 months was selected to exceed the anticipated median PFS and to ensure feasibility. The bevacizumab dose of 15 mg/kg every 3 weeks was selected based on the approved combination with carboplatin and paclitaxel for advanced non–small cell lung cancer.
- Most adverse events were reported during chemotherapy. All but one gastrointestinal (GI) perforation/fistula occurred during chemotherapy. Exceptions included hypertension, proteinuria, and pain, which were more commonly reported during the extended phase in patients receiving maintenance bevacizumab.
- This cohort had relatively poor prognosis with 40% with suboptimal stage III and 26% with stage IV disease.
- The maximum separation in the PFS curves (PC vs PCB+B) occurred at 15 months with convergence of the curves 9 months later. This convergence of PFS curves was also seen in the ICON7 trial (which used 12 months of maintenance bevacizumab). There was no convergence of PFS curves in the OCEANS trial (for recurrent ovarian cancer) in which bevacizumab was used until disease progression and not discontinued at a predefined time. This suggests that the magnitude of benefit may correlate directly with treatment duration and is consistent with preclinical studies that demonstrate regrowth of tumor upon discontinuation of anti-VEGF therapy (Bagri et al. 2010).
- The improvement in PFS was consistent across different subgroup analyses (Figure 2C in manuscript).

- There was no reduction in quality of life with the addition of bevacizumab.
- There was no improvement in OS, but the ability to detect a difference may be limited by later crossover to receiving bevacizumab or other anti-VEGF agents.
- Bevacizumab increased the risk of hypertension, which appeared to be cumulative, but this tended to be controlled with medical therapy and did not lead to many treatment discontinuations.
- The lack of survival difference between control and bevacizumab initiation suggests that bevacizumab must be continued as a maintenance therapy to delay disease progression.
- The change in primary endpoint from OS to PFS is a major limitation of this study. The authors note that the GCIG supports the use of PFS as a primary endpoint for trials evaluating front-line therapy because of the influences of postprogression therapy on OS (Stuart et al. 2011).

MITO-7 (Pignata, Lancet Oncol 2014)

REFERENCE

- Pignata S, et al. Carboplatin plus paclitaxel once a week versus every 3 weeks in patients with advanced ovarian cancer (MITO-7): a randomised, multicentre, open-label, phase 3 trial. *Lancet Oncol.* 2014;15(4): 396-405. PMID: 24582486. (Pignata et al. 2014)

TRIAL SPONSORS

- MITO-7 (Multicentre Italian Trials in Ovarian Cancer)
- ENGOT-OV-10 (European Network of Gynaecological Oncological Trial Groups)
- GCIG (Gynecologic Cancer InterGroup) Trial

RATIONALE FOR TRIAL

- Standard paclitaxel-carboplatin chemotherapy every 3 weeks is toxic and causes alopecia, neurotoxicity, and fatigue.
- Weekly paclitaxel may reduce toxicity by decreasing the peak concentrations and increase efficacy by reducing tumor regrowth and providing an antiangiogenic effect.
- Weekly paclitaxel in patients with recurrent ovarian cancer resulted in fewer hematologic and neurologic side effects.

- This trial sought to investigate whether weekly carboplatin and paclitaxel is more effective than the every 3-week regimen.

PATIENT POPULATION
- N = 822.
- Recruited from 67 institutions in Italy and France from November 2008 to March 2012.
- Women older than 18 years.
- Stage IC to IV epithelial ovarian, fallopian tube, or peritoneal cancer.
- ECOG performance status 0 to 2.
- Life expectancy of at least 3 months.
- Adequate bone marrow, kidney, and liver function.
- Excluded if clinically relevant heart disease or other contraindication to treatment.
- Randomization after initial surgery and staging.

TREATMENT DETAILS

Arm 1: Standard Regimen Every 21 Days
- Paclitaxel starting dose 175 mg/m^2 infused over 3 hours.
- Carboplatin AUC 6 mg/mL per minute, Calvert formula, creatinine clearance estimated by Cockcroft-Gault formula.
- Hematologic parameters to treat were more restrictive than in the weekly treatment with WBC >3000//µL, ANC >1500/µL, platelets >100,000/µL.
- Dose reduction of all drugs by 20% if ANC <500/µL or platelets <50,000/µL for 7 days or longer.
- Dose reduction by 25% for grade 2 neuropathy.
- Treatment discontinuation for prolonged toxic effects causing treatment delay of 2 weeks or longer.

Arm 2: Weekly Regimen
- Paclitaxel 60 mg/m^2 infused over 1 hour weekly for 18 weeks.
- Carboplatin AUC 2 mg/mL per minute infused over 30 minutes for 18 weeks.
- Hematologic parameters to treat—WBC >3000/µL, ANC >1000/µL, platelets >75,000/µL.
- Dose reduction of all drugs by 20% if ANC <500/µL or platelets <50,000/µL for 7 days or longer.
- Dose reduction by 25% for grade 2 neuropathy.

- Treatment discontinuation for prolonged toxic effects causing treatment delay of 2 weeks or longer.

Surgery
- Interval debulking surgery was allowed after 3 cycles.

ASSESSMENTS
- Baseline CT or nuclear magnetic resonance (NMR) and CA125.
- Imaging after 3 and 6 cycles of chemotherapy, response assessed by RECIST version 1.0 (French centers did not image after 3 cycles if clinical suspicion of progression was absent).
- Quality of life assessed by FACT-O version 4.
    - FACT-O/TOI (trial outcome index) calculated by adding scores from physical, functional, and ovarian cancer-specific subscales.
- Neurotoxicity assessed by FACT/GOG-Ntx.
- Adverse events graded according to CTCAE version 3.0.

ENDPOINTS
- Quality of life, measured by FACT-O/TOI score (primary endpoint).
- PFS (co-primary endpoint). In 2010, PFS was added as co-primary endpoint after publication of the JGOG NOVEL trial showed 11-month prolongation of PFS.
- Overall survival.
- Toxic effects.
- Proportion of patients who achieved an objective response (complete or partial response).

STATISTICAL CONSIDERATIONS

Sample Size
- Sample size of 350 patients calculated to find a difference between arms in FACT-O/TOI changes between baseline and 9 weeks of 0.30 with α of 0.05 and power of 80%.
- Sample size adjusted to 810 patients to detect a 0.75 hazard ratio of progression (median PFS from 18 to 24 months) with α of 0.05 and an interim analysis of efficacy after half of events had occurred.

CONCLUSION OF TRIAL
- Weekly carboplatin and paclitaxel.
    - Does not improve progression-free survival.

Table 2.23 Results of MITO-7

Treatment arm	Every 3 weeks N=404	Weekly N=406	Statistics
Patient characteristics			
Median age (range)	59 (29-83)	60 (23-87)	
No residual	41%	41%	
≤1 cm residual	12%	12%	
>1 cm residual	23%	23%	
No surgery	25%	24%	
Stage IC	6%	8%	
Stage II	8%	8%	
Stage III	63%	58%	
Stage IV	23%	27%	
Serous	72%	67%	
Endometrioid	8%	12%	
Clear cell	6%	5%	
Mucinous	2%	2%	
Other	12%	14%	
Grade 3	71%	66%	
Treatment delivery			
Interval debulking	20%	17%	
Received all treatment	90%	83%	
Stopped for toxicity	4%	8%	
At least 1 delay	62%	79%	
Dose reduction	36%	19%	
Carboplatin dose intensity	82.7%	76.6%	
Paclitaxel dose intensity	86.8%	79.1%	
Efficacy			
PFS (95% CI)	17.3 months (15.2-20.2)	18.3 months (16.8-20.9)	HR 0.96, P=NS
24-month survival	78.9%	77.3%	HR 1.20, P=NS
Objective response rate	58.8%	56.2%	
Toxicity			
FACT-O/TOI	QOL scores declined after every chemotherapy cycle	QOL scores declined after week 1, then stabilized	
Deaths	N=3	N=5	
Worse with q 3 weeks			
G3-4 neutropenia	50%	42%	
Febrile neutropenia	3%	0.5%	
≥G2 neuropathy	17%	6%	
≥G2 hair loss	59%	29%	
Worse with weekly			
≥G2 pulmonary	3%	5%	

CI, confidence interval; FACT-O/TOI, Functional Assessment of Cancer Therapy—Ovarian/Trial Outcome Index; HR, hazard ratio; NS, not significant; PFS, progression-free survival; QOL, quality of life.

- Better toxicity profile and better quality of life.
  - Less adherence to treatment schedule, challenging regimen.
- Carboplatin and paclitaxel every 3 weeks.
  - More frequent and severe hematologic toxicity, vomiting, neuropathy, hair loss.

COMMENTS

- Differences between NOVEL and MITO-7 every 3-week treatment arms.
- Frequency and severity of toxicities were higher in NOVEL trial.
  - G3-4 neutropenia—88% vs 50%.
  - Thrombocytopenia—38% vs 7%.
  - Anemia—44% vs 8%.
- Suggests possible genetic reasons for drug sensitivity.
- Similar PFS for q 3-week treatment arm across studies, but PFS differed in the weekly regimens.
- Dose of weekly paclitaxel was 80 mg/m^2 in NOVEL compared to 60 mg/m^2 in MITO-7. Dose density may be needed to improve outcomes.
- Carboplatin every 3 weeks may be more efficacious than carboplatin every week; weekly carboplatin may antagonize the effects of paclitaxel.

CHAPTER 3

Advanced Stage Epithelial Ovarian Cancer

Timing of Surgery and Interval Cytoreduction

Two trials have addressed the utility of a second attempt at surgical cytoreduction (following 3 rounds of chemotherapy) when the first attempt leaves a residual disease burden of greater than 1 cm (suboptimal cytoreduction). The EORTC-GCG 55865 trial demonstrated a survival advantage to second cytoreduction while the GOG 152 trial showed no benefit. Because the residual disease burden was higher among patients in the EORTC trial, these seemingly contradictory results have been reconciled with the caveat that patients who had a maximal first cytoreduction attempt (ie, GOG 152 patient population) are those who would not benefit from a second surgery. The EORTC 55971 and CHORUS trials suggest that there is no difference between primary cytoreduction (followed by 6 cycles of chemotherapy) and neoadjuvant chemotherapy (3 cycles) and interval cytoreduction (followed by 3 cycles of chemotherapy). Both of these trials were conducted in patients with a high baseline tumor burden.

EORTC-GCG 55865 (van der Burg, NEJM 1995)

REFERENCE

- van der Burg ME, et al. The effect of debulking surgery after induction chemotherapy on the prognosis in advanced epithelial ovarian cancer. Gynecological Cancer Cooperative Group of the European Organization for Research and Treatment of Cancer. *N Engl J Med.* 1995;332(10):629-634. PMID: 7845426. (van der Burg et al. 1995)

TRIAL SPONSOR

- Gynecological Cancer Cooperative Group of the European Organization for Research and Treatment of Cancer (EORTC)

RATIONALE FOR TRIAL

- Reasons for cytoreductive surgery in ovarian cancer.
  - Large tumors have poor central blood supply.
  - Areas with slow growth rate are relatively insensitive to cytotoxic therapy (Skipper 1974).
  - Smaller tumors are better perfused and have a higher growth rate and chemotherapy more effectively diffuses into the tumors.
  - Removal of large tumors also reduces the likelihood of drug-resistant clones developing (Goldie and Coldman 1979).
  - Smaller tumors require fewer cycles of chemotherapy, which also reduces the probability of drug resistance developing.
- The value of cytoreductive surgery on survival is controversial.
  - Nonrandomized studies demonstrate that patients with optimal cytoreduction have better survival than patients left with larger residual lesions (Vogl et al. 1983; Omura et al. 1989; Neijt et al. 1991). These studies are subject to bias as patients with difference surgical outcomes also have different baseline prognostic factors.
  - Other studies have demonstrated that among patients with optimal cytoreduction, those with large masses before cytoreduction still have worse survival than patients with small lesions prior to surgery (Hacker et al. 1983; Hoskins et al. 1992).
  - It is not settled whether cytoreduction influences survival among patients with the same-size tumors.
- It is not clear whether debulking surgery after induction chemotherapy influences survival.
  - While some studies report similar survival among patients with induction chemotherapy and optimal cytoreduction and patients with optimal primary cytoreduction (Neijt et al. 1984; Wils et al. 1986; Jacob et al. 1991; Potter et al. 1991), other studies report inferior survival for those patients undergoing induction chemotherapy (Neijt et al. 1987; Neijt et al. 1991) that is closer to the survival of patients undergoing suboptimal cytoreduction.

- The EORTC initiated a randomized phase 3 trial in 1987 to assess the influence of debulking surgery after induction chemotherapy on survival in ovarian cancer.

PATIENT POPULATION

- N=425, 391 underwent randomization.
- Patients enrolled from March 1987 to May 1993.
- Biopsy-proven epithelial ovarian cancer, International Federation of Gynecology and Obstetrics (FIGO) stage IIB to IV, with residual lesions >1 cm after cytoreductive surgery that occurred no more than 6 weeks before treatment began.
- Performance status of 0 to 2.
- Age less than 75 years.
- Adequate bone marrow and renal function.

TREATMENT DETAILS

- After randomization, all patients received 3 cycles of chemotherapy.
  - Cyclophosphamide 750 mg/m^2.
  - Cisplatin 75 mg/m^2.
  - Treatment every 3 weeks.
- After the third cycle, patients underwent clinical assessment.
  - Patients with progression or contraindication to surgery were removed from the study.
  - Patients with clinical response or stable disease were randomized to undergo interval debulking or no debulking.

Arm 1: No Debulking Surgery
Arm 2: Debulking Surgery

- Surgery scheduled within 28 days of the third cycle of chemotherapy.
- Maximal cytoreduction to include (if not previously done) hysterectomy, bilateral salpingo-oophorectomy, and infracolic omentectomy.

Additional Chemotherapy

- Resumed within 4 weeks of surgery.
- At least 6 total cycles of cyclophosphamide and cisplatin.
- Decision to continue beyond 6 cycles was at the discretion of the center.
- Patients with a complete clinical response preferably had a "second-look" operation, regardless of randomization arm.

ASSESSMENTS

- Clinical response assessed according to World Health Organization (WHO) response criteria.
  - Complete response was the absence of tumor at surgery.
- Clinical evaluation with physical exam, imaging (computed tomography [CT] scan or sonography or both), and cancer antigen 125 (CA125) was performed after the third and sixth cycles of chemotherapy.
- After therapy, patients were seen every 2 months for 2 years, then indefinitely thereafter per each center's policy.

ENDPOINTS

- Overall survival (OS) calculated from the day chemotherapy was started to death, regardless of cause.
- Progression-free survival (PFS) was calculated from the day chemotherapy was started until the time of progression or death.

STATISTICAL CONSIDERATIONS

Stratification Factors

- Patients were stratified with a minimization technique to account for institution, performance status, and clinical response.

Sample Size

- Accrual target of 440 patients to have 80% probability of detecting a 30% reduction in the risk of death using a 2-tailed log-rank test at an α of 0.05 (George and Desu 1974).
- Interim analyses were performed yearly per EORTC policy (Buyse 1993).
- A difference in survival was seen in September 1991, October 1992, February 1993, and April 1993. At this time, the group decided to stop enrolling patients.

Statistical Tests

- Kaplan-Meier estimates used to calculate survival and progression-free survival.
- Log-rank test used to compare survival across treatment groups.
- Cox regression analyses and stratified analyses were used to adjust treatment comparisons for known prognostic factors (Cox 1972).

Table 3.1 Results of EORTC-GCG 55865

Treatment arm	No debulking surgery N=138	Debulking surgery N=140	Statistics
Patient characteristics			
Median age (range)	Not stated	Not stated	59 (32-74) whole group
Largest baseline tumor			
1-2 cm	4%	6%	
2-5 cm	20%	25%	
5-10 cm	24%	20%	
>10 cm	32%	28%	
Unknown, >2 cm	20%	21%	
Stage IIB	4%	6%	
Stage III	75%	71%	
Stage IV	21%	23%	
Serous	56%	59%	
Endometrioid	10%	7%	
Mucinous	4%	8%	
Clear cell	4%	1%	
Other	26%	25%	
Ovary in situ	31%	29%	
Carcinomatosis	43%	46%	
Ascites	72%	78%	
Response after 3 cycles			
Complete response	17%	18%	
Partial response	55%	54%	
Stable disease	28%	28%	
Treatment delivery			
No interval debulking	100%		
Interval debulking		93%	
No residual		38%	
Optimal <1 cm		26%	
Suboptimal ≥1 cm		36%	
Six cycles of chemotherapy	84%	84%	
Stop chemotherapy early for			
Progression	3%	5%	
Toxicity	2%	3%	
Refusal to continue	5%	4%	
Unknown	6%	4%	
Dose reduction	37%	36%	
Dose delay	49%	48%	

Table 3.1 Results of EORTC-GCG 55865 *(continued)*

Treatment arm	No debulking surgery N=138	Debulking surgery N=140	Statistics
Median time cycle 1 to 6	17.5 weeks	21 weeks	
Consolidation chemotherapy	51%	36%	
Second-look surgery	51%	52%	
Efficacy			
Clinical response	70%	84%	
Second look			
Complete response	33%	37%	
Partial response	37%	28%	
Stable disease	6%	2%	
Progression	6%	8%	
Median OS	20 months	26 months	HR 0.69, $P=.01$
Median PFS	13 months	18 months	$P=.01$
Toxicity			
Bowel injury		3%	
Bladder injury		2%	
EBL >500 mL		22%	
Fever		4%	
Ileus		1%	
Urinary tract infection		4%	
Wound infection		2%	
Deep venous thrombosis		1%	
Lung embolism		2%	

EBL, estimated blood loss; HR, hazard ratio; NS, not significant; PFS, progression-free survival; OS, overall survival.

CONCLUSION OF TRIAL

- Interval debulking surgery after induction chemotherapy significantly lengthened progression-free and overall survival.

COMMENTS

- The beneficial effect of surgery on survival was seen throughout the follow-up period.
- The survival benefit was greatest when excluding patients with stage IV disease.

- Survival was comparable between patients with suboptimal interval cytoreduction and patients who did not undergo debulking surgery. Either patients with suboptimal cytoreduction did not benefit from surgery or patients who did not undergo surgery might have benefited from surgery.
- In multivariate analysis, all subgroups benefited from debulking surgery.
- There were no severe morbidities or deaths associated with interval debulking surgery. Therefore, the 6-month improvement in overall survival outweighs the risks of surgery in this trial.

GOG 152 (Rose, NEJM 2004)

REFERENCE

- Rose PG, et al. Secondary surgical cytoreduction for advanced ovarian carcinoma. *N Engl J Med*. 2004;351(24):2489-2497. PMID: 15590951. (Rose et al. 2004)

TRIAL SPONSOR

- Gynecologic Oncology Group (GOG)

RATIONALE FOR TRIAL

- The EORTC trial demonstrated an improvement in progression-free survival and overall survival in patients who underwent suboptimal primary debulking followed by secondary surgery after 3 cycles of induction chemotherapy (van der Burg et al. 1995).
- This trial was designed to determine whether secondary cytoreductive surgery influences survival among patients with suboptimal primary cytoreduction and treatment with cisplatin and paclitaxel.

PATIENT POPULATION

- N = 550 enrolled, 424 randomized.
- Enrollment between June 1994 and January 2001.

Inclusion Criteria

- Stage III or IV ovarian cancer with residual tumor >1 cm after a maximum effort.
- In March 1996, patients with stage IV disease (malignant pleural effusion or resected anterior abdominal wall tumor) were made ineligible

based on the report from the EORTC trial of greatest benefit when stage IV patients were excluded (van der Burg et al. 1995).
- GOG performance status of 0 to 2.
- Life expectancy of at least 8 weeks.
- Lab requirements.
  - Leukocyte count >3000/mm^3.
  - Platelet count >100,000/mm^3.
  - Granulocyte count >1500/mm^3.
  - Serum creatinine <2.0 mg/dL.
  - Bilirubin <1.5 times upper limit of normal.
  - Serum aspartate aminotransferase (AST), alanine aminotransferase (ALT), and alkaline phosphatase <3 times upper limit of normal.

Exclusion Criteria
- Prior cancer, chemotherapy, or radiotherapy.
- Low malignant potential tumors.
- Nonepithelial cancers.
- Active infection.
- Hepatitis.
- Gastrointestinal bleeding.
- History of congestive heart failure, myocardial infarction, unstable angina, or abnormal cardiac conduction within the preceding 6 months.

TREATMENT DETAILS

Chemotherapy
- Chemotherapy with paclitaxel and cisplatin, consistent with prior GOG protocols (McGuire et al. 1996; Muggia et al. 2000; Ozols et al. 2003).
- Paclitaxel 130 mg/m^2 intravenous (IV) over 24 hours.
- Cisplatin 75 mg/m^2 IV.
- Premedications to avoid paclitaxel hypersensitivity reactions and antiemetics administered.
- Administered every 21 days for total of 6 cycles.
- Dose modifications.
  - Paclitaxel—reduced to 110 mg/m^2 for neutropenic fever, grade 4 thrombocytopenia, or grade 3 to 4 mucositis or diarrhea. In April 1997, to be consistent with other GOG protocols, paclitaxel also reduced for grade 4 neutropenia, and granulocyte colony-stimulating factor was to be administered for recurrent episodes. Reduced to 90 mg/m^2 for persistent grade 3 to 4 adverse events.

- Cisplatin—reduced to 50 mg/m^2 for grade 2 neuropathy, tinnitus, or symptomatic hearing loss. Discontinued for grade 3 to 4 neuropathy or persistent elevation in serum creatinine above 2.0 mg/dL.
- Patients were removed from study for treatment delay of more than 2 weeks.

Randomization
- After 3 cycles of chemotherapy (patients with no progression and no extraperitoneal tumor >1 cm).

Arm 1
- No surgery.

Arm 2
- Secondary surgical cytoreduction was performed as soon as possible after hematologic recovery and within 6 weeks of completion of third cycle of chemotherapy through laparotomy with maximal effort to resect all gross tumor.
- Additional chemotherapy was administered as soon as possible but no more than 6 weeks after secondary surgery.

ASSESSMENTS
- Pretreatment.
  - History, physical examination, determination of race and performance status, electrocardiography, complete blood count, renal and liver function tests, urinalysis, imaging (CT scan of the abdomen and pelvis, chest radiography), CA125 levels.
- Three weeks after third cycle of chemotherapy.
  - Evaluation for response with physical examination and CT of abdomen and pelvis (unless CT findings were normal at study entry and CA125 had returned to normal). Patients without progression and with residual extraperitoneal tumor no more than 1 cm in diameter were randomized.
- Toxicity graded according to GOG Common Toxicity Criteria and summarized as the maximal reported grade.

Reassessments
- Six to 9 weeks after completing protocol therapy: history, physical exam, evaluation of GOG performance status, complete blood count, electrolytes, renal and liver function tests, CT of abdomen and pelvis, chest radiography, CA125.

- Every 3 months for 2 years, semiannually for 3 years, yearly thereafter.

ENDPOINTS

- Planned analysis was log-rank test stratified according to the clinical response after 3 cycles of chemotherapy.
- PFS and OS assessed to compare results to the EORTC study.
  - Progression defined as clinically evident increase in disease or CA125 ≥100 U/mL, confirmed by retesting 2 weeks later (or a doubling of the nadir CA125 levels in a patient whose CA125 values did not normalize).
  - Survival measured from date of randomization.

STATISTICAL CONSIDERATIONS

Stratification Factors

- Within each parent institution, patients were stratified by response to first 3 cycles of chemotherapy and by measurable disease at study entry.

Sample Size

- Enrollment of at least 400 patients. A 29% reduction in death rate with secondary cytoreduction was considered clinically significant. This is equivalent to an 11% increase in the proportion of patients who survival more than the expected median of 2.8 years. Assuming proportional hazards, the study would have an 81% chance of detecting this treatment effect (hazard ratio [HR], 1.40) with a 1-sided type I error of .05.
- An interim analysis scheduled to be performed after 60 deaths reported in the chemotherapy-alone arm.
- Final analysis scheduled to occur after at least 225 deaths reported.

Statistical Tests

- *P* values reported in publication are 2-sided.

CONCLUSION OF TRIAL

- In this trial, in patients with suboptimal cytoreduction after a maximal effort at primary surgery, chemotherapy plus secondary surgery does not improve survival compared to chemotherapy alone. This is in contrast to previously reported findings from EORTC, which found secondary cytoreduction to improve survival.

Table 3.2 Results of GOG 152

Treatment arm	Chemotherapy alone N=208	Secondary surgery N=216	Statistics
Patient characteristics			
Median age (range)	57 (27-81)	58 (24-81)	
Measurable disease	70%	70%	
Residual tumor			
1-2 cm	12%	12%	
2-5 cm	44%	43%	
5-10 cm	38%	33%	
>10 cm	6%	12%	
Stage III	96%	93%	
Stage IV	4%	7%	
Serous	76%	76%	
Endometrioid	5%	8%	
Mucinous	1%	<1%	
Clear cell	1%	2%	
Other	16%	13%	
Grade 1	10%	9%	
Grade 2	39%	39%	
Grade 3 or clear cell	50%	52%	
Treatment delivery			
No interval debulking	97%		
Interval debulking		93%	
Optimal <1 cm		70%	
Suboptimal ≥1 cm		30%	
Six cycles of chemotherapy	98%	93%	
Median time cycle 3 to 4	21 days	45 days	$P<.001$
Consolidation chemotherapy	12%	10%	
Efficacy			
Median OS	33.7 months	33.9 months	HR 0.99 (95% CI, 0.79-1.24)
Median PFS	10.7 months	10.5 months	HR 1.07 (95% CI, 0.87-1.31)
Toxicity			
≥G2 neuropathy	26%	16%	$P=.01$
G3-4 gastrointestinal	4%	7%	
G4 pulmonary event	N=0	N=2	
G4 cardiovascular event	N=1	N=3	

CI, confidence interval; G, grade; HR, hazard ratio; PFS, progression-free survival; OS, overall survival.

COMMENTS
- There was no effect of secondary surgery on overall survival in different subgroups based on maximal residual tumor after initial cytoreduction, age, performance status, or presence of absence of measurable disease before chemotherapy.
- Factors associated with survival.
  - Tumor diameter >1 cm before primary surgery. HR, 1.71 (95% confidence interval [CI], 1.21-2.42, $P = .003$).
- Factors not associated with survival.
  - Suboptimal secondary cytoreduction. HR 1.25 (95% CI, 0.79-2.00; $P = .34$).
- Patients undergoing secondary cytoreduction had a longer delay between cycles 3 and 4 of chemotherapy as well as a lower rate of grade 2 or higher peripheral neuropathy, suggesting the respite may have lessened the neurologic adverse effects.
- Differences between GOG and EORTC studies.
  - Amount of residual tumor was less in GOG compared to EORTC, suggesting a greater effort at primary cytoreduction in the GOG trial. Tumor <5 cm was achieved after primary surgery in about 55% in GOG compared to about 28% in EORTC.
  - GOG study used the more efficacious combination of paclitaxel and cisplatin, whereas EORTC used cyclophosphamide and cisplatin.
  - The frequency and timing of clinical evaluations may have influenced differences in survival (Eisenhauer et al. 1997).
- There are hurdles to evaluating surgical interventions (Reynolds 1999).
  - Differences in surgical aggressiveness are difficult to quantify.
  - Significance of number or tumor deposits and the definition of optimal residual disease are controversial.
  - There is a high degree of interobserver variability with tumor measurements (Prefontaine et al. 1994).
- Patients who undergo initial cytoreduction by a nongynecologic oncologist (ie, a general surgeon or an obstetrician-gynecologist) might benefit from a secondary cytoreduction.
- The utility of neoadjuvant chemotherapy is being investigated, but the value is uncertain as survival among patients who have a complete response to chemotherapy is shorter for those who begin with bulky disease (Rubin et al. 1999).

EORTC 55971 (Vergote, NEJM 2010)

REFERENCE

- Vergote I, et al. Neoadjuvant chemotherapy or primary surgery in stage IIIC or IV ovarian cancer. *N Engl J Med*. 2010;363(10):943-953. PMID: 20818904. (Vergote et al. 2010)

TRIAL SPONSORS

- EORTC–Gynaecological Cancer Group (EORTC-GCG)
- National Cancer Institute of Canada (NCIC) Clinical Trials Group

RATIONALE FOR TRIAL

- Primary cytoreduction surgery is considered standard of care for advanced ovarian cancer despite a lack of evidence from randomized, controlled trials to support this practice.
- A meta-analysis of 835 patients suggested that neoadjuvant chemotherapy was associated with worse outcome than primary cytoreduction (Bristow and Chi 2006).
- This was a randomized controlled trial to assess the outcomes of primary debulking surgery followed by platinum-based chemotherapy compared to platinum-based neoadjuvant chemotherapy with interval cytoreduction in patients with advanced ovarian cancer.

PATIENT POPULATION

- N = 718 enrolled.
- Patients enrolled between September 1998 and December 2006.
- Biopsy-proven stage IIIC or IV invasive epithelial ovarian cancer, fallopian tube cancer, or primary peritoneal cancer.
- If biopsy was not available, a fine-needle aspiration was acceptable under the following conditions: presence of a pelvic mass, presence of metastases outside the pelvis of at least 2 cm (noted during surgery or on CT scan), regional lymph node metastases or proof of stage IV disease, and ratio of CA125/carcinoembryonic antigen (CEA) >25.
    - If CA125/CEA <25, then results of a barium enema or colonoscopy, gastroscopy or radiologic examination of the stomach, and mammogram had to be negative for primary tumor.
- If biopsy was performed during laparoscopy or laparotomy, no further procedures could have been performed during surgery.
- WHO performance status of 0 to 2.

- Absence of serious disabling diseases that would be contraindications to therapy.
- No CT or laparoscopic scoring systems were used to select patients.

TREATMENT DETAILS

Arm 1
- Primary debulking + at least 6 cycles of platinum-based chemotherapy.
  - Interval debulking surgery was permitted if stable disease or response documented. However, after GOG 152 was published (Rose et al. 2004), interval debulking was not recommended in patients who did not have optimal cytoreduction despite a maximal surgical effort at the time of primary debulking.

Arm 2
- Three cycles of neoadjuvant platinum-based chemotherapy + interval debulking + chemotherapy.

Chemotherapy Details
- Recommended regimen was paclitaxel 175 mg/m^2 IV over 3 hours followed by carboplatin area under the curve (AUC) 6 IV over 1 hour.
- Other allowed regimens include cisplatin 75 mg/m^2 IV or carboplatin AUC 5.

ASSESSMENTS
- Imaging (preferable CT scan) was performed prior to each surgical procedure, within 1 week prior to cycle 1 of chemotherapy, and in the third week of chemotherapy cycles 3 and 6.
- Tumor response evaluated by WHO criteria (Miller et al. 1981).
- EORTC quality-of-life questionnaire (QLQ)–C30 and QLQ-Ov28 questionnaires at 5 time points.
- Second-look surgery was allowed but not recommended.

ENDPOINTS
- Overall survival (primary endpoint).
- Progression-free survival.
- Quality of life.
- Adverse events were considered postoperative if they occurred within 28 days of surgery.

STATISTICAL CONSIDERATIONS

Stratification Factors
- Patients stratified by institution, method of biopsy (image-guided laparoscopy, laparotomy, or fine-needle aspiration), tumor stage (IIIC or IV), and largest preoperative tumor size excluding ovaries (≤5 cm, 5-10 cm, 10-20 cm, >20 cm).

Sample Size
- Based on a prior EORTC trial evaluating interval debulking surgery, patients with suboptimal primary debulking and interval debulking surgery had an expected survival of 26 months (van der Burg et al. 1995). Patients with optimal debulking to residual <1 cm had a median survival of 36 months (Vergote et al. 1998). The median survival of the whole group was estimated to be 31 months. In total, 498 events in 704 patients were required to show noninferiority with an α of 0.05, power of 80%, and accrual time of 4 years and a minimum follow-up period of 3 years. A hazard ratio of <1.25 was considered noninferior.

Statistical Tests
- Kaplan-Meier method to estimate OS and PFS.
- Log-rank test to compare survivals with a noninferiority ratio of 0.8.
- Cox proportional hazards model for multivariate time-to-event analysis with univariate screening followed by a stepwise variable-selection procedure.
- Log-rank test for trend used to compare adverse events between treatment groups.
- Because of an allegation of ethical irregularities at one of the centers, all patients from that center were excluded from the analysis.

CONCLUSION OF TRIAL
- Survival was similar between upfront debulking followed by adjuvant chemotherapy and neoadjuvant chemotherapy with interval debulking surgery. No advantages were seen for either approach with respect to survival, adverse effects, quality of life, or postoperative morbidity or mortality.

COMMENTS
- This was a population with bulky baseline disease with 61.6% with metastatic lesions >10 cm and 74.5% with lesions >5 cm, which may partially account for the poor survival outcomes in the trial.

Table 3.3 Results of EORTC 55971

Treatment arm	Primary debulking N=336	Neoadjuvant chemotherapy N=334	Statistics
Patient characteristics			
Median age (range)	62 (25-86)	63 (33-81)	
Largest baseline tumor			
0-2 cm	1.2%	3.0%	
2-5 cm	26.8%	25.4%	
5-10 cm	26.8%	26.3%	
>10 cm	39.0%	41.0%	
Stage IIIC	76.5%	75.7%	
Stage IV	22.9%	24.3%	
Serous	65.5%	58.1%	
Endometrioid	3.3%	1.5%	
Mucinous	2.4%	3.3%	
Clear cell	1.8%	1.2%	
Other	27.1%	35.9%	
Method of biopsy			
Laparotomy	3.6%	3.6%	
Laparoscopy	31.0%	34.7%	
Image guidance	22.6%	15.9%	
Fine-needle aspiration	42.3%	45.8%	
Missing data	0.6%	0	
Type of chemotherapy			
Platinum-taxane	78.4%	87.9%	
Platinum only	8.1%	6.2%	
Other	6.8%	5.9%	
No chemotherapy	6.8%	0	
Residual tumor			
None	19.4%	51.2%	
≤1 cm	22.2%	29.5%	
1-2 cm	11.7%	5.8%	
>2 cm	41.3%	11.9%	
Missing	5.4%	1.7%	
Efficacy			
Median OS	29 months	30 months	HR 0.98 (95% CI, 0.84-1.13)
Median PFS	12 months	12 months	HR 1.01 (95% CI, 0.89-1.15)
Toxicity			
Postoperative death	2.5%	0.7%	
G3/4 hemorrhage	7.4%	4.1%	
Infection	8.1%	1.7%	
Venous complications	2.6%	0%	

CI, confidence interval; HR, hazard ratio; PFS, progression-free survival; OS, overall survival.

- Optimal debulking rates (to <1 cm residual) was 41.6% for patients undergoing upfront debulking surgery and 80.6% for patients undergoing neoadjuvant chemotherapy and interval debulking surgery. These rates are similar to other trials evaluating surgery for stage IIIC and IV ovarian cancers (O'Malley et al. 2003; Crawford et al. 2005; Heintz et al. 2006; Schrag et al. 2006; Vernooij et al. 2008; du Bois et al. 2009; Marth et al. 2009).
- There was no trend in favor of primary debulking surgery, even in countries with high rates of optimal primary debulking surgery. This may be due to the strong correlation between rates of optimal primary debulking and rates of optimal interval debulking within each country ($r = 0.92$).
- The most frequent sites of residual tumor after both types of surgery were the diaphragm, abdominal peritoneum, and pelvis (pouch of Douglas, uterus, bladder, rectum, and sigmoid).
- In patients with baseline tumors <5 cm, overall survival was slightly better with primary surgery than neoadjuvant chemotherapy (HR, 0.64; 95% CI, 0.45-0.93).
- In descending order, the strongest predictors for improved overall survival in Cox regression analyses were absence of residual tumor after surgery ($P < .0001$), stage IIIC disease ($P = .001$), small tumor size at baseline ($P = .001$), and histology (endometrioid, serous, mixed, undifferentiated, mucinous, clear cell) ($P = .005$).
- Complete resection of all macroscopic disease is the single most important prognostic factor for ovarian cancer survival. This has been shown in many prior studies and was confirmed in this EORTC trial.
- A possible limitation of neoadjuvant chemotherapy may be the resulting fibrosis, which may hinder complete resection of macroscopic disease.
- This trial only evaluates patients with stage IIIC and IV disease. The standard of care for stage IIIB and earlier stage ovarian cancer is still primary cytoreductive surgery.

CHORUS (Kehoe, Lancet 2015)

REFERENCE

- Kehoe S, et al. Primary chemotherapy versus primary surgery for newly diagnosed advanced ovarian cancer (CHORUS): an open-label, randomised, controlled, non-inferiority trial. *Lancet.* 2015;386(9990):249-57. PMID: 26002111. (Kehoe et al. 2015)

TRIAL SPONSORS

- UK Medical Research Council Clinical Trials Unit (MRC CTU) Gynaecological Cancer Trial Steering Committee

RATIONALE FOR TRIAL

- Primary cytoreduction followed by platinum-based chemotherapy is the international standard of care for advanced ovarian cancer.
- Observational studies consistently report better survival with smaller residual tumor after cytoreduction (Griffiths 1975; van der Burg et al. 1995; Bristow et al. 2002; Winter et al. 2007; Winter et al. 2008; du Bois et al. 2009; Polterauer et al. 2012), but no randomized trials exist. Even in specialty centers, many women will be left with suboptimal bulky residual tumor after surgery.
- An alternative treatment strategy is to use primary chemotherapy followed by delayed surgery. Observational studies suggest that this strategy increases rates of optimal cytoreduction and reduces surgical complications (Vergote et al. 1998; Hou et al. 2007), but data are conflicting, with 2 meta-analyses demonstrating conflicting results (Bristow and Chi 2006; Kang and Nam 2009).
- The CHORUS trial was designed to evaluate primary chemotherapy and delayed surgery with the hypothesis that survival outcomes would be similar and that surgical morbidity would be reduced compared to a primary surgery approach.

PATIENT POPULATION

- N=552 randomized, 550 included in analysis.
- Enrollment between March 2004 and August 2010.
- Women with clinical or imaging evidence of a pelvic mass with metastases consistent with stage III or IV ovarian, fallopian tube, or peritoneal cancer (Benedet et al. 2000).
  - If CA125/CEA ratio was <25, gastrointestinal primary needed to be ruled out prior to study entry.
  - Histological or cytological diagnosis was not required before randomization.

TREATMENT DETAILS

Arm 1
- Primary debulking surgery followed by 6 cycles of chemotherapy.
  ○ After randomization, histological or cytological confirmation of diagnosis was required through laparoscopic or imaging-guided biopsy or fine-needle aspiration of tumor or effusion.
  ○ In women with more than 1 cm residual disease after primary surgery, interval debulking surgery was allowed after 3 cycles of chemotherapy.

Arm 2
- Primary chemotherapy × 3 cycles, delayed debulking surgery, 3 cycles of chemotherapy.

Chemotherapy Details
- Regimen was decided before random assignment and based on patient fitness, choice, and usual local practice.
  ○ Carboplatin AUC 5 or AUC 6 with paclitaxel 175 mg/m^2 every 3 weeks.
  ○ Alternative carboplatin combination regimen.
  ○ Carboplatin AUC 5 or AUC monotherapy.
- Chemotherapy was started within 6 weeks after surgery in both treatment groups.

Surgery Details
- Done in 64 centers by specialist gynecological oncologists accredited by the Royal College of Obstetricians and Gynaecologists (RCOG).
- All surgeons operate on at least 15 patients with ovarian cancer each year.
- Intent of surgery was tumor debulking to no macroscopic residual disease.

Surgical Procedures
- Recommended procedures included midline incision; cytology; thorough inspection of abdomen, pelvis, upper abdomen, diaphragm, and retroperitoneal spaces; hysterectomy; bilateral salpingo-oophorectomy; and omentectomy.
- If FIGO stage IIIB or less, then pelvic and para-aortic nodes were to be sampled.

- Ultra-radical procedures included multiple resections of small or large bowel, diaphragm stripping, splenectomy, partial cystectomy, and complete pelvic or para-aortic lymphadenectomy. These procedures were recommended if they would assist with the goal of optimal debulking.
- The volume of disease was assessed and recorded by the surgeon at the start and end of the operation. Disease volume was recorded as the largest diameter of disease in 13 areas: diaphragm, liver surface, paracolic gutters, omentum, intestines, peritoneal surface, pelvis, adnexa, pelvic and para-aortic lymph nodes, spleen, and liver.

ASSESSMENTS

At Screening
- Clinical assessment, imaging (CT or magnetic resonance imaging [MRI]) of abdomen and pelvis, chest radiograph), CA125 and CEA measurements.

During Chemotherapy
- At each cycle, assessments included clinical review and measurement of CA125.

After Protocol Treatment
- Clinical review and CA125 every month for 9 months, then every 3 months for 2 years, every 6 months for 3 years, then annually until death, withdrawal from study, or study completion.

Imaging
- Done after 3 cycles of chemotherapy and after completion of therapy.
- During follow-up, imaging was triggered by clinical symptoms or a rise in CA125 concentrations.

Disease Progression
- Defined according to WHO criteria.
- During follow-up, progression could also be defined by a rise in CA125 concentrations according to GCIG criteria (Vergote et al. 2000).

Quality of Life
- EORTC Quality of Life Questionnaire Core–36 (QLQC-30) and the ovarian cancer-specific questionnaire (QLQ-Ov28) (Fayers 2001) were completed before randomization, after 3 and 6 cycles of chemotherapy, and at 6 and 12 months after treatment assignment.

Adverse Events
- Graded according to the National Cancer Instituted Common Terminology Criteria for Adverse Events (CTCAE) version 3.0 at each chemotherapy cycle and after.

ENDPOINTS
- Overall survival (primary endpoint).
  - OS was defined as time from randomization until death. Data were censored at the time survivors were last known to be alive.
- PFS.
  - PFS was defined as time of randomization until the date of first progression or death, whichever occurred first. For patients without progression or death, data were censored at the time of last visit.
  - Analysis included only progression events that were confirmed radiologically or clinically.
  - A secondary analysis was performed that also included progression events based on CA125 elevation without clinical or radiologic confirmation.
- Quality of life.

STATISTICAL CONSIDERATIONS

Stratification Factors
- Patients were stratified according to center, largest radiological tumor size, FIGO stage, and prespecified chemotherapy regimen.

Sample Size
- Sample size calculation was based on noninferiority.
- Three-year survival rate was estimated at 50% for primary surgery.
- The noninferiority boundary was selected to exclude a detriment of more than 6% with primary chemotherapy with a 10% (1-sided) level of significance.
- The upper bound of the 1-sided 90% CI for the hazard ratio had to be less than 1.18.
- CHORUS was designed with the intention of combining results with the EORTC 55971 trial (Vergote et al. 2010) in a later meta-analysis. The combined sample size was calculated to give a total of 1250 women in the 2 trials with 90% power. CHORUS had 65% power for comparison between the 2 treatment groups.

- The predefined trigger for analysis was when the final enrolled patient had completed 2 years of follow-up.

Statistical Tests

- Stratified log-rank test used to compare treatment groups, adjust for variables used to stratify the random assignments.
- Cox proportional hazards models were used to calculate hazard ratios adjusting for stratification factors.
- Proportional hazards assumptions were assessed with the Grambsch-Therneau test (Grambsch and Therneau 1994).
- Analysis of covariance was used to assess global quality of life at 6 and 12 months with adjustment for baseline scores. Only cases with complete information were included in the analysis. For comparisons of mean scores between treatment groups, a difference of 10 points was considered clinically meaningful. For comparisons of mean scores between individuals, a difference of 5 points was considered meaningful (Osoba et al. 1998).

CONCLUSION OF TRIAL

- Primary chemotherapy is noninferior to primary surgery in patients with advanced stage III and IV ovarian cancer with high tumor burden.

COMMENTS

- There were no subgroups that benefited more or less from primary chemotherapy.
- Debulking to <1 cm residual disease was achieved in 41% with primary surgery and 73% with primary chemotherapy ($P = .001$). Debulking to no macroscopic residual was achieved in 17% with primary surgery and 39% with primary chemotherapy ($P = .001$).
- Volume of residual disease was prognostic in both groups (data are in appendix of paper).
- Quality of life was slightly higher for patients receiving primary chemotherapy than patients receiving primary surgery at 6 at 12 months. Improvement of global quality of life of at least 5 points was higher in patients receiving primary chemotherapy at 6 and 12 months, but the differences were not significant.
- The median survival of 22 to 24 months was lower than expected. Some potential explanations:
  ◦ Older median age of patients (65 years).

Table 3.4 Results of CHORUS

Treatment arm	Primary surgery N=276	Primary chemotherapy N=274	Statistics
Patient characteristics			
Median age (range)	66 (26-87)	65 (34-88)	
Median tumor size			
0-2 cm	5%	5%	
2-5 cm	21%	22%	
5-10 cm	40%	40%	
10-20 cm	29%	29%	
>20 cm	3%	3%	
Unmeasurable	3%	2%	
Stage III	75%	75%	
Stage IV	25%	25%	
Serous, high grade	74%	71%	
Serous, low grade	4%	4%	
Serous, not specified	10%	12%	
Endometrioid	4%	2%	
Mucinous	1%	2%	
Clear cell	2%	6%	
Other	5%	1%	
Well differentiated	6%	6%	
Moderately differentiated	19%	14%	
Poorly differentiated	75%	79%	
Type of chemotherapy			
Carboplatin-paclitaxel	75%	77%	
Other carboplatin combo	1%	<1%	
Carboplatin only	24%	23%	
Residual tumor			
None	18%	39%	
≤1 cm	24%	34%	
>1 cm	58%	27%	
Treatment delivery			
Started as allocated	91%	92%	
Received postoperative chemotherapy	77%		
Received delayed surgery		79%	
Median duration of treatment	22 weeks	22 weeks	
Median operative time	120 minutes	120 minutes	
Received 6 cycles of chemotherapy	82%	79%	
Chemotherapy delays	37%	28%	
Carboplatin dose modification	38%	39%	
Taxol dose modification	26%	28%	

Table 3.4 Results of CHORUS *(continued)*

Treatment arm	Primary surgery N=276	Primary chemotherapy N=274	Statistics
Efficacy			
Median OS	22.6 months	24.1 months	HR 0.87, NS
Median PFS	10.7 months	12.0 months	HR 0.91, NS
Toxicity			
Surgical			
G3/4 adverse events	24%	14%	$P=.007$
G3/4 hemorrhage	3%	6%	
Postoperative deaths	6%	<1%	$P=.001$
Hospitalization <14 days	80%	93%	$P<.001$
Chemotherapy			
G3/4 toxicity	49%	40%	$P=.06$
G3/4 neutropenia	20%	16%	

G, grade; HR, hazard ratio; NS, not significant; PFS, progression-free survival; OS, overall survival.

- ○ 77% of tumors were poorly differentiated.
- ○ 19% of patients had performance status of 2 or 3.
- There have been no randomized trials that compare standard to ultraradical surgery (Ang et al. 2011). It is not known whether patients in this trial would have benefited from more aggressive attempts at debulking surgery.
- Postoperative mortality, delayed discharge after surgery, and grade 3/4 surgical morbidities were all higher in the group undergoing primary surgery.
- Based on ICON3 (International Collaborative Ovarian Neoplasm Group 2002), the addition of paclitaxel is not considered mandatory in upfront chemotherapy, and 23% to 24% of patients in this trial received single-agent carboplatin.

CHAPTER 4

Epithelial Ovarian Cancer

Maintenance Therapy

Maintenance therapy is the use of additional chemotherapy, biologic therapy, or other treatment approaches after a patient has achieved remission with the goal of prolonging remission and delaying recurrence. Many different agents have been studied and have not demonstrated a benefit. This chapter is by no means comprehensive but rather highlights 2 phase III trials conducted by the GOG. The GOG 178/SWOG 9701 study compared 3 vs 12 cycles of maintenance paclitaxel in patients with advanced ovarian cancer and found a progression-free survival advantage with 12 cycles. GOG 175 included patients with early-stage ovarian cancer who received 3 cycles of paclitaxel and carboplatin chemotherapy and demonstrated no advantage to the administration of 24 weekly cycles of low-dose paclitaxel maintenance therapy compared to observation. In both trials, there was greater toxicity with the longer administration of paclitaxel.

GOG 178/SWOG 9701 (Markman, JCO 2003)

REFERENCE

- Markman M, et al. Phase III randomized trial of 12 vs 3 months of maintenance paclitaxel in patients with advanced ovarian cancer after complete response to platinum and paclitaxel-based chemotherapy: a Southwest Oncology Group and Gynecologic Oncology Group trial. *J Clin Oncol*. 2003;21(13):2460-2465. PMID: 12829663. (Markman et al. 2003a)

TRIAL SPONSORS

- Southwest Oncology Group (SWOG)
- Gynecologic Oncology Group (GOG)

RATIONALE FOR TRIAL

- Initial therapy for ovarian cancer is 5 to 6 courses of platinum/taxane (McGuire et al. 1996; Piccart et al. 2000).
- There are limited randomized trial data to support the use of additional consolidation chemotherapy in ovarian cancer (Hakes et al. 1992; Bertelsen et al. 1993; Lambert et al. 1997) or other malignancies (Einhorn et al. 1989, Polychemotherapy for early breast cancer... 1998).
- Randomized experience suggests possible utility for prolonged treatment with paclitaxel in ovarian cancer (Einzig et al. 1992; Markman et al. 1996; Zanotti et al. 2000).
- This trial hypothesized that more prolonged treatment with paclitaxel in patients who responded to front-line therapy that included paclitaxel would benefit from both time to disease progression and overall survival.

PATIENT POPULATION

- N=277 entered trial.
- Accrual from 1997 until September 2001.
- Histologically confirmed stage III/IV epithelial ovarian cancer, fallopian tube cancer, or primary peritoneal cancer.
- Treatment with 5 to 6 cycles of platinum/paclitaxel with clinical complete response, defined as no cancer-related symptoms, normal physical examination, normal computed tomography (CT) scan of the abdomen/pelvis, normal chest x-ray, and cancer antigen 125 (CA125) level ≤35 U/mL.
- Optimal or suboptimal residual disease. Suboptimal was defined as residual disease ≥1 cm in diameter after exploratory laparotomy.
- Ineligible.
    - Prior treatment on a SWOG or GOG front-line regimen where trial endpoint was progression-free survival (PFS) or overall survival (OS).
    - Grade 2 or higher persistent neuropathy from prior therapy.

TREATMENT DETAILS

Treatment Arms
- Arm 1: paclitaxel 175 mg/m^2 over 3 hours every 28 days for 3 cycles.
- Arm 2: paclitaxel 175 mg/m^2 over 3 hours every 28 days for 12 cycles.

Taxol Dose Reduction
- Dose reduction to 135 mg/m^2 for
  - Grade 4 neutropenia.
  - Grade 3 or 4 thrombocytopenia.
  - Grade 2 neuropathy.

Taxol Dose Reescalation
- Not permitted.

Supportive Measures
- Prophylactic granulocyte colony-stimulating factor for recurrent grade 4 neutropenia in subsequent cycles.

Parameters to Treat
- Recovery from all toxicities to grade 1 or less.

Treatment Delay
- Maximum delay for toxicity was 2 weeks.

Treatment Discontinuation
- Persistent grade 4 neutropenia despite dose reduction and prophylactic granulocyte colony-stimulating factor use.
- Grade 3 or higher neuropathy.

Trial Modification
- In March 2001, more patients were electing to discontinue treatment on the 12-cycle arm (n = 10) compared to the 3-cycle arm (n = 3) due to the development of grade 2 and grade 3 peripheral neuropathy.
- Because the aim was to evaluate total treatment duration rather than the total dose administered, the paclitaxel dose was reduced to 135 mg/m^2 for both arms.
- First-level dose reduction for toxicity was to 100 mg/m^2.

ASSESSMENTS

- All patients were followed monthly for 1 year.
  - History, physical exam, toxicity evaluation, complete blood cell count with differential, and serum CA125 were obtained at each visit.

- After 1 year, patients were followed at regular intervals until death.
- Disease recurrence was defined as appearance of a new lesion or effusion, reappearance of any lesion that had disappeared, or development of tumor-related symptoms.

ENDPOINTS

- PFS (measured from date of registration to date of first recurrence or death) (primary endpoint).
- OS (measured from date of registration until date of death).

STATISTICAL CONSIDERATIONS

Stratification Factors

- Prior treatment with paclitaxel for ≥24 hours vs <24 hours.
- Optimal stage III vs suboptimal stage III vs stage IV.
- Age ≤65 years vs age >65 years.

Sample Size

- Sample size estimation was based on PFS. The median PFS after a clinical complete response to induction therapy for the control arm was estimated to be 16 months for stage IV or suboptimal stage III disease and 24 months for patients with optimal stage III disease (Alberts et al. 1996; McGuire et al. 1996; Muggia et al. 2000).
- Assuming equal numbers of patients in the 2 strata, 450 patients needed to be entered in the trial over 5 years. With uniform accrual, 2 additional years' follow-up, exponential survival distribution, and a 1-sided log-rank test at a .05 significance level, there was approximately 85% power to detect a hazard ratio (HR) of 1.33 in PFS.
- With 225 patients per arm, the power to detect an absolute 15% difference in the incidence rate of any toxicity is at least 93% using a 1-sided .05 test.

Interim Analysis

- Interim analysis was planned to guard against extreme findings of either excessive toxicity or a substantial improvement in efficacy. These were planned for when:
  ◦ 225 eligible patients were entered.
  ◦ When 50% and 75% of the estimated events had been observed.

Early Termination

- The decision for early termination was to be made by the SWOG Data and Safety Monitoring Committee. Evidence for early termination of the study included:

Table 4.1 Results of GOG 178/SWOG 9701

Treatment arm	Paclitaxel 3 cycles N = 128	Paclitaxel 12 cycles N = 134	Statistics
Patient characteristics			
Median age	58.5 years	58 years	
Optimal, stage III	66%	66%	
Suboptimal stage III	20%	20%	
Stage IV	14%	14%	
Prior paclitaxel ≥24 hours	14%	13%	
Prior paclitaxel <24 hours	86%	87%	
Histology	Not stated	Not stated	
Treatment delivery	Not stated	Not stated	
Efficacy (interim analysis at 50% enrollment)			
Median PFS	21 months	28 months	HR 2.31 (95% CI, 1.08-4.94)
Median OS (immature)			
Toxicity			
Grade 4 neutropenia	10%	4%	
Grade 2 neuropathy	14%	18%	
Grade 3 neuropathy	1%	5%	

CI, confidence interval; HR, hazard ratio; PFS, progression-free survival; OS, overall survival.

- The null hypothesis of no difference in PFS.
- The alternative hypothesis (that the progression hazard ratio of the control arm over the prolonged paclitaxel arm is 1.33 or greater) was rejected at the .005 level.

CONCLUSION OF TRIAL

- Twelve additional cycles of paclitaxel maintenance chemotherapy (135 mg/m^2) after complete response to platinum/paclitaxel chemotherapy prolongs the duration of progression-free survival in patients with advanced ovarian cancer.

COMMENTS

- Because of the early closure of this study, all patients in this report initiated treatment at the 175-mg/m^2 dose level, but the protocol dose was reduced to 135 mg/m^2 for excessive toxicity at the initial dose.

- The only major difference between the 2 arms for toxicity was neuropathy. The trial did not prospectively evaluate the duration of therapy. Information is not available regarding symptom duration after discontinuation of therapy.
- The interim analysis at 50% enrollment was performed in September 2001, when 54 PFS had occurred among 222 patients. The SWOG Data Safety and Monitoring Committee recommended study closure in October 2001 based on a PFS advantage of 28 months vs 21 months for 12 cycles vs 3 cycles of paclitaxel maintenance therapy.
- Data from this trial suggest that there is a higher hazard for disease progression after treatment is stopped.
  - The hazard ratio for progression posttreatment vs during treatment was 5.80 (95% confidence interval [CI], 2.09-16.10).
  - The hazard ratio for progression posttreatment vs during treatment when analyzed for the 12-cycle arm only was 9.17 (95% CI, 2.47-34.0).
  - These data were generated in an exploratory analysis adding a treatment-stop indicator to the Cox model, which also included treatment and stratification factors. The value of the treatment-stop indicator is time dependent and starts at 0 and changes to 1 at 28 days after treatment is stopped. Patients with disease progression during therapy have a value of 0 for this indicator throughout.
- The authors discuss 4 points raised by this trial.
- First, why did the control arm receive 3 cycles of therapy rather than no further treatment?
  - This control arm was chosen over concern that patients would not agree to participate in a trial where one arm received no further therapy. Patients being recruited to the trial would be told:
  - Approximately 75% of women in this clinical situation would recur (McGuire et al. 1996; Muggia et al. 2000; Piccart et al. 2000).
  - If disease recurs, there is no evidence that any second-line regimen has the potential to provide cure.
  - Paclitaxel is a part of the regimen that has led to a complete clinical response and was tolerated (otherwise, they would not be a candidate for the trial).
  - There is evidence that paclitaxel can be given safely for extended periods (Markman et al. 1996).
  - Extending the duration of paclitaxel administration could expose tumor during active cycling (Rowinsky and Donehower 1995) or provide an antiangiogenic effect with continued intermittent drug exposure (Browder et al. 2000).

- There was further concern that a patient might choose not to participate in the trial and would instead ask her oncologist to administer maintenance paclitaxel as the drug was commercially available at the time of trial initiation.
- Next, was it appropriate to consider PFS as the primary endpoint rather than OS?
  - The investigators designing this trial considered prolongation of PFS without impairment in overall quality of life would be a highly clinically relevant goal, especially in a disease like ovarian cancer, where multiple second-line therapies affect overall survival independent of initial treatment (Gordon et al. 2001). Quality of life was not formally assessed in this trial. The authors note that the rate of neurotoxicity observed in this trial is within what is generally considered to be acceptable in clinical practice (Rowinsky and Donehower 1995; McGuire et al. 1996; Neijt et al. 2000). Using a lower dose of paclitaxel in future studies and in clinical practice would make the issue of neuropathy an even lesser concern. The authors also speculate that the duration rather than the dose of paclitaxel resulted in the beneficial impact of treatment, and reducing the dose of paclitaxel may result in further enhancement of the therapeutic ratio (no change in efficacy and reduced toxicity). However, the current trial offers no data on either the efficacy or toxicity of any regimen starting at a lower dose level than 175 mg/m^2.
- Next, why did the SWOG Data and Safety Monitoring Committee close this study prematurely, considering the negative impact this would have on determining an overall survival effect?
  - The committee is a federally mandated review panel whose purpose is to independently evaluate the results of ongoing studies and to determine whether a trial should be discontinued for excessive toxicity or for extremely favorable or unfavorable results (Smith et al. 1997). Based on the improvement in PFS with 12 months of paclitaxel therapy, the study was closed to allow patients randomized to 3 months of treatment to consider receiving additional courses of therapy.
- Finally, what are the implications of the exploratory analysis that suggests there is an acceleration of recurrence risk shortly after completing maintenance therapy?
  - The authors suggest that this effect was not due to the inevitable risk of recurrence with the passage of time or from the early discontinu-

ation of therapy (from toxicity or refusal) in patients with unrecognized symptoms of early disease progression. This leads the authors to speculate that even longer maintenance therapy (2 or 3 years) may have an even greater impact. The treatment effect could be due to the persistent chemosensitivity of slowly dividing tumor cells to a cycle-specific agent or due to an antiangiogenic effect of intermittent drug exposure (Rowinsky and Donehower 1995; Browder et al. 2000). However, this approach would have to be balanced against the impacts of neurotoxicity, continued alopecia, and risk of secondary malignancy (eg, secondary acute leukemia) (Greene et al. 1982).
- Has the standard of care been changed based on these trial results?
  - No. This trial provides no evidence of a favorable impact on overall survival. Entry into the trial required a complete clinical response following first-line chemotherapy and no significant preexisting peripheral neuropathy, which limits the generalizability of these trial results to the general advanced ovarian cancer population. The decision of whether to use maintenance paclitaxel should balance the favorable impact on progression-free survival with the risk of treatment-related toxicity.

GOG 175 (Mannel, Gynecol Oncol 2011)

REFERENCE

- Mannel RS, et al. A randomized phase III trial of IV carboplatin and paclitaxel × 3 courses followed by observation versus weekly maintenance low-dose paclitaxel in patients with early-stage ovarian carcinoma: a Gynecologic Oncology Group Study. *Gynecol Oncol.* 2011;122(1):89-94. PMID: 21529904. (Mannel et al. 2011)

TRIAL SPONSOR

- Gynecologic Oncology Group (GOG)

RATIONALE FOR TRIAL

- Consensus on the treatment of low-risk early-stage ovarian cancer.
  - Patients with fully staged IA or IB disease with grade 1 or 2 non–clear cell histology have greater than 90% survival with surgery alone (Young et al. 1990).
- Consensus on treatment of high-risk early-stage ovarian cancer.

- Patients with stage IA or IB and unfavorable histology including grade 3 and clear cell, stage IC, or stage II disease have a recurrence risk of 25% to 45% with adjuvant therapy (Young et al. 1990; Vergote et al. 1992; Bolis et al. 1995; Trimbos et al. 2003a, 2003b; Young et al. 2003; Bell et al. 2006).
- The 2004 Gynecologic Cancer Intergroup (GCIG) Ovarian Cancer Consensus Conference recommended that these patients receive at least 3 cycles of carboplatin chemotherapy (du Bois et al. 2005b).
- The Gynecologic Oncology Group (GOG) chose carboplatin and paclitaxel as the standard arm based on data from advanced disease, which demonstrates the superiority of cisplatin/paclitaxel over cisplatin/cyclophosphamide and the therapeutic equivalence of carboplatin to cisplatin (McGuire et al. 1996; Ozols et al. 2003; Bell et al. 2006).
- GOG 157 compared 3 vs 6 cycles of carboplatin area under the curve (AUC) 6 and paclitaxel 175 mg/m^2 every 3 weeks in the high-risk early-stage ovarian cancer population. There was no significant difference in recurrence-free or overall survival, and grade 3 and 4 neurotoxicity increased from 2% to 11% with the increased courses of chemotherapy. This led the GOG to recommend 3 cycles of chemotherapy as the standard arm.
• In patients with advanced ovarian cancer, GOG 178/SWOG 9701 demonstrated a significant increase in progression-free survival for patients receiving 12 cycles of monthly maintenance paclitaxel 175 mg/m^2 compared to 3 cycles after complete remission (Markman et al. 2003a). There was no difference in overall survival, possibly due to crossover effect since the control arm received 3 cycles of maintenance therapy.
• Rationale for using a frequent low dose of paclitaxel as a maintenance therapy approach.
  - Lower dose paclitaxel exerts an antiangiogenic effect in mouse models (Klauber et al. 1997). Extrapolation from mouse dosing and phase I trials suggests that paclitaxel 40 mg/m^2 weekly may have an equivalent effect in humans.
  - Katsumata et al. (2009) reported a survival benefit to weekly paclitaxel dosing in advanced ovarian cancer therapy.
• GOG 175 was designed to evaluate the impact of maintenance paclitaxel dosed at 40 mg/m^2 weekly for 24 weeks in patients with high-risk early-stage ovarian cancer.
  - Lower weekly dose could exert an antiangiogenic effect.

- Total monthly dose of 160 mg/m^2 is almost 20% higher than the tolerable monthly dose of 135 mg/m^2 in GOG 178/SWOG 9701.

PATIENT POPULATION

- N = 571 enrolled.
- Enrollment from September 1998 to December 2006.
- Epithelial ovarian cancer.
  - Allowable histologies: serous, mucinous, endometrioid, clear cell, transitional cell, mixed epithelial, Brenner, and undifferentiated carcinoma.
- Completely resected early-stage high-risk ovarian cancer.
  - Stage IA or IB grade 3 or clear cell subtype, any stage IC, or any stage II.
  - Definitive surgical staging by GOG guidelines—included total abdominal hysterectomy, bilateral salpingo-oophorectomy, resection of all gross disease, infracolic omentectomy, selective pelvic and para-aortic lymph node dissection, peritoneal biopsies from the pelvis and bilateral paracolic gutters, biopsy or cytology from the right diaphragm, and aspiration of free fluid or abdominal washing for cytology.
  - Entry into the trial within 6 weeks for staging surgery.
- Adequate bone marrow, renal, and liver function.
- Ineligible.
  - Borderline tumors.
  - Another invasive malignancy in the past 5 years.
  - GOG performance status of 4 or more.

TREATMENT DETAILS

- All patients received 3 cycles of paclitaxel 175 mg/m^2 intravenous (IV) over 3 hours and carboplatin AUC 6 IV every 21 days, then:

Treatment Arms
- Arm 1: Observation.
- Arm 2: Paclitaxel 40 mg/m^2 over 1 hour weekly for 24 weeks.

Carboplatin Dosing
- Calvert formula for AUC calculations.
- Creatinine clearance calculated using the method of Jelliffe.
- Dose of carboplatin was recalculated for each cycle.

Paclitaxel Dosing
- Maximum body surface area (BSA) or 2.0.
- Standard pretreatment regimen with dexamethasone, diphenhydramine, and cimetidine.
- Monthly pretreatment complete blood count (CBC) and physical exam prior to each monthly maintenance cycle.

Treatment Modifications
- Applied in a sequential manner using delay, dose reduction, and addition of granulocyte colony stimulating factor (G-CSF).
- Minimum counts for treatment: absolute neutrophil count (ANC) $\geq$1500 cells/mm^3 and platelets $\geq$100,000 cells/mm^3.
- No dose modifications for uncomplicated nadirs.
- Dose reduction for grade 4 thrombocytopenia, febrile neutropenia, delay >2 weeks.
- G-CSF used for recurrent delays or neutropenic precautions after appropriate dose reductions.

ASSESSMENTS
- Weekly blood counts.
- Physical exam prior to each of the initial 3 cycles.
- After completion of chemotherapy, patients were evaluated quarterly for 2 years, semi-annually for 3 years, then annually thereafter.
  - Recurrence defined as any clinical or radiographic evidence of new tumor.
  - CA125 elevation alone was not considered enough evidence for recurrence.

ENDPOINTS
- Recurrence rate (primary endpoint).
- Time to recurrence.
- Overall survival.

STATISTICAL CONSIDERATIONS

Sample Size
- Study was designed to provide 85% chance of detecting a true 50% decrease in the recurrence rate with a type I error of .05 for a 1-tail test (Schoenfeld 1981). The expected effect size is an increase in the 5-year recurrence-free proportion from 77% to 88%. The study provided

guidelines to compensate for possible early withdrawal of patients and loss of statistical power.

Interim Analysis
- An interim analysis was scheduled when at least 30 recurrences were reported among the control group (3 cycles of carboplatin and paclitaxel) to assess for either extreme differences or futility.

Statistical Tests
- Log-rank test was used to assess the study hypothesis that recurrence rates would be equivalent (Mantel 1966).
- Data were locked in January 2010.

CONCLUSION OF TRIAL
- The addition of 24 weeks of weekly paclitaxel at 40 mg/m^2 to 3 cycles of carboplatin and paclitaxel does not improve outcomes in patients with high-risk early-stage epithelial ovarian cancer but does lead to a significant increase in toxicity (neuropathy, infection, dermatologic events, and possibly cardiovascular events).

COMMENTS
- Five-year survival by stage.
  ◦ Stage I: 88.8%.
  ◦ Stage II: 78.9%.
- Attrition was approximately 1% per week during maintenance paclitaxel therapy, with 79% of patients completing the entire 24 weeks of additional treatment.
- The 5-year recurrence-free survival of this trial falls within the expected and previously reported ranges.
  ◦ 75% to 80% with adjuvant melphalan, intraperitoneal phosphorous-32, cisplatin, carboplatin, and cisplatin plus cyclophosphamide (Young et al. 1990; Vergote et al. 1992; Bolis et al. 1995; Trimbos et al. 2003a, 2003b; Young et al. 2003).
  ◦ 74.6% with 3 cycles of adjuvant carboplatin and paclitaxel in GOG 157 (Bell et al. 2006).
  ◦ 79.9% with 6 cycles of adjuvant carboplatin and paclitaxel in GOG 157 (Bell et al. 2006).
  ◦ 76.8% with 3 cycles of adjuvant CT and observation in this trial.
  ◦ 80.0% with 3 cycles of adjuvant CT and 24 weeks of maintenance Taxol in this trial.

Table 4.2 Results of GOG 175

Treatment arm	CT × 3 cycles N = 268	CT × 3 cycles, T × 24 weeks N = 274	Statistics
Patient characteristics			
Median age	56.0	55.1	
Stage I	72.8%	70.8%	
Stage II	27.2%	29.2%	
Serous	29.1%	26.6%	
Endometrioid	20.5%	20.8%	
Mucinous	6.7%	4.7%	
Clear cell	30.6%	32.1%	
Other	13.1%	15.7%	
Grade 1	14.2%	10.2%	
Grade 2	25.7%	21.9%	
Grade 3	29.5%	35.8%	
Clear cell (no grade)	30.6%	32.1%	
Treatment delivery			
Completed 3 cycles CT	97%	96%	
Completed 12 weeks T	NA	86%	
Completed 24 weeks T	NA	79%	
Reason for discontinuation			
Progression	0%	2.2%	
Patient refusal	1.5%	9.5%	
Toxicity	0.8%	6.9%	
Other reason	0.8%	1.8%	
Efficacy			
5-year recurrence rate	23.2%	20.4%	HR 0.81 (95% CI, 0.57-1.15)
5-year survival	85.4%	86.2%	HR 0.78 (95% CI, 0.52-1.17)
Toxicity			
Worse with maintenance			
≥G2 neuropathy	6.0%	15.5%	$P < .001$
G3/4 peripheral neuropathy	0.7%	4.4%	$P = .012$
≥G2 infection, fever	8.7%	19.9%	$P < .001$
≥G2 dermatologic events	52.1%	70.8%	$P < .001$
≥G2 cardiovascular events	3.8%	8.1%	$P = .04$
Secondary cancer	N = 11	N = 10	

CI, confidence interval; CT, carboplatin+paclitaxel HR, hazard ratio; NA, not applicable T, paclitaxel.

- An exploratory analysis of GOG 157 suggested that patients with serous histology had significantly reduced risk of recurrence with 6 vs 3 cycles of adjuvant CT (HR, 0.33; 95% CI, 0.14-0.77) (Chan et al. 2010). Benefit was not seen in the serous subtype in this study comparing maintenance weekly paclitaxel to observation (HR, 0.82; 95% CI, 0.44-1.54).
- The lack of benefit demonstrated in this trial could be attributed to histology.
    ◦ The patient population in this trial is not representative of a population that might be predicted to benefit from extended paclitaxel treatment. The preponderance of clear cell, mucinous, and low-grade tumors in this trial may have affected treatment benefit as these tumors have shown poor response to standard carboplatin and paclitaxel treatment in multiple trials (Takano et al. 2007; Kurman and Shih Ie 2008; Yoshida et al. 2009).

CHAPTER 5

Recurrent Epithelial Ovarian Cancer

Patients with recurrent epithelial ovarian cancer can be treated with a number of different treatment options that are generally selected based on time since last platinum therapy and other patient and treatment regimen characteristics. Patients with platinum-resistant cancer are usually treated with single-agent chemotherapy with paclitaxel, topotecan, pegylated liposomal doxorubicin (PLD) (Topotecan versus Paclitaxel study, Doxil Study 30-49, Gemcitabine versus PLD study), or these selected agents in combination with trabectadin or bevacizumab (OVA-301, AURELIA). Patients with platinum-sensitive cancer are generally treated with multiagent regimens, including platinum+paclitaxel (ICON4/AGO-OVAR2.2), carboplatin+PLD (CALYPSO), or carboplatin+gemcitabine (AGO-OVAR, NCIG CTG, EORTC GCG trial) with or without bevacizumab (OCEANS).

Topotecan Versus Paclitaxel (ten Bokkel, JCO 1997)

REFERENCE

- ten Bokkel Huinick W, et al. Topotecan versus paclitaxel for the treatment of recurrent epithelial ovarian cancer. *J Clin Oncol.* 1997;15(6):2183-2193. PMID: 9196130. (ten Bokkel Huinink et al. 1997)

TRIAL SPONSOR

- Supported by a grant from SmithKline Beecham Pharmaceuticals, Collegeville, PA

RATIONALE FOR TRIAL

- Standard front-line therapy at this time is cyclophosphamide combined with a platinum analogue, but the majority of patients relapse and die of progressive disease (Neijt et al. 1991; Cannistra 1993; Ozols 1994; McGuire et al. 1996).
- In small phase II studies of patients with recurrent disease, second-line agents have yielded response rates ranging from 8% to 26%. Treatment options include:
  - Hexamethylmelamine (Vergote et al. 1992).
  - Ifosfamide (Baker et al. 1993).
  - Etoposide (Baker et al. 1993; Hoskins and Swenerton 1994).
- There is an urgent need to develop new treatment strategies with non-cross-resistant chemotherapy in recurrent ovarian cancer.
- Paclitaxel has been studied in recurrent ovarian cancer.
  - Response rates range from 22% to 37% in small, nonrandomized studies (McGuire et al. 1989; Einzig et al. 1992; Thigpen et al. 1994).
  - In a large, randomized, international study evaluating 2 different doses (175 mg/m^2 vs 135 mg/m^2) and 2 different dosing schedules (3 hours vs 24 hours), responses confirmed by independent review ranged from 14% to 24% (Eisenhauer et al. 1994). At the approved dose of 175 mg/m^2 over 3 hours every 21 days, the response rate was 15%.
  - In the front-line setting, cisplatin and paclitaxel were found to be superior to cisplatin and cyclophosphamide (McGuire et al. 1996; Piccart et al. 2000).
- Topotecan (Hycamtin) has been studied.
  - Water-soluble, semisynthetic analogue of camptothecin, an alkaloid antitumor agent isolated from the *Camptotheca acuminata* tree from South China.
  - Inhibits topoisomerase I, an enzyme that binds to double-stranded DNA and leads to a single-strand break in front of the replication fork and relieves DNA torsion caused by replication.
  - Topotecan and other camptothecin analogues bind to the topoisomerase I–DNA complex and interfere with the process of DNA breakage and resealing. This blocks the progress of the replication fork and results in DNA breaks and cell death (Hertzberg et al. 1989; Hsiang et al. 1989).

- ○ Preclinical data suggest that topotecan could be given intermittently over multiple days (Houghton et al. 1992).
- ○ Three phase I studies concluded the maximum tolerated dose is 1.5 mg/m^2/d on 5 consecutive days in a 21-day cycle without the use of growth factor support. The dose-limiting toxicity was myelosuppression (Rowinsky et al. 1992; Saltz et al. 1993; Verweij et al. 1993).
- ○ Phase II studies demonstrate response rates ranging from 14% to 25% in recurrent ovarian cancer (abstract: Armstrong et al. 1995).
- This was a phase III study designed to compare the efficacy and toxicity of topotecan (1.5 mg/m^2 intravenous [IV] over 30 minutes on 5 consecutive days every 21 days) to paclitaxel (175 mg/m^2 IV over 3 hours every 21 days) in patients with recurrent ovarian cancer who progressed after 1 platinum-based chemotherapy regimen.

PATIENT POPULATION
- N=235 enrolled, 226 included in the intent-to-treat analysis.
- Stage III/IV, histologically confirmed epithelial ovarian carcinoma.
- Failed first-line therapy with a platinum-based chemotherapy regimen.
- Measurable disease—at least 1 bidimensionally measurable lesion on computed tomography (CT) or magnetic resonance imaging (MRI) scan, ultrasound, or physical exam.
- At least 4 weeks from prior surgery, hormonal therapy, radiotherapy or chemotherapy, and initiation of study drug.
- Eastern Cooperative Oncology Group (ECOG) performance status ≤2.
- Adequate bone marrow function: white blood cells (WBC) ≥3500/µL, neutrophil count ≥1000/µL, and platelet count ≥100,000/µL.
- Normal liver function: bilirubin ≤2.0 mg/dL.
- Normal renal function: creatinine level ≤1.5 mg/dL or creatinine clearance >60 mL/min.
- Ineligible:
  - ○ More than 1 prior chemotherapy regimen.
  - ○ Prior topotecan or paclitaxel.

TREATMENT DETAILS

Arm 1: Topotecan
- Premedications: none initially, but antiemetics could be added as indicated.
- Starting dose: 1.5 mg/m^2 IV over 30 minutes for 5 consecutive days every 21 days.

- Dose reduction for toxicity to minimum dose of 1.0 mg/m^2/d.
- Due to the limited experience with topotecan in this population, dose could also be escalated to 2.0 mg/m^2/d.
- Treatment withdrawn for >2-week delay at the minimum dose due to medication or toxicity.

Arm 2: Paclitaxel
- Premedications: dexamethasone, H$_1$ receptor antagonist, H$_2$ receptor antagonist.
- Starting dose: 175 mg/m^2 IV over 3 hours every 21 days.
- Dose reduction for toxicity to minimum dose of 135 mg/m^2.
- Treatment withdrawn for >2-week delay at the minimum dose due to medication or toxicity.

Supportive Measures
- To maintain dose-intensity and a 21-day treatment cycle, prophylactic granulocyte colony-stimulating factor (G-CSF) could be added starting with second cycle of therapy (on day 6 following topotecan or on day 2 following paclitaxel) if the patient experienced any of the following:
  - Grade 4 neutropenia with fever or infection.
  - Grade 4 neutropenia that lasted more than 7 days.
  - Grade 3 neutropenia that required a delay in treatment.

Duration of Treatment Depended on Response
- Patients with a complete response (CR) or partial response (PR) could continue treatment until progression or for 6 months past the maximum response.
- Patients with progression were removed from the study.
- Patients with best response of stable disease after 6 courses could be removed from the study or switched to the alternate regimen.

ASSESSMENTS
- Responses were determined by the World Health Organization (WHO) criteria.
  - All responses required independent review and confirmation by a radiologist blinded to treatment regimen.
  - CR was defined as the complete disappearance of all measurable and assessable disease on 2 separate scans at least 4 weeks apart.
  - PR was defined as a 50% reduction in the sum of products of the perpendicular diameters of all measurable lesions for at least 4 weeks and no new lesions or progression of assessable disease.

- Progressive disease (PD) was defined as a 25% increase in a single measurable lesion, reappearance of measurable disease, worsening of assessable disease, or the development of a new metastatic lesion.
  - Stable disease (SD) was any measurement not fulfilling the criteria for response or progression and lasting at least 8 weeks.
  - Nonassessable disease was defined as nonmeasurable lesions with an elevated cancer antigen (CA125) tumor marker.
- Toxicities measured by the National Cancer Institute (NCI) Common Toxicity Criteria (CTC).

ENDPOINTS

- Response rate.
- Duration of response measured from time of initial documented response to first sign of disease progression.
- Time to progression measured from time of first study drug administration to documented progression or initiation of third-line therapy.
- Time to response measured from time of first study drug administration to initial response.
- Survival measured from time of first study drug administration to death.

STATISTICAL CONSIDERATIONS

Stratification Factors

- Age: <65 or ≥65 years.
- Ascites: present or absent.
- Response to prior platinum-based therapy: resistant, early, interim, or late relapse (van der Burg et al. 1991; Markman et al. 1992).
  - Resistant disease defined as not having response to initial chemotherapy or having an initial PR or CR and then progressing while still on therapy.
  - Early relapse defined as CR or PR and relapse within 3 months.
  - Interim relapse defined as CR or PR and relapse within 3 to 6 months.
  - Late relapse defined as CR or PR and relapse more than 6 months after chemotherapy. This group is recognized as potentially platinum sensitive and responsive to reintroduction of platinum therapy.

Statistical Tests

- Kaplan-Meier estimates were obtained for each efficacy end point and presented in life-table format over 4-week intervals.

Table 5.1 Results of Topotecan Versus Paclitaxel Trials

Treatment arm	Topotecan N=112	Paclitaxel N=114	Statistics
Patient characteristics			
Median age (range)	59.2 (29-85)	58.3 (29-79)	
Relapse <6 months	54%	52%	
Prior chemotherapy			
Cyclophosphamide	66.0%	69.0%	
Carboplatin	55.0%	61.0%	
Cisplatin	54.0%	51.0%	
Epirubicin	8.0%	5.3%	
Doxorubicin	8.1%	9.6%	
Etoposide	1.8%	0.9%	
Other	0%-1.8%	0%-1.8%	
Tumor diameter			
<5 cm	48.2%	46.5%	
≥5 cm	50.0%	51.8%	
Serous	51.8%	51.8%	
Endometrioid	8.9%	13.2%	
Mucinous	5.4%	5.3%	
Undifferentiated	16.1%	7.0%	
Other	17.9%	22.8%	
Grade 1	5.0%	7.0%	
Grade 2	20.5%	25.4%	
Grade 3	50.0%	43.9%	
Grade 4	8.9%	10.5%	
Unknown grade	15.2%	13.2%	
Treatment delivery			
Target dose maintained	90%	98%	
Median dose intensity	2.3 mg/m^2/wk	56.3 mg/m^2/wk	
Treatment on schedule	77%	92%	
Delays beyond 7 days	5%	3%	
Efficacy			
Overall response rate	20.5%	13.2%	NS
CR	4.5%	2.6%	
PR	16.1%	10.5%	
Duration of response	32.1 weeks	19.7 weeks	RR 0.42, NS
Time to progression	23.1 weeks	14.0 weeks	RR 0.58, $P=.002$
Time to response	9 weeks	6 weeks	RR 0.48, $P=.041$
Median OS	61 weeks	43 weeks	RR 1.21, NS

(continued)

Table 5.1 Results of Topotecan Versus Paclitaxel Trials   *(continued)*

Treatment arm	Topotecan N=112	Paclitaxel N=114	Statistics
Toxicity			
Greater with topotecan			
G4 neutropenia	79%	23%	$P<.01$
G4 thrombocytopenia	25%	2%	$P<.01$
G4 anemia	4%	3%	NS
Infection	15%	4%	
Sepsis	5%	2%	
G-CSF prophylaxis	23%	3%	
G-CSF treatment	7%	1%	
Platelet transfusions	3%	0%	
Blood transfusions	27%	4%	
Nausea	63.5%	44.8%	
Vomiting	41.1%	30.8%	
Fever	28.6%	17.7%	
Greater with paclitaxel			
Alopecia	75.9%	93.0%	
Arthralgia	6.4%	31.5%	
Myalgia	3.6%	28.0%	
Neuropathy	0.9%	15.8%	

CR, complete response; G-CSF, granulocyte colony-stimulating factor; NS, not significant; OS, overall survival; PR, partial response; RR, relative risk.

- Cox regression was used to compare time-to-event outcomes.
- A model that included treatment and the 3 stratification covariates was used to compare treatment effects.
- Hazards ratios (HRs) with 95% confidence intervals (CIs) were reported.

CONCLUSION OF TRIAL

- Compared to paclitaxel, topotecan has a higher response rate and longer time to progression in patients with recurrent epithelial ovarian cancer.

COMMENTS

- Choice of paclitaxel as the comparison arm was based on prior studies suggesting response rates of 22% to 37% with paclitaxel in patients who had not responded to first-line platinum (McGuire et al. 1989; Einzig et al. 1992; Thigpen et al. 1994). The regimen of 175 mg/m^2 over 3 hours was chosen due to ease of administration, less toxicity,

and no other regimen with proven greater efficacy (Eisenhauer et al. 1994).
- Topotecan toxicities:
  - 79% had grade 4 neutropenia.
  - 25% had grade 4 thrombocytopenia.
  - Hematologic toxicity was short duration and noncumulative (lack of progressively lower hematologic nadirs on subsequent rounds of therapy).
  - Dose reductions and use of G-CSF resulted in effective prevention of significant clinical sequelae from hematologic toxicities.
  - Only 5.4% had grade 3 diarrhea and no one had grade 4 diarrhea. Incidence of diarrhea is lower with topotecan compared to other topoisomerase I inhibitors.
  - There were no dose-limiting nonhematologic toxicities in this study.
- Topotecan appears to be at least as active as paclitaxel in this paclitaxel-naïve population, but paclitaxel is better tolerated.

Doxil Study 30-49 (Gordon, JCO 2001; Gordon, Gyn Onc 2004)

REFERENCES

- Gordon AN, et al. Recurrent epithelial ovarian carcinoma: a randomized phase III study of pegylated liposomal doxorubicin versus topotecan. *J Clin Oncol.* 2001;19(14):3312-3322. PMID: 11454878. (Gordon et al. 2001)
- Gordon AN, et al. Long-term survival advantage for women treated with pegylated liposomal doxorubicin compared with topotecan in a phase 3 randomized study of recurrent and refractory epithelial ovarian cancer. *Gynecol Oncol.* 2004;95(1):1-8. PMID: 15385103. (Gordon et al. 2004)

TRIAL SPONSOR

- ALZA Corp, Mountain View, CA

RATIONALE FOR TRIAL

- Patients with recurrent ovarian cancer are treated with the goals of palliation and optimization of quality of life as the probability of cure is remote.

- Treatment options that lack cross-resistance to front-line therapies of platinum and paclitaxel (McGuire et al. 1996) are needed for recurrent or refractory disease.
  - Options include topotecan, oral etoposide, and gemcitabine (Shapiro et al. 1996; Bookman et al. 1998; Rose et al. 1998a).
  - At the time of this trial, topotecan is the only approved agent for recurrent ovarian cancer. Topotecan has response rates that range from 13% to 33% depending on platinum sensitivity (Kudelka et al. 1996; Swisher et al. 1997; Bookman et al. 1998; McGuire et al. 2000).
- Pegylated liposomal doxorubicin (PLD).
  - Received Food and Drug Administration (FDA) approval in June 1999 for use on patients with disease refractory to paclitaxel and platinum-based chemotherapy.
  - Encapsulation of doxorubicin in pegylated liposomes decreases the toxicities attributed to high peak levels of doxorubicin (nausea, vomiting, cardiotoxicity) (Gordon et al. 2000), alters the pharmacokinetic profile of doxorubicin, and enhances the therapeutic benefit.
  - Compared to doxorubicin, PLD has a smaller volume of distribution, a larger area under the curve (AUC), slower clearance, and longer elimination half-life of approximately 55 hours (Greene et al. 1983; Eksborg et al. 1986).
  - Pegylated liposomes are small (approximately 100 nm in diameter), which allows them to pass through endothelial gaps and leaky membranes in tumors (Jain 1987; Dvorak et al. 1988).
  - A phase II study using PLD in patients with platinum-resistant and refractory ovarian cancers demonstrated overall response rates of 16.9% and 18.3% in the overall and refractory populations with median times to progression of 19.3 weeks and 17 weeks, respectively. Toxicities included stomatitis, palmar-plantar erythrodysesthesia (PPE), and skin lesions and were easily managed with dosing modifications (Gordon et al. 2000).
- Given the promising results of PLD in phase I/II studies, this trial was performed to compare PLD to topotecan in patients with recurrent epithelial ovarian cancer.

PATIENT POPULATION

- N=481 randomized, 474 at least partially treated.
- Enrollment from May 1997 to March 1999 from 104 sites in the United States and Europe.

Inclusion Criteria
- Age ≥18 years.
- Measurable or measurable and assessable disease.
  - Measurable defined as bidimensionally measurable lesion(s) by plain x-ray with at least 1 diameter ≥0.5 cm or by CT, MRI, or other imaging scan with both diameters ≥2 cm.
  - Assessable diseased defined as unidimensionally measurable lesion(s), mass(es) with margins not clearly defined, lesion(s) with both diameters ≤0.5 cm, lesion(s) with diameter smaller than the distance between cuts, palpable lesion(s) with either diameter ≤2 cm, malignant ascites, or pleural effusion with CA125 ≥100 U/mL in the absence of cirrhosis.
- Recurrence after first-line platinum-based chemotherapy.
- Adequate bone marrow function (platelets ≥100,000/mm^3, hemoglobin ≥9 g/dL, absolute neutrophil count ≥1500 cells/mm^3).
- Adequate renal function (serum creatinine ≤2.5 mg/dL).
- Adequate liver function (aspartate aminotransferase [AST] ≤2 times the upper limit of normal, alkaline phosphatase ≤2 times the upper limit of normal, bilirubin equal to or greater than the upper limit of normal).
- Adequate cardiac function (left ventricular ejection fraction [LVEF] ≥50% or the institutional normal).
- Karnofsky performance status ≥60%.
- Disease-free period of >5 years from prior malignancies (excluding curatively treated basal cell carcinoma, squamous cell carcinoma of the skin, carcinoma in situ of the cervix).

Exclusion Criteria
- Pregnant or breastfeeding.
- Life expectancy of ≤3 months.
- Prior radiation therapy to greater than one-third of hematopoietic sites.
- History of cardiac disease that met the criteria for class 2 or higher by the New York State Heart Association Classification system.
- Uncontrolled systemic infection.
- Receipt of investigational agent within 30 days of first dose of study drug.
- Prior PLD or topotecan therapy.
- Receipt of chemotherapy within 29 days of first dose of study drug (or within 42 days for nitrosurea or mitomycin).
- Concurrent use of investigational or antineoplastic agents during the study.

TREATMENT DETAILS

Arm 1: Pegylated Liposomal Doxorubicin (PLD).
- 50 mg/m^2 IV over 1 hour every 28 days.
- Dose modifications for PPE, hematologic toxicity, elevated bilirubin, or stomatitis (Gordon et al. 2000).
- Dose reduced by 25% for all other grade 3 and 4 events until resolution to grade 2 or lower.
- Prophylactic cytokine administration not recommended during first cycle of drug but allowed in subsequent cycles for any grade 4 neutropenia >7 days or failure of absolute neutrophil count (ANC) to recover within 22 days or febrile neutropenia.
- Treatment continued for up to 1 year in the absence of disease progression or evidence for sustained clinical benefit.
- Patients who completed 6 months of PLD were considered to have completed the protocol.

Arm 2: Topotecan
- 1.5 mg/m^2/d IV over 30 minutes daily on days 1 to 5 every 21 days.
- G-CSF could be administered from day 6 at the discretion of the treating physician for severe neutropenia. Prophylactic cytokine administration not recommended during first cycle of drug but allowed in subsequent cycles for any grade 4 neutropenia >7 days or failure of ANC to recover within 22 days or febrile neutropenia.
- For severe neutropenia during a cycle, dose was reduced by 0.25 mg/m^2 for subsequent courses.
- For moderate renal impairment (creatinine clearance 20-39 mL/min), dose reduction to 0.75 mg/m^2 recommended. No dose adjustment needed for mild renal impairment (creatinine clearance 40-60 mL/min).
- Treatment continued for up to 1 year in the absence of disease progression or evidence for sustained clinical benefit.
- Patients who completed 8 cycles of topotecan were considered to have completed the protocol.

Treatment Discontinuation
- Disease progression.
- Serious or intolerable adverse events precluding further treatment.
- Inability to tolerate study drug despite dose modification.
- LVEF <45% or a 20% decrease from baseline.
- Patient's decision to withdraw from participation.
- Need for radiation treatment.

ASSESSMENTS
- Radiographic imaging (chest x-ray, CT, or MRI) at baseline and every 8 weeks.
- Response based on objective tumor measurements.
  - CR defined as complete disappearance of all measurable and assessable disease, no new lesions, and no disease-related symptoms. CR confirmed at least 4 weeks later by imaging to confirm the response.
  - PR documented in patients with ≥50% decrease in sum of the products of bidimensional perpendicular diameters of all measurable lesions; no progression of assessable disease and no new lesions. PR confirmed at least 4 weeks later by imaging to confirm the response.
  - PD in patients with ≥50% increase in the sum of bidimensionally measured lesions over the smallest sum obtained at best response; reappearance of any lesion that had disappeared; clear worsening of any assessable disease; failure to return for evaluation because of death or deteriorating condition; appearance of any new lesion or site.
  - SD in any patient that did not meet criteria for CR, PR, or PD.
- LVEF by multiple gated acquisition scan or echocardiogram at baseline and 4 weeks after the last dose of study drug for all patients; after every 2 cycles of PLD after cumulative dose >300 mg/m^2.
- Physical examination, chemistries, and CA125 at baseline and before every cycle.
- Complete blood count performed weekly.
- Toxicity assessed by the National Cancer Institute Common Toxicity Criteria (grade 1, mild; grade 2, moderate; grade 3, severe; grade 4, life-threatening).
- Quality of life assessed by the European Organization for Research and Treatment of Cancer (EORTC) Quality of Life Questionnaire (QLQ-C30) (Aaronson et al. 1993) at baseline, during every cycle, and 4 weeks after the last treatment dose.
  - Includes 6 domains (physical functioning, role functioning, cognitive functioning, emotional functional, social functioning, and global quality of life) and 8 symptoms scales (fatigue, pain, nausea/vomiting, dyspnea, insomnia, appetite loss, constipation, diarrhea).
  - Twelve weeks was the first study time point when quality of life (QOL) could be assessed at the same time for the 2 groups. Less than 50% of patients were completing questionnaires by this time point (approximately 100 patients in each arm available for assessment).

The main reasons for discontinuation were disease progression and death.

ENDPOINTS

- Time to progression (primary endpoint).
- Overall survival.
- Response rate.
- Time to response.
- Duration of response.
- Safety and toxicity.

STATISTICAL CONSIDERATIONS

Stratification Factors
- Platinum sensitivity.
- Presence or absence of bulky disease (defined as tumor mass >5 cm).

Sample Size
- In total, 350 patients allowed 80% probability that the 95% 1-sided confidence limit of the hazard ratio of topotecan to PLD would not fall below 0.757 (80% power to demonstrate statistical equivalence between the 2 groups). Based on 2 additional mitigating factors, the trial was designed to enroll 460 patients, depending on the accessibility rate.
- Two interim analyses were planned, requiring enrollment of approximately 5% more patients.
- It was anticipated that 20% of patients might not be assessable for efficacy endpoints.

Statistical Tests
- Cochran-Mantel-Haenszel test used to compare baseline differences for categorical data, adjusting for platinum sensitivity and bulky disease.
- Three-way analysis of variance was used to compare continuous variables with effects for treatment, platinum sensitivity, bulky disease, and all 2-way interactions involving the treatment group.
- Kaplan-Meier method used to estimate PFS and OS rates.
- Stratified log-rank test used to compare survival between treatment arms.
- Cochran-Mantel-Haenszel use to compare response rates, stratified by platinum sensitivity and bulky disease.
- Quality-adjusted time without symptoms and toxicity used to evaluate the impact of treatment on both length and quality of life (Gelber et al. 1995).

Table 5.2 Results of Doxil Study 30-49

Treatment arm	PLD N=239	Topotecan N=235	Statistics
Patient characteristics			
Median age (range)	60 (27-87)	60 (25-85)	
Time from prior chemotherapy, median (range)	7 months (0.9-82.1)	6.7 months (0.5-109.6)	
Initial stage Stage I Stage II Stage III Stage IV	5% 5% 73% 17%	6% 3% 70% 20%	
Histology Grade	Not reported Not reported	Not reported Not reported	
Sum of lesions (cm^3), median (range)	20 (1-441)	20 (1-296)	
Platinum sensitive	46%	47%	
Platinum refractory	54%	53%	
Bulky disease present	46%	47%	
Bulky disease absent	54%	53%	
Prior platinum/taxane	74%	72%	
Treatment delivery			
Total number of dosing cycles	1164	1349	
Cumulative dose, mg/m^2	200 (47-1301)	36 (3-165)	
Mean cycle dose, mg/m^2	50 (34-58)	7 (3-10)	
Mean cycle length, days	30 (27-56)	24 (20-38)	
Efficacy			
2001 publication			
CR+PR	19.7%	17.0%	NS
SD	32.2%	40.4%	NS
Median PFS	16.1 weeks	17.0 weeks	NS
Platinum sensitive	28.9 weeks	23.3 weeks	P=.037
Platinum resistant	9.1 weeks	13.6 weeks	NS
Median OS	60 weeks	56.7 weeks	NS
Platinum sensitive	108.0 weeks	71.1 weeks	P=.008
Platinum resistant	35.6 weeks	41.3 weeks	NS
2004 publication			
Median OS	62.7 weeks	59.7 weeks	HR 1.21 (95% CI, 1.00-1.48)
Platinum sensitive	107.9 weeks	70.1 weeks	HR 1.43 (95% CI, 1.07-1.92)

(continued)

Table 5.2 Results of Doxil Study 30-49 *(continued)*

Treatment arm	PLD N=239	Topotecan N=235	Statistics
Platinum resistant	Not reported	Not reported	HR 1.06 (95% CI, 0.82-1.39)
Toxicity			
Worse with PLD			
Any grade PPE	49%	1%	$P<.001$
Any grade stomatitis	40%	15%	$P<.001$
Worse with topotecan			
G3/4 neutropenia	12%	77%	$P<.001$
G3/4 anemia	5%	28%	$P<.001$
G3/4 thrombocytopenia	1%	34%	$P<.001$
G3/4 leukopenia	10%	50%	$P<.001$
Alopecia	16%	49%	$P=.007$
G-CSF	4.6%	29.1%	
Erythropoietin	6.3%	23.1%	
Blood transfusions	14.9%	57.8%	
Dosing modifications	57.3%	78.3%	
Sepsis	N=0	N=9 (3.8%)	
Treatment-related deaths	N=0	N=3	

CI, confidence interval; CR, complete response; G-CSF, granulocyte colony-stimulating factor; HR, hazard ratio; NS, not significant; OS, overall survival; PFS, progression-free survival; PLD, pegylated liposomal doxorubicin; PPE, palmar-plantar erythrodysesthesia; PR, partial response; SD, stable disease.

CONCLUSION OF TRIAL

- PLD has comparable efficacy, a favorable safety profile, and convenient dosing, which supports its role as a treatment option in patients with recurrent ovarian cancer. Long-term follow-up demonstrates a survival benefit to PLD compared to topotecan, which is most pronounced among patients with platinum-sensitive recurrent disease.

COMMENTS FROM 2001 STUDY

- There was no evidence of a relationship between cumulative PLD dose and change in LVEF.
- Sixty-one patients received cumulative dose >300 mg/m^2 PLD.
  - Three of 61 had ≥20% decrease in LVEF.
  - Three of 61 had postbaseline LVEF <45% (2 started study with LVEF <45%).
  - No patients had clinical signs or symptoms of congestive heart failure.
- Fourteen patients received cumulative dose >450 mg/m^2 PLD.

- At 12 weeks, there were no differences in quality of life between the 2 groups.
- Treatment options for recurrent ovarian cancer are limited and response rates are modest.
- Intravenous chemotherapy.
  - Ifosfamide: 20% (Sutton et al. 1989).
  - Hexamethylmelamine: 14% (Vergote et al. 1992).
  - Oral etoposide: 26% (Hoskins and Swenerton 1994).
  - Gemcitabine: 19% (Lund et al. 1994; Friedlander et al. 1998).
  - Vinorelbine: 20% (Bajetta et al. 1996).
- Intraperitoneal chemotherapy.
- Hormonal therapy.
- Secondary cytoreductive surgery.
- Radiotherapy.
- High-dose chemotherapy with stem cell support.
- In the recurrent setting, combination chemotherapy has not proven to be more effective but is associated with higher toxicity. Median survival times are limited, ranging from 6 to 16 months (Bajetta et al. 1996; ten Bokkel Huinink et al. 1997; Bookman et al. 1998). Palliation and quality of life are important priorities in this setting.
- Overall, PFS and OS were similar between the 2 groups, but in subgroup analysis, PLD was superior to topotecan in PFS and OS among platinum-sensitive patients.
  - Data on subsequent therapies were not collected, but topotecan was commercially available at the time while PLD was not yet approved.
  - PLD was associated with less marrow toxicity and may have allowed more subsequent doses of marrow-toxic drugs.
  - PLD may prevent the development of multidrug resistance (Oudard et al. 1991; Thierry et al. 1992).
- Topotecan administration was associated with more grade 4 hematologic toxicities, including fatal toxicities. Grade 4 neutropenia has been observed in 79% to 94% of patients treated with topotecan in other trials (Swisher et al. 1997; ten Bokkel Huinink et al. 1997; Bookman et al. 1998).
- PLD was generally well tolerated in this trial.
  - The most common treatment-related adverse events were stomatitis and PPE.
  - Only 5.3% of dose modifications were due to stomatitis.

- PPE is a cutaneous reaction typically involving the palms of the hands and soles of the feet.
  - PPE typically begins with a 3- to 5-day period of paresthesias followed by edema and erythema and possibly with severe pain and cracking of the skin.
  - Discontinuation of therapy results in desquamation followed by reepithelialization of the affected areas.
  - PPE can be prevented and managed by early recognition and dose modification (decreasing the dose or lengthening the dosing interval) (Uziely et al. 1995; Lopez et al. 1999; Gordon et al. 2000).
  - Topical dimethyl sulfoxide or pyridoxine have been used to manage PPE (Vail et al. 1998; Lopez et al. 1999), although there is no definitive evidence that pharmacologic therapy is effective.
  - PPE typically develops 1 to 3 weeks after repeated dosing of PLD (Gabizon and Muggia 1997).
  - The long half-life and small liposomes of PLD are theorized to result in accumulation of the drug in the skin (Gabizon and Muggia 1997).
  - The primary approach to preventing PPE includes observation for early signs.
- The tolerability of PLD makes it a good candidate treatment for long-term use.
- The lack of hematologic toxicity makes PLD a candidate for combined treatment with other agents.
- PLD is dosed less frequently than other drugs, which makes it more convenient for administration.
- PLD has a favorable safety profile and overall comparable efficacy, making it a good candidate treatment for patients who have progressed after front-line platinum-containing chemotherapy.

COMMENTS FROM 2004 STUDY

- Comparison of this study to ICON4 (Parmar et al. 2003).
  - In patients with platinum-sensitive disease, median OS was 107.9 weeks with PLD in this study compared to 116 weeks (29 months) with combination platinum/taxane in ICON4.
  - In ICON4, approximately 40% of patients received prior taxane therapy. In this study, 73% of patients received prior taxane.
  - In ICON4, almost 75% of patients had a platinum-free interval of >12 months, compared to 23% of patients in this study. The probability

of response increases with increasing treatment-free intervals (Gore et al. 1990; Markman et al. 1991).
- Results of this analysis as well as the convenience in administration (1-hour infusion every 28 days) and the safety profile suggest that PLD is the treatment of choice among nonplatinum agents for patients with recurrent ovarian cancer, particularly in those with platinum-sensitive disease.

ICON4/AGO-OVAR 2.2 (Parmar, Lancet 2003)

REFERENCE
- Parmar MK, et al. Paclitaxel plus platinum-based chemotherapy versus conventional platinum-based chemotherapy in women with relapsed ovarian cancer: the ICON4/AGO-OVAR-2.2 trial. *Lancet*. 2003;361 (9375):2099-106. PMID: 12826431. (Parmar et al. 2003)

TRIAL SPONSORS
- ICON4 was coordinated by the Instituto Mario Negri, Milan, Italy (IRFMN) and the Medical Research Council's Clinical Trials Unit, London, UK (MRC CTU)
- Arbeitsgemeinschaft Gynaekologische Onkologie Studiengruppe Ovarialkarzinom (AGO-OVAR) 2.2 was coordinated by AGO, Karlsruhe, Germany

RATIONALE FOR TRIAL
- At the time of ovarian cancer relapse, the probability of response to retreatment is based on the platinum-free interval (Markman et al. 1991).
  ○ Patients with platinum-sensitive disease (relapse >6 months from last platinum therapy) would generally be retreated with another platinum agent.
  ○ Patients with platinum-resistant disease (relapse <6 months from last platinum therapy) rarely respond to further platinum therapy and would be treated with an alternative agent such as paclitaxel.
- It is not known whether the addition of paclitaxel to platinum therapy for platinum-sensitive relapse would improve outcomes. Paclitaxel has a different mode of action from platinum drugs. In observational studies, the combination has been reported to have response rates of up to 90% (Rose et al. 1998b; Dizon et al. 2002).

- This trial is a randomized controlled trial to evaluate the efficacy of paclitaxel plus platinum versus platinum alone in patients with platinum-sensitive relapsed ovarian cancer.

PATIENT POPULATION
- N = 802.
- Enrolled between January 1996 and March 2002 from 119 hospitals in 5 countries to 1 of 3 protocols, each of which had slightly different eligibility criteria.
- One trial coordinated by the MRC CTU for hospitals in the United Kingdom, Norway, and Switzerland.
    - Allowed to have more than 1 line of prior chemotherapy, which included platinum plus or minus paclitaxel.
    - Measurable disease was not required.
    - Diagnosis of relapsed disease could be based on CA125 elevation alone.
- One trial coordinated by the IRFMN in Italy.
    - Only 1 prior line of chemotherapy, which was platinum plus or minus paclitaxel.
    - Measurable disease was required.
- One trial coordinated by the AGO.
    - Only 1 prior line of chemotherapy, which must have been cisplatin plus paclitaxel or carboplatin plus paclitaxel.
    - Measurable disease was not required.
- Epithelial ovarian cancer requiring chemotherapy.
- Previously received platinum-based chemotherapy with relapse more than 6 months from last platinum (>12 months for the Italian ICON4 group).
- No concomitant or prior malignant disease likely to interfere with treatment or outcomes.

TREATMENT DETAILS

Arm 1: Conventional Platinum-Based Chemotherapy
- Carboplatin.
    - Dose based on area under the curve (AUC) method of Calvert (Calvert et al. 1989) with a minimum of 5 (glomerular filtration rate [GFR] + 25). GFR was determined by a radioisotope method or 24-hour urine collection.

- If GFR was assessed by the Cockcroft formula, the dose was a minimum of 6 (GFR+25).
- Cisplatin.
  - Minimum dose of 75 mg/m^2 if given as single agent.
  - Minimum dose of 50 mg/m^2 if given in combination with other agents.
  - Protocol treatments included carboplatin, CAP (cyclophosphamide, Adriamycin, cisplatin), carboplatin+cisplatin, cisplatin+doxorubicin, cisplatin alone, and carboplatin+nontaxane.

Arm 2: Paclitaxel+Platinum
- ICON4 protocol: paclitaxel 175 mg/m^2 IV over 3 hours followed by carboplatin or cisplatin as dosed above.
- AGO protocol: paclitaxel 185 mg/m^2 IV over 3 hours followed by carboplatin or cisplatin as dosed above.
- Protocol treatments included paclitaxel+carboplatin, paclitaxel+cisplatin, paclitaxel+carboplatin+cisplatin, and paclitaxel alone.

ASSESSMENTS BASED ON PROTOCOL
- MRC protocol (ICON4)—assigned at least 6 cycles.
- IRFMN protocol (ICON4)—assigned at least 3 cycles, further 3 cycles based on results of response assessment.
- AGO protocol—assigned 6 to 8 cycles with response assessments done after second and fourth cycles.
- Quality of life collected for MRC and AGO protocols on slightly different schedules.

ENDPOINTS
- Overall survival (primary endpoint).
- Progression-free survival.
  - Elevated CA125 in the absence of radiologic evidence of disease was not considered progression.
- Quality of life.

STATISTICAL CONSIDERATIONS

Stratification Factors
- Stratification for ICON4 protocol included center, age, last chemotherapy received, time since completion of last chemotherapy, and intended platinum treatment. Platinum treatment had to be specified before randomization.

- Stratification for the AGO protocol included time since completion of last chemotherapy and whether the patient underwent secondary debulking surgery.

Sample Size
- Original was based on the assumption that the 2-year survival would be around 5% for the control group and would increase by 5% to 10% in the experimental group. Accrual target of 800 patients was set to detect this difference with 95% power at the 5% significance level, corresponding to a hazard ratio of 0.77.
- In 2001, the data monitoring and ethics committee noted the 2-year survival in the control group was much higher than originally predicted at approximately 50%. In the revised calculation, accrual of 800 patients would allow detection of an 11% difference in 2-year survival (from 50% to 61%) with 90% power at the 5% significance level, corresponding to a hazard ratio of 0.71.

Statistical Tests
- Kaplan-Meier curves for overall and progression-free survival.
- Mantel-Cox log rank test to compare survival.
- χ^2 to test for differences in effect size in different subgroups.
- Mann-Whitney nonparametric test used to compare quality-of-life measures: worst score and area under the curve for the first 6 months.

CONCLUSION OF TRIAL
- Paclitaxel plus platinum chemotherapy improves survival and progression-free survival in patients with platinum-sensitive recurrent ovarian cancer compared to conventional platinum-based chemotherapy alone. The benefit is seen even in the subset of patients who received prior front-line treatment with paclitaxel and platinum.

COMMENTS
- There was no evidence that the effect of combination treatment was any different in the subgroup of patients that had received prior paclitaxel+platinum (about 40% of the population).
- Differences in subsequent treatment at the time of progression: 31% in the conventional treatment arm received paclitaxel; 8% in the paclitaxel+platinum arm received further taxane-based treatment.
- Myelosuppression was greater in the conventional platinum chemotherapy arm, supporting prior reports suggesting a myeloprotective effect of paclitaxel (van Warmerdam et al. 1997).

Table 5.3 Results of ICON4/AGO-OVAR 2.2

Treatment arm	Platinum N=410	Paclitaxel+ platinum N=392	Statistics
Patient characteristics			
Median age	59.2	60.0	
Time from prior chemotherapy			
6-12 months	27%	23%	
≥12 months	73%	77%	
No. of prior chemotherapies			
1	93%	90%	
2	6%	6%	
3 or more	1%	4%	
Last chemotherapy			
Paclitaxel/carboplatin	34%	34%	
Carboplatin	31%	30%	
CAP	18%	16%	
Paclitaxel/cisplatin	5%	7%	
Other platinum	10%	11%	
Other nonplatinum	1%	3%	
Intended platinum			
Carboplatin	83%	85%	
Cisplatin	17%	15%	
Stage	Not stated	Not stated	
Histology	Not stated	Not stated	
Treatment delivery			
Received ≥6 cycles	66%	79%	
Received <6 cycles	30%	19%	
Efficacy			
2-year OS	50%	57%	
Median OS	24 months	29 months	HR 0.82 (95% CI, 0.69-0.97)
1-year PFS	40%	50%	
Median PFS	9 months	12 months	HR 0.76 (95% CI, 0.66, 0.89)
CR or PR	54%	66%	$P=.06$
Toxicity			
Worse with platinum			
Hematologic	46%	29%	
G2-4 nausea/vomiting	40%	35%	
Worse with combo			
G2-4 neurologic	1%	20%	
Alopecia	25%	86%	
No difference			
Infection	14%	17%	
Renal	9%	8%	
G2-3 mucositis	6%	7%	

CAP, cyclophosphamide+Adriamycin/doxorubicin+cisplatin; CI, confidence interval; CR, complete response; HR, hazard ratio; PFS, progression-free survival; PR, partial response; OS, overall survival.

AGO-OVAR, NCIC CTG, EORTC GCG Trial (Pfisterer, JCO 2006)

REFERENCE

- Pfisterer J, et al. Gemcitabine plus carboplatin compared with carboplatin in patients with platinum-sensitive recurrent ovarian cancer: an intergroup trial of the AGO-OVAR, the NCIC CTG, and the EORTC GCG. *J Clin Oncol*. 2006;24(29):4699-4707. PMID: 16966687. (Pfisterer et al. 2006a)

TRIAL SPONSOR

- Gynecologic Cancer Intergroup
  - AGO-OVAR
  - National Cancer Institute of Canada Clinical Trials Group
  - European Organisation for Research and Treatment of Cancer (EORTC) Gynecologic Cancer Group

RATIONALE FOR TRIAL

- The majority of patients with ovarian cancer relapse and die within 5 years. Patients with recurrence are classified as having platinum-sensitive or platinum-resistant disease based on the time interval from last therapy to recurrence (Gore et al. 1990; Markman et al. 1991).
- For patients with platinum-sensitive disease, standard therapy is retreatment with a single-agent platinum compound, and carboplatin is the drug of choice due to its favorable therapeutic profile.
- The ICON4/AGO-OVAR2.2 was a pooled analysis of 3 randomized controlled trials that demonstrated that retreatment with platinum and taxane results in superior PFS and OS compared to treatment with platinum alone in patients with platinum-sensitive recurrent ovarian cancer (Parmar et al. 2003). Global quality of life did not differ between the arms, but 20% of patients treated with platinum/taxane experienced grade 2 to 4 neurotoxicity compared to 1% of patients receiving platinum alone. This may underestimate the true incidence of neurotoxicity as many patients had not received taxane in the first-line setting. The OVAR2.2 portion of the study had been discontinued early due to concern that retreatment with paclitaxel would lead to excessive neuropathy. A large proportion of potentially eligible patients could not be entered due to persisting neurotoxicity from first-line therapy.

- In the AGO-OVAR study evaluating first-line cisplatin/paclitaxel vs carboplatin/paclitaxel, 83% and 75% of patients developed grade 1 to 4 neurotoxicity that slowly resolved (du Bois et al. 2003). However, 20% of patients continued to have persistent neuropathy for 2 or more years.
- These data underscore the need for an alternative platinum-based combination with less risk of neuropathy.
- Gemcitabine is a nucleoside analogue that has single-agent activity in phase II studies of recurrent ovarian cancer, including in patients who have received prior platinum and/or taxane (Lund et al. 1994; Lund and Neijt 1996; Shapiro et al. 1996).
- The AGO-OVAR group conducted a phase I/II study of carboplatin plus gemcitabine in patients with platinum-sensitive recurrent ovarian cancer to identify recommended doses. This trial demonstrated a high response rate of 62.5% and acceptable toxicity (du Bois et al. 2001).
- This trial is a phase III investigation comparing the efficacy of carboplatin and gemcitabine against carboplatin alone in patients with platinum-sensitive recurrent ovarian cancer.

PATIENT POPULATION

- N=366 enrolled.
- Enrolled between September 1999 and April 2002.
- Recurrent ovarian cancer at least 6 months from completion of first-line platinum-based chemotherapy.
- Measurable or assessable lesions per Southwest Oncology Group criteria (Green and Weiss 1992).
- ECOG performance status of 0, 1, or 2.
- Adequate bone marrow reserve and renal function.
  - ANC ≥1500/μL.
  - Platelets ≥100,000/μL.
  - Estimated glomerular filtration rate >50 mL/min.
- No serious concomitant systemic disorders incompatible with the study.
- Estimated life expectancy of 12 weeks or longer.

TREATMENT DETAILS

Arm 1: Standard Chemotherapy
- Carboplatin AUC 5 mg/mL/min IV on day 1.

Arm 2: Experimental Chemotherapy
- Gemcitabine plus carboplatin (du Bois et al. 2001).

- Gemcitabine 1000 mg/m² IV on days 1 and 8.
- Carboplatin AUC 4 mg/mL/min IV on day 1.

Dosing Details
- Carboplatin dosed by Calvert formula (Calvert et al. 1989). AUC calculation was based on GFR calculation based on the formula of Jelliffe (Jelliffe 1973).
- Patients received treatment every 21 days for 6 cycles with the option to receive a maximum of 10 cycles at the investigator's discretion. Treatment was discontinued for progressive disease or unacceptable toxicity.

Dose Modifications
- Treatment could be postponed for a maximum of 2 weeks for toxicity, including ANC ≤1500/µL and platelets ≤100,000/µL. Longer toxicity-related delays resulted in treatment discontinuation.
- For ANC 1000 to 1500/µL or platelets 75,000 to 100,000/µL, gemcitabine day 8 reduced 50%.
- For ANC ≤1000/µL or platelets ≤75,000/µL, gemcitabine day 8 omitted.
- For G3 nonhematologic toxicities (excluding nausea and vomiting), dose modifications or study discontinuation were at the investigator's discretion.
- For toxicity-related treatment delays of >1 week, ANC 500/µL for more than 5 days or ANC <100/µL for more than 3 days, febrile neutropenia, platelets <25,000/µL, and grade 3 or 4 nonhematologic toxicities (other than nausea or vomiting), successive dose reductions by 1 dose level.
- Carboplatin dose reductions.
  - Dose level 1: carboplatin AUC 4.
  - If additional dose reductions required, patients were discontinued.
- Gemcitabine plus carboplatin.
  - Dose level 1: gemcitabine 800 mg/m².
  - Dose level 2: omission of day 8 gemcitabine.

ASSESSMENTS

- Baseline assessment: medical history, physical examination, blood counts, chemistries, and radiologic studies to establish tumor burden.
- Blood counts were obtained on days 1 and 8 of each cycle.
- Quality of life was assessed by the EORTC QLQ-C30 and QLQ-OV28, version 2 (Aaronson et al. 1993; Greimel et al. 2003).
  - QOL assessed within 2 weeks before enrollment, before each cycle.

- Toxicity was assessed before each cycle and 30 days after last treatment.
- Patient assessment was performed before random assignment, before each cycle during treatment, and every 2 to 3 months after treatment for at least 2 years.
  - Progressive disease was based on clinical and/or radiologic evaluation.
  - Progressive disease was not based on CA125 elevation alone.

ENDPOINTS

- PFS, defined as time from date of randomization to date of disease progression or death from any cause (primary endpoint).
- Duration of response was measured from date of first response to date of disease progression or death due to any cause.
- Overall survival was measured from the date of random assignment to the date of death from any cause.
- Response was measured according to Southwest Oncology Group criteria (Green and Weiss 1992).
- Quality of life.
- Toxicity, graded according to the National Cancer Institute Common Toxicity Criteria version 2 (Trotti et al. 2000).

STATISTICAL CONSIDERATIONS

Stratification Factors
- Platinum-free interval (6-12 months vs ≥12 months).
- First-line therapy (platinum/paclitaxel vs other platinum-based therapy).
- Bidimensionally measurable disease (yes vs no).

Sample Size
- Target enrollment was 350 patients. Based on historical data, it was expected that between 300 and 350 patients with disease progression would be observed. Based on the AGO-OVAR phase I/II study (du Bois et al. 2001), the expected median PFS for gemcitabine and carboplatin was 8.5 months compared to a median PFS for carboplatin alone of 6 months. The constant HR was 0.71 with a significance level of .05; the study had 85% power using the log-rank comparison of PFS.
- The study was not powered to detect differences in OS. To detect a 25% improvement of 25% (assuming an HR of 0.8), power would have been 55% with an α of 0.05 and 352 deaths.

Table 5.4 Results of AGO-OVAR, NCIC, CTG EORTC GCG Trial

Treatment arm	Carboplatin N=178	Carboplatin+ gemcitabine N=178	Statistics
Patient characteristics			
Median age (range)	58 (21-81)	59 (36-78)	
Time from prior chemotherapy			
<6 months	0%	0.6%	
6-12 months	39.9%	39.9%	
≥12 months	60.1%	59.6%	
Prior platinum/taxane	71.3%	70.2%	
Stage IA-IIA	7.9%	9.0%	
Stage IIB-IIIB	19.1%	21.4%	
Stage IIIC	60.1%	54.5%	
Stage IV	12.4%	15.2%	
Histology	Not specified	Not specified	
Grade 1	7.3%	8.4%	
Grade 2	27.5%	28.7%	
Grade 3	49.4%	43.8%	
Undifferentiated	3.9%	5.6%	
Unknown grade	11.8%	13.5%	
Treatment delivery			
% planned carboplatin	98.2%	96.2%	
% planned gemcitabine day 1		92.8%	
% planned gemcitabine day 8		63.4%	
D/C for heme toxicity	4.0%	5.1%	
Efficacy			
Overall response	30.9%	47.2%	$P=.0016$
Complete response	6.2%	14.6%	
Partial response	24.7%	32.6%	
Stable disease	38.8%	38.2%	
Progressive disease	16.3%	7.9%	
Median PFS	5.8 months	8.6 months	HR 0.72 (95% CI, 0.58-0.90)
Median OS	17.3 months	18.0 months	HR 0.96, NS
Median DOR	7.3 months	8.4 months	$P=NS$
Toxicity			
Worse in carboplatin/gemcitabine			
G3/4 anemia	8.0%	27.4%	$P<.001$
G3/4 neutropenia	12.0%	70.3%	$P<.001$
G3/4 thrombocytopenia	11.4%	34.9%	$P<.001$

Table 5.4 Results of AGO-OVAR, NCIC, CTG EORTC GCG Trial *(continued)*

Treatment arm	Carboplatin N=178	Carboplatin + gemcitabine N=178	Statistics
No difference			
Febrile neutropenia	0%	1.1%	NS
G1-4 neuropathy, motor	4.0%	6.3%	NS
G1-4 neuropathy, sensory	26.9%	29.7%	NS
G1/2 alopecia	17.8%	49.2%	

CI, confidence interval; D/C, discontinue; DOR, duration of response; HR, hazard ratio; NS, not significant; PFS, progression-free survival.

Statistical Tests

- Kaplan-Meier estimations were used for time-to-event parameters.
- Log rank χ^2 tests used to compare the distribution between groups.
- Univariate Cox models were fitted for each covariate and PFS.
  - Covariates included age (≤60 vs >60 years), performance status (0 vs 1-2), prior platinum therapy (platinum plus nonpaclitaxel vs platinum plus paclitaxel), disease status (bidimensionally measurable vs assessable), and duration of platinum-free interval (6-12 months vs >12 months).
- Unadjusted normal approximation for the difference of 2 binomial proportions used to compare response rates.
- Paired *t* test and analysis of variance (ANOVA) were used to analyze changes in QLQ-C30 and QLQ-OV38 baseline scores within and between arms.

CONCLUSION OF TRIAL

- Gemcitabine and carboplatin significantly improve PFS and response rate without worsening quality of life in patients with platinum-sensitive ovarian cancer.

COMMENTS

- In the Cox proportional hazards model, the improved PFS was maintained in patients who had received prior platinum-taxane as first-line therapy and in patients with a short platinum-free interval of less than 12 months.
- Quality of life did not differ between treatment arms.

- Postprogression therapy: no major differences between carboplatin or carboplatin/gemcitabine.
  - Platinum: 23% vs 29%.
  - Topotecan: 21% vs 29%.
  - Anthracyclines: 18% vs 15%.
  - Etoposide: 4% vs 12%.
  - Alkylating agents: 20% vs 12%.
  - Taxanes: 7% vs 1%.
  - Gemcitabine: 6% vs 0%.
- Because epithelial ovarian cancer often behaves like a chronic illness, there is an urgent need to identify active platinum-based combinations that do not have the same cumulative neurotoxicity of platinum and taxane.
- Carboplatin and gemcitabine are feasible and increase progression-free survival and response rates in patients with platinum-sensitive ovarian cancer, irrespective of factors such as prior taxane exposure and platinum-free interval.
- This study did not show a benefit to OS, but it was not designed or powered to do so. Because the OS outcome reflects all treatments administered and not just the treatment received during a trial, PFS has been considered an important endpoint in ovarian cancer patients.
- Carboplatin and gemcitabine were associated with greater hematologic toxicity, but it was tolerable and associated with infrequent sequelae such as febrile neutropenia and no detrimental effect to quality of life.
- Compared to treatment with taxanes, carboplatin and gemcitabine were associated with a better toxicity profile with less neuropathy and alopecia. This treatment combination represents a treatment option for patients with platinum-sensitive ovarian cancer recurrence.

Gemcitabine Versus PLD (Mutch, JCO 2007)

REFERENCE

- Mutch DG, et al. Randomized phase III trial of gemcitabine compared with pegylated liposomal doxorubicin in patients with platinum-resistant ovarian cancer. *J Clin Oncol.* 2007;25(19):2811-2818. PMID: 17602086. (Mutch et al. 2007)

TRIAL SPONSOR

- Eli Lilly & Co.

RATIONALE FOR TRIAL
- There are limited treatment options for patients with platinum-resistant ovarian cancer that has progressed within 6 months of prior platinum treatment.
  - These patients are typically treated sequentially with single-agent regimens, including topotecan, gemcitabine, and pegylated liposomal doxorubicin (PLD).
  - Treatment choice depends on possibility of efficacy, cumulative adverse effects, and optimal sequencing of agents.
- PLD is approved by the US Food and Drug Administration (FDA) for use in patients with progressive or recurrent ovarian cancer after platinum-based chemotherapy. Single-agent PLD has equivalent efficacy and safety to topotecan (Gordon et al. 2001) and is commonly used in patients with platinum-resistant ovarian cancer.
- Gemcitabine has been extensively studied in phase II studies as a single agent (Lund and Neijt 1996; Friedlander et al. 1998; D'Agostino et al. 2003; Markman et al. 2003b) and in combination regimens (Greggi et al. 2001; Goff et al. 2003; Rose et al. 2003; Raspagliesi et al. 2004; Tewari et al. 2004; Ferrandina et al. 2005; Rose 2005) and is active and generally well tolerated.
- This phase III trial was designed to compare the efficacy and safety of gemcitabine to PLD in patients with platinum-resistant recurrent ovarian cancer.

PATIENT POPULATION
- N = 195 randomized.
- Patients enrolled between July 2002 and May 2004 from 44 independent sites in the United States.

Inclusion Criteria
- Age ≥18 years.
- Documented pathologic diagnosis of epithelial ovarian, fallopian tube, or primary peritoneal carcinoma.
- Prior platinum-based chemotherapy.
- No more than 2 prior regimens.
- Platinum resistance was based on the most recent exposure to a platinum-containing regimen and was defined as progressive disease within 6 months of completing therapy.
- Measurable disease (Therasse et al. 2000) or CA125 ≥100 U/mL.

- Zubrod performance status of 0 to 2.
- Adequate bone marrow reserve and hepatic and neurologic function.

Exclusion Criteria
- Prior radiation to the breast, head, or neck within the past 3 years.
- Any prior abdominal or pelvic radiation therapy.
- Tumors of low malignant potential.
- Prior PLD or gemcitabine treatment.
- Tamoxifen use (concurrent low-dose corticosteroid or hormone replacement therapy was allowed).

TREATMENT DETAILS

Arm 1
- PLD 50 mg/m^2 IV over 60 minutes on day 1 every 28 days.
- Treatment continued until progressive disease or unacceptable toxicity.

Arm 2
- Gemcitabine 1000 mg/m^2 IV over 30 to 60 minutes on days 1 and 8 every 21 days.
- Treatment continued until progressive disease or unacceptable toxicity.

Crossover to Other Therapy Allowed
- At progressive disease.
- At toxicity requiring withdrawal after reversal to grade 1 or less.
- At a cumulative PLD dose of 500 mg/m^2.

Dose Modifications
- Dose/cycle delay or reduction.
- Cytokines were allowed for neutropenia >7 days or febrile neutropenia.
- Dose adjustments were based on ANC counts, platelets, and nonhematologic toxicities.
- Therapy could be resumed after toxicities resolved to grade 2 or less.

ASSESSMENTS
- Patients allowed with measurable and/or assessable disease.
- CT scan evaluated by Response Evaluation Criteria in Solid Tumors (RECIST) criteria (Therasse et al. 2000).
    - Baseline within 28 days of enrollment.
    - Gemcitabine: CT before every fourth 21-day cycle.
    - PLD: CT before every third 28-day cycle.
- CA125 assessable disease.
    - Progression defined by Rustin criteria (Rustin et al. 2001).

- Quality of life assessed by Functional Assessment of Cancer Therapy–Ovarian (FACT-O) (Basen-Engquist et al. 2001).
- Safety evaluated using the National Cancer Institute Common Toxicity Criteria, version 2.0.

ENDPOINTS

- PFS, defined as time from random assignment to PD or death (primary endpoint).
- OS.
- Disease control rate (DCR), defined as percentage of patients with confirmed complete response, partial response, or stable disease.

STATISTICAL CONSIDERATIONS

Sample Size

- Calculation was based on Freedman's method (Freedman 1982). Assuming a constant hazard ratio of 0.625, 148 events (progressions or death) were needed to have 80% power to detect a difference between the treatment arms with a 2-sided α of .05.

Statistical Tests

- Log-rank test to compared PFS between the 2 arms.
- Kaplan-Meier method (Kaplan and Meier 1958) to estimate survival curves.
- Multiple Cox regression model to explore the impact of prognostic factors on survival.
- Descriptive statistics for quality-of-life data.
- Two-sided Fisher's exact test to compare incidences of toxicities.

CONCLUSION OF TRIAL

- Although this was not designed as an equivalency trial, gemcitabine seemed to have a comparable therapeutic index to pegylated liposomal doxorubicin in patients with platinum-resistant ovarian cancer, and single-agent gemcitabine could be considered an acceptable treatment alternative.

COMMENTS

- Impact of prognostic factors on survival.
  - Stepwise Cox regression model ($P = .20$ for entry, $P = .10$ to stay), including age, number of prior chemotherapies, number of prior platinum regimens, response to prior platinum therapy, disease

Table 5.5 Results of Gemcitabine Versus PLD

Treatment arm	Gemcitabine N=99	PLD N=96	Statistics
Patient characteristics			
Median age (range)	59 (38-85)	62 (28-83)	
Time from prior chemotherapy	3.5 months	4.3 months	
No. of prior chemotherapies			
1	60.6%	67.7%	
2	39.4%	32.3%	
Response to platinum			
Response: CR+PR	46.5%	45.8%	
Nonresponse: SD+PD	53.5%	54.2%	
Measurable disease	65.7%	62.5%	
CA125 only	34.3%	37.5%	
Stage	Not reported	Not reported	
Histology	Not reported	Not reported	
Grade	Not reported	Not reported	
Treatment delivery			
Median No. of cycles (range)	4 (1-21)	3 (1-13)	
Median No. of doses	8	3	
Mean dose intensity	90.8%	92.4%	
% cycles with reduction	14.5%	9.0%	
Crossover	N=64 (PLD)	N=66 (gemcitabine)	
Efficacy			
Median PFS	3.6 months	3.1 months	NS
Median OS	12.7 months	13.5 months	NS
Median time to failure	2.7 months	2.5 months	NS
ORR, initial treatment	6.1%	8.3%	NS
SD, initial treatment	54.5%	38.5%	
DCR, initial treatment	60.6%	46.9%	$P=.63$
ORR, crossover	7.6%	4.7%	NS
DCR, crossover	63.6%	45.3%	$P=.52$
Toxicity—initial treatment	Gemcitabine (N=99)	PLD (N=96)	
Higher with gemcitabine			
Grade 2-4 constipation	25	9	$P=.004$
Grade 2-4 nausea/vomiting	28	12	$P=.008$
Grade 2-4 fatigue	36	23	$P=.043$
Grade 3-4 neutropenia	38	18	$P=.003$
Higher with PLD			
Grade 2-3 PPE	0	19	$P<.0001$
Grade 2-3 mucositis	3	15	$P=.003$

Table 5.5 Results of Gemcitabine Versus PLD *(continued)*

Treatment arm	Gemcitabine N=99	PLD N=96	Statistics
No difference			
Grade 2-4 dyspnea	20	10	NS
Grade 2-4 neuropathy	3	8	NS
Grade 2-4 rash	5	5	NS
Grade 3-4 thrombocytopenia	6	5	NS
Grade 3-4 anemia	3	2	NS
Febrile neutropenia	4	4	NS
Toxicity—crossover treatment	PLD (N=64)	Gemcitabine (N=66)	
Grade 2-4 fatigue	22	38	$P=.009$
Grade 2-3 PPE	11	13	NS
Grade 3-4 neutropenia	12	27	$P=.007$
Febrile neutropenia	7	3	NS

CA125, cancer antigen 125; CR, complete response; DCR, disease control rate; NS, not significant; ORR, overall response rate; OS, overall survival; PFS, progression-free survival; PLD, pegylated liposomal doxorubicin; PPE, palmar-plantar erythrodysesthesia; PR, partial response; SD, stable disease.

measurability at baseline, and baseline CA125 and baseline Zubrod performance status.
- PFS: only baseline CA125 was a significant predictor. Patients with a higher than median CA125 level had a higher risk of progression and death.
- OS: both baseline CA125 and performance status were significant prognostic factors.
- Quality-of-life analysis.
  - Study was not able to examine changes in QOL from baseline to study end.
  - Post hoc analysis of baseline QOL and treatment outcome demonstrated that higher baseline FACT-O scores were associated with lower hazard for death (HR, 0.54; $P=.003$).
- Identification of agents active against platinum-resistant ovarian cancer is a priority.
  - Second-line agents should lack cross-resistance.
  - Second-line agents should have a favorable toxicity profile due to the palliative nature of therapy.
- Limited number of randomized studies evaluating single agents in platinum-resistant ovarian cancer (ten Bokkel Huinink et al. 1997; Piccart et al. 2000; Bolis et al. 2001; Gordon et al. 2001; du Bois et al.

2002; Gore et al. 2002; Rosenberg et al. 2002; Buda et al. 2004; ten Bokkel Huinink et al. 2004) have shown no statistically significant differences in therapeutic index with the exception of treatments considered nonstandard, including treosulfan and luteinizing hormone-releasing hormone analogues (du Bois et al. 2002).
  - ten Bokkel phase III study suggested that topotecan and paclitaxel are equivalent, but this was in patients who did not receive prior taxane therapy (ten Bokkel Huinink et al. 2004).
  - Largest randomized phase III trial in this patient population compared topotecan and PLD (Gordon et al. 2001). There was no survival benefit to either agent. Only 74% of patients treated with PLD received prior taxane therapy. Patients receiving topotecan had significantly more grade 3 and 4 hematologic toxicity.
- This study demonstrates comparable efficacy between gemcitabine and PLD with response rates in line with prior studies evaluating PLD (Gordon et al. 2000; Gordon et al. 2001) and gemcitabine (Lund and Neijt 1996; Friedlander et al. 1998; D'Agostino et al. 2003; Markman et al. 2003b; Rose et al. 2003; Rose 2005).
- Gemcitabine trends toward a higher rate of stable disease, an important efficacy measure in platinum-resistant patients.
- There were no differences in PFS or OS in this study. OS should be interpreted with caution due to the crossover study design. Furthermore, this trial was not designed as an equivalency trial, and so caution must be exercised in interpreting the results.
- Toxicity.
  - Twenty percent of patients who crossed over from PLD to gemcitabine experienced PPE during gemcitabine administration. Based on the timing of this toxicity, much of this is attributed to latent or delayed toxicity from initial PLD administration.
  - A phase II study reported lower rates of grade 2 PPE (12%) when dosing PLD at 40 mg/m^2 every 28 days (Markman et al. 2000). No grade 3 or 4 events were observed. However, the median number of cycles was 2 (range, 1-12 cycles), and 12% of patients had dose adjustments.
- This is the second largest population of platinum-resistant ovarian cancer patients studied in a phase III randomized trial. This trial includes almost exclusively patients previously treated with platinum and taxane and therefore reflects current clinical practice patterns.
- Gemcitabine is an option to consider for taxane-pretreated platinum-resistant ovarian cancer patients.

OVA-301 (Monk, JCO 2010)

REFERENCE

- Monk BJ, et al. Trabectedin plus pegylated liposomal doxorubicin in recurrent ovarian cancer. *J Clin Oncol.* 2010;28(19):3107-3114. PMID: 20516432. (Monk et al. 2010)

TRIAL SPONSORS

- Johnson & Johnson Pharmaceutical Research & Development, Raritan, NJ
- PharmaMar, Madrid, Spain

RATIONALE FOR TRIAL

- Recurrent ovarian cancer is a clinical challenge with limited numbers of compounds with clinical activity. The only approved drugs by the US FDA are carboplatin, cisplatin, paclitaxel, altretamine, topotecan, PLD, and gemcitabine (in combination with carboplatin).
- Clinical trials to identify new agents for recurrent ovarian cancer have been hampered by several factors, including
  - Slow accrual.
  - Nonstandardized endpoint reporting (CA125, tumor response, progression-free survival, overall survival).
  - The FDA partnered with the American Society of Clinical Oncology (ASCO) and the American Association for Cancer Research (AACR) in 2006 to evaluate surrogate endpoints for ovarian cancer and concluded that PFS might be an acceptable endpoint (Bast et al. 2007). The panel posed the question as to what degree of PFS improvement would be clinically meaningful and recommended that studies should also be designed to evaluate the OS outcome.
- Trabectedin is a synthetically produced antineoplastic agent that was originally isolated from the marine tunicate *Ecteinascidia turbinata*.
  - Trabectedin exerts its antineoplastic effect by binding to the minor groove of DNA, bending DNA toward the major groove, disrupting transcription, and leading to G_2-M cycle arrest and apoptosis (Carter and Keam 2007).
  - Trabectedin is more effective in cells that have a functioning transcription-coupled nucleotide excision repair system.

- ○ This compound has encouraging single-agent activity in recurrent ovarian cancer and is tolerable (Sessa et al. 2005; Krasner et al. 2007; von Mehren et al. 2008).
- ○ In vitro studied demonstrate synergy between trabectedin and pegylated liposomal doxorubicin (Takahashi et al. 2001; Meco et al. 2003).
- This phase III randomized multicenter trial was performed to assess the efficacy of PLD vs PLD plus trabectedin in patients with relapsed ovarian cancer.

PATIENT POPULATION

- N = 672 enrolled.
- Enrolled between April 2005 and May 2007 from 124 centers in 21 countries.

Inclusion Criteria
- Age ≥18 years.
- Histologically confirmed epithelial ovarian, fallopian tube, or primary peritoneal carcinoma.
- One prior platinum-based chemotherapy regimen only followed by persistence, recurrence, or progression.
  - ○ Platinum resistant: platinum-free interval (PFI) <6 months.
  - ○ Platinum sensitive: PFI ≥6 months.
- Measurable disease by RECIST.
- ECOG performance status ≤2.
- Adequate bone marrow function: hemoglobin ≥9 g/dL, ANC ≥1500/μL, platelets ≥100,000/μL.
- Adequate renal function: serum creatinine ≤1.5 mg/dL or creatinine clearance ≥60 mL/min.
- Creatine phosphokinase less than or equal to upper limit of normal (ULN).
- Adequate liver function: total bilirubin ≤1.5× ULN, direct bilirubin less than or equal to ULN, total alkaline phosphatase (ALP) ≤1.5× ULN, AST and alanine aminotransferase (ALT) ≤2.5× ULN.
- Adequate cardiac function: LVEF within institutional limits.
- Interval between prior treatment and study initiation.
  - ○ ≥4 weeks for radiation or experimental therapy.
  - ○ ≥2 weeks for hormonal therapy.
  - ○ ≥3 weeks for chemotherapy or biologic therapy.

Exclusion Criteria
- Platinum refractory—disease progression during front-line therapy.
- Women of childbearing potential and not using adequate contraception.

TREATMENT DETAILS

Stratification Factors
- ECOG performance status (0 to 1 vs 2).
- Platinum sensitivity (sensitive vs resistant).

Arm 1: PLD
- Treatment on day 1 of a 4-week cycle.
- PLD 50 mg/m^2 IV over 90 minutes.
- Maximum of 2 dose reductions allowed.
- PLD could be reduced to 37.5 mg/m^2, then to 28 mg/m^2.

Arm 2: PLD + Trabectedin
- Treatment on day 1 of a 3-week cycle.
- IV dexamethasone 20 mg (or equivalent) (Donald et al. 2003) 30 minutes prior to treatment.
- PLD 30 mg/m^2 IV over 90 minutes.
- Trabectedin 1.1 mg/m^2 IV over 3 hours through a central venous catheter.
- Maximum of 2 dose reductions for each drug allowed.
- Trabectedin could be reduced to 0.9 mg/m^2, then to 0.75 mg/m^2.
- PLD could be reduced to 25 mg/m^2, then to 20 mg/m^2.

Additional Treatment Details
- Treatment continued until disease progression or confirmation of complete response and could be continued for 2 or more cycles beyond confirmed CR.
- Colony-stimulating factors were permitted after cycle 1 per ASCO guidelines (Smith et al. 2006).
- Additional antiemetics could be added per the investigator's discretion.

Dose Reductions
- One level for neutrophils <500/μL with temperature ≥38.5°C or infection.
- One level for neutrophils <500/μL lasting >5 days.
- One level for platelets ≤25,000/μL.
- One level for grade ≥3 nausea/vomiting (despite adequate treatment).

- PLD reduction for stomatitis.
- PLD reduction for first occurrence of hand-foot syndrome (HFS) and day 15 transaminase elevation.
- Trabectedin reduction for first occurrence of grade ≥2 ALP elevation.
- PLD reduction for grade ≥1 HFS after first occurrence of grade 3 to 4 HFS.
- Trabectedin reduction of conjugated bilirubin more than ULN.
- Trabectedin reduction for second occurrence of grade ≥1 ALP elevation.
- One level reduction of both drugs if grade ≥3 transaminase elevations on day 15 recovered to grade 1 or less by day 1 of the next cycle or within 3 weeks after that date.
- Both drugs terminated if grade ≥3 transaminase elevations on day 15 and no recovery to grade 1 or less by day 1 of the next cycle or within 3 weeks.

ASSESSMENTS

- Disease assessments at screening and every 8 weeks thereafter.
  - Independent radiology review by RECIST criteria (Therasse et al. 2000).
  - Secondary analyses of PFS based on independent oncologist and investigator's assessments.
  - Both independent radiologists and oncologists were blinded to treatment assignment.
- Evaluation of LVEF.
  - Every 2 cycles for patients with cardiac history or total cumulative anthracycline dose more than 360 mg/m^2.
  - At treatment discontinuation for all patients.
- Complete blood count (CBC) and chemistries every week.
- Safety evaluated by National Cancer Institute Common Terminology Criteria for Adverse Events (CTCAE), version 3.0.
- Quality-of-life questionnaires at screening, day 1 of each cycle, and at treatment end.
  - EORTC QLQ-C30 (Aaronson et al. 1993).
  - EORTC QLQ-OV28 (ovarian cancer module) (Greimel et al. 2003).

ENDPOINTS

- PFS (primary endpoint).
- OS.

- Overall response rate (ORR; response maintained ≥4 weeks by RECIST).
- Duration of response (date from first documentation of response to date of progression or death).
- Safety.
- QOL.

STATISTICAL CONSIDERATIONS

Sample Size

- In total, 650 patients were to be enrolled over 2 years and 415 PFS events were required to test a statistical difference assuming a median PFS of 16 weeks for PLD and 22 weeks for trabectedin/PLD with 90% power and 2-sided α of .05.
- OS analysis was to be performed when 520 deaths were observed to allow for testing of a statistical difference assuming a median OS of 63 weeks for PLD and 83 weeks for PLD/trabectedin with 90% power and a 2-sided α of .05.
- In December 2006, after the FDA/ASCO/AACR public workshop evaluating endpoints for ovarian cancer clinical trials (Bast et al. 2007), the endpoints were changed to a single primary endpoint of PFS. OS was made a secondary endpoint. Sample size remained unchanged. This occurred when 440 subjects had been enrolled and before central radiology review.

Statistical Tests

- Kaplan-Meier method was used to estimate survival.
- The log-rank test was used to compare survival.
- The stratified log-rank test was used to compare PFS between treatment arms while adjusting for ECOG PS and platinum sensitivity (Kaplan and Meier 1958).
- A Cox proportional hazards model was used to compare treatment arms while adjusting by prognostic factors as a secondary analysis (Cox 1972).

CONCLUSION OF TRIAL

- Trabectedin combined with PLD improves PFS compared to PLD alone with acceptable toxicity in patients with recurrent ovarian cancer.

Table 5.6 Results of OVA-301

Treatment arm	PLD N=335	PLD/ trabectedin N=337	Statistics
Patient characteristics			
Median age (range)	58 (27-87)	56 (26-82)	
Time from prior chemotherapy			
<6 months	35%	35%	
6-12 months	28%	37%	
≥12 months	37%	29%	
Prior taxane	81%	80%	
Prior consolidation chemotherapy	10%	8%	
Serous	69%	67%	
Endometrioid	5%	7%	
Mucinous	1%	1%	
Clear cell	5%	4%	
Other	21%	21%	
Grade 1	3%	5%	
Grade 2	18%	17%	
Grade 3	52%	52%	
Unknown grade	27%	25%	
Treatment delivery			
Median cumulative trabectedin dose (range)	NA	5.6 mg/m^2 (1-23)	
Median cumulative PLD dose (range)	216 mg/m^2 (3-1061)	154.4 mg/m^2 (15-630)	
Efficacy			
Median PFS	5.8 months	7.3 months	HR 0.79 (95% CI, 0.64-0.96)
Platinum sensitive	7.5 months	9.2 months	HR 0.73 (95% CI, 0.56-0.95)
Platinum resistant	3.7 months	4.0 months	NS
Overall survival	Immature	Immature	
Toxicity			
More common with PLD/T			
Grade 3/4 neutropenia	22.4%	62.7%	
Grade 3/4 ALT elevations	0.3%	30.9%	
Colony-stimulating factors	17%	42%	
Congestive heart failure	N=1	N=6	
More common with PLD			
Hand-foot syndrome	19.7%	3.9%	
Mucosal inflammation	5.8%	2.1%	
Stomatitis	5.1%	0.9%	

Table 5.6 Results of OVA-301 *(continued)*

Treatment arm	PLD N = 335	PLD/ trabectedin N = 337	Statistics
Death during treatment	N = 8	N = 11	
Progressive disease	N = 6	N = 6	
Adverse event	N = 1	N = 5	
Unknown cause	N = 1	N = 0	

ALT, alanine aminotransferase; CI, confidence interval; HR, hazard ratio; NA, not applicable; NS, not significant; PFS, progression-free survival; OS, overall survival; PLD, pegylated liposomal doxorubicin; PLD-T, pegylated liposomal doxorubicin + trabectedin.

COMMENTS

- Incidence of dose reductions was similar between arms.
- Cycle delays were more common with PLD/trabectedin.
  - Drug-related adverse events were the most common reason for cycle delay in both arms.
  - HFS was most common reason for treatment termination or dose adjustment for PLD alone.
  - Neutropenia was most common reason for treatment termination or dose adjustment for PLD/trabectedin.
- Treatment effect with PLD/trabectedin was seen across different subgroups.
- OS data are immature at the time of publication.
- ORR was higher with trabectedin/PLD (Appendix Table A2 in manuscript), $P = .008$.
- Response duration did not differ between arms.
- Duration of disease stabilization was improved with the combination, $P = .0106$.
- Proportion of patients receiving subsequent ovarian cancer therapy was similar in both groups.
- There were no differences in quality of life using mixed-effects models to predict baseline and follow-up scores as a function of treatment, days after baseline and interaction between treatment and days after baseline.
- Toxicities.
  - The criteria for Hy's law (concurrent increase in both transaminases and bilirubin) (Temple 2006), which predicts severe liver toxicity, were met for 3 patients (0.9%) receiving PLD/trabectedin. Liver toxicity resolved in all 3 cases and was never severe.

- Nonplatinum monotherapy.
  - Preferred treatment for patients with platinum-resistant disease.
  - Also considered in patients with platinum-sensitive disease as a potential means of increasing the benefit of subsequent platinum-based treatment.
- Prior to this trial, 4 positive randomized phase III trials in second-line treatment of recurrent ovarian cancer have led to regulatory approval of a drug or a change in treatment paradigm.
  - Topotecan vs paclitaxel trial demonstrated efficacy of topotecan (ten Bokkel Huinink et al. 1997).
  - Topotecan vs PLD trial demonstrated improved efficacy, conventional dosing, and a favorable safety profile for PLD, supporting regulatory approval for PLD for both platinum-resistant and platinum-sensitive ovarian cancer (Gordon et al. 2001; Gordon et al. 2004).
  - ICON4/AGO-OVA 2.2 trial comparing single-agent platinum to platinum + paclitaxel demonstrated prolonged PFS and OS for combination therapy (Parmar et al. 2003).
  - AGO-OVAR, NCIC CTG, and EORTC GCG trials comparing carboplatin to carboplatin + gemcitabine showed improvement in PFS with the combination treatment (Pfisterer et al. 2006a).
- This current trial differs from these prior trials in that it combines nonplatinum agents and demonstrates superiority in PFS with the combination regimen.
- Because most women with recurrent ovarian cancer die of their disease, measures such as quality of life, convenience, and safety are as important as efficacy in evaluating a regimen.
  - Findings of this trial and others demonstrate that doublets are more toxic than monotherapies, and this must be weighed in the benefit-risk ratio when choosing a therapy.

CALYPSO (Pujade-Lauraine, JCO 2010)
Caelyx in Platinum Sensitive Ovarian Patients

REFERENCE

- Pujade-Lauraine E, et al. Pegylated liposomal doxorubicin and carboplatin compared with paclitaxel and carboplatin for patients with platinum-sensitive ovarian cancer in late relapse. *J Clin Oncol.* 2010;28(20):3323-3329. PMID: 20498395. (Pujade-Lauraine et al. 2010)

TRIAL SPONSORS

- Gynecologic Cancer Intergroup Trial of Groupe d'Investigateurs Nationaux pour l'Etude des Cancers Ovariens (GINECO)
  - Arbeitsgemeinschaft Gynakologische Onkologie Studiengruppe Ovarialkarzinom (AGO-OVAR)
  - Nordic Society Gynecologic Oncology (NSGO)
  - Australia New Zealand Gynaecological Oncology Group (ANZGOG)
  - National Cancer Institute of Canada Clinical Trials Group (NCIC-CTG)
  - Arbeitsgemeinschaft Gynaekologische Onkologie (AGO) Austria
  - European Organisation for Research and Treatment of Cancer (EORTC)
  - Multicenter Italian Trials in Ovarian Cancer (MITO)
  - Mario Negri Gynecologic Oncology (MaNGO)

RATIONALE FOR TRIAL

- A pooled analysis of 3 randomized controlled trials from AGO-OVAR and ICON showed improved PFS and OS in patients with platinum-sensitive recurrent ovarian cancer treated with paclitaxel and carboplatin compared to platinum alone (Parmar et al. 2003). A GEICO phase II study demonstrated a significant improvement in time to tumor progression in patients treated with paclitaxel and carboplatin compared to carboplatin alone (Gonzalez-Martin et al. 2005).
- Retreatment with paclitaxel and carboplatin is limited by the risk of cumulative peripheral neuropathy. In addition, grade 2 alopecia (total hair loss) occurs in 80% of patients.
- Carboplatin and gemcitabine improve PFS and response rates in platinum-sensitive recurrent ovarian cancer, but OS is not improved compared to carboplatin alone in a phase III trial (Pfisterer et al. 2006a). Hematologic toxicities are greater. There remains a need for other active carboplatin combinations.
- PLD is an active drug against ovarian cancer in the second-line setting (Gordon et al. 2001; Gordon et al. 2004; Ferrandina et al. 2008). PLD has equivalent to superior activity in this setting compared to other agents such as paclitaxel or gemcitabine (ten Bokkel Huinink et al. 1997; Ferrandina et al. 2008).
- A phase II study showed the combination of PLD 30 mg/m^2 followed by carboplatin AUC 5 every 4 weeks is safe and efficacious with a high

response rate of 63% and median PFS and OS of 9.4 months and 32.0 months, respectively (Ferrero et al. 2007).
- This phase III trial was designed to compare the efficacy of PLD/carboplatin every 4 weeks vs standard paclitaxel and carboplatin every 3 weeks.

PATIENT POPULATION

- N = 976 enrolled.
- Enrollment from April 2005 to September 2007.
- Cancer of ovary, fallopian tube, or extra-ovarian papillary serous tumor with disease progression >6 months after receiving first- or second-line platinum-based chemotherapy.
- Prior taxane therapy was required.
- Measurable disease according to RECIST or CA125 assessable disease according to Gynecologic Cancer InterGroup criteria or histologic proven relapse (Therasse et al. 2000; Vergote et al. 2000).
- ECOG performance status of 0, 1, or 2.
- Life expectancy of at least 12 weeks.
- Adequate bone marrow, renal, and hepatic function.
- Exclusion: preexisting more than grade 1 neuropathy.

TREATMENT DETAILS

Arm 1: Paclitaxel and Carboplatin
- Paclitaxel 175 mg/m^2 IV on day 1.
- Carboplatin AUC 5 IV on day 1 based on Calvert formula using glomerular filtration rate calculated from serum creatinine values by Cockcroft and Gault method (Cockroft and Gault 1976).
- Treatment administered every 3 weeks for 6 courses in the absence of unacceptable toxicity or disease progression.
- In the event of partial response or stable disease, patients were allowed to stay on treatment until disease progression.

Arm 2: Pegylated Liposomal Doxorubicin and Carboplatin
- PLD 30 mg/m^2 IV on day 1.
- Carboplatin AUC 5 IV.
- Treatment administered every 4 weeks for 6 courses in the absence of unacceptable toxicity or disease progression.
- In the event of partial response or stable disease, patients were allowed to stay on treatment until disease progression.

Treatment Plan and Dose Modification
- All patients received antiemetics, including a serotonin antagonist and a corticosteroid. Patients receiving paclitaxel received premedications to prevent hypersensitivity reactions.
- Guidelines for dose delay and reduction are in the appendix of the manuscript (Smith et al. 2006).

ASSESSMENTS
- Baseline:
  - History and physical examination, including a gynecologic examination, laboratory studies including CA125, radiographic imaging (CT scan, ultrasound, MRI, or site-specific radiography) within 4 weeks of study entry.
  - Baseline electrocardiogram (ECG) for patients receiving paclitaxel.
  - Baseline left ventricular ejection fraction by ECG or multigated angiography for patients receiving PLD.
- Before each cycle:
  - Clinical, hematologic, and biochemical assessments, including evaluation for toxic events as assessed by the NCI CTCAE.
  - For patients receiving PLD, a left ventricular ejection fraction measurement was performed before each course of therapy if cumulative anthracycline dose was >450 mg/m^2.
- At 3 month intervals during treatment:
  - CA125.
  - Quality-of-life evaluations by EORTC QLQ C30 version 3.0 and OV-28 version 1 (Aaronson et al. 1993; Greimel et al. 2003).
- Follow-up after treatment discontinuation:
  - Clinical examination, including gynecologic examination, CA125, and adverse event evaluation every 3 months for 2 years and every 6 months thereafter for 5 years.
  - Quality-of-life evaluation every 3 months for 1 year from the date of enrollment.
- Definition of disease progression was based on RECIST and GCIG modifications and included clinical or imaging signs of any new lesions, increase in measurable and/or nonmeasurable tumor defined by RECIST, CA-125 elevation defined by GCIG criteria, health status deterioration attributable to disease, and death of any cause before progression was diagnosed (Therasse et al. 2000; Vergote et al. 2000).

ENDPOINTS
- PFS (primary endpoint).

STATISTICAL CONSIDERATIONS

Stratification Factors
- Patients stratified by therapy-free interval (6-12 vs >12 months), measurable disease (yes vs no), center.
- Based on method of random assignment, a slight imbalance in treatment allocation was observed but treatment arms were well balanced for baseline characteristics and stratification factors.

Sample Size
- Designed as a 2-arm parallel noninferiority trial. Calculations were based on the results of ICON4/AGO-OAR 2-2, which showed a 23% relative benefit for PFS and OS favoring paclitaxel and carboplatin (Parmar et al. 2003). A sample size of 898 evaluable patients with 745 progressions was estimated for a noninferiority margin with an HR of 1.23 at 15 months or a 7.9% absolute difference at 12 months with 90% power and a 1-sided confidence interval of 95%.

Statistical Tests
- Cox proportional hazards were used to calculate hazard ratios for survival.
- Kaplan-Meier curves and the log-rank test were used to compare survival curves.
- χ^2 and Wilcoxon rank-sum tests were used as appropriate for toxicity comparisons.

CONCLUSION OF TRIAL
- Pegylated liposomal doxorubicin and carboplatin were associated with a statistically significant improvement in PFS and lower toxicity compared to paclitaxel and carboplatin in patients with platinum-sensitive ovarian cancer.

COMMENTS
- This is one of the largest trials to be conducted in relapsed/recurrent ovarian cancer to date.
- In addition to demonstrating an improvement in PFS, CD (carboplatin and PLD) produced less severe toxicities, including less carboplatin hypersensitivity reactions and less peripheral neuropathy and less alopecia compared to CP (carboplatin and paclitaxel).

Table 5.7 Results of CALYPSO

Treatment arm	Paclitaxel and carboplatin (CP) N=507	PLD and carboplatin (CD) N=466	Statistics
Patient characteristics			
Median age (range)	61 (27-82)	60.5 (24-82)	
Time from prior chemotherapy			
<6 months	0%	0%	
6-12 months	36.1%	35%	
≥12 months	63.9%	65%	
No. of prior chemotherapies			
1	82.6%	87.6%	
Carboplatin	98.1%	96.8%	
Taxane	96.7%	97.1%	
2	17.3%	12.4%	
Stage I/II	13.0%	12.3%	
Stage III/IV	84.2%	85.8%	
Serous	72.2%	71.7%	
Endometrioid	6.9%	8.2%	
Mucinous	1.6%	1.9%	
Clear cell	2.6%	3.0%	
Other	16.7%	15.2%	
Grade 1	4.5%	6.2%	
Grade 2	25.2%	21.5%	
Grade 3	53.3%	55.1%	
Unknown grade	17.0%	17.2%	
Measurable disease	63.3%	60.3%	
Tumor size >5 cm	17.7%	19.1%	
Surgery for this relapse	19.6%	18.7%	
Treatment delivery			
Completed 6 cycles	77%	85%	$P<.001$
Completed 9 cycles	7%	8%	
Median duration of treatment	16 weeks	21 weeks	
Delay >7 days	5%	7%	
D/C for toxicity	15%	6%	$P<.001$
Efficacy			
Median PFS	9.4 months	11.3 months	HR 0.82 (95% CI, 0.72-0.94)
Progression by RECIST	80%	79%	
Progression by CA125	20%	21%	

(continued)

Table 5.7 Results of CALYPSO *(continued)*

Treatment arm	Paclitaxel and carboplatin (CP) N=507	PLD and carboplatin (CD) N=466	Statistics
Toxicity			
Deaths during protocol	N=1	N=5	
Worse with CP			
G3/4 nonheme toxicity	36.8%	28.4%	$P<.001$
≥G2 neurosensory	26.9%	4.9%	$P<.001$
≥G2 arthralgia/myalgia	19.2%	4.0%	$P<.001$
Allergic/hypersensitivity	18.8%	5.6%	$P<.001$
Alopecia	83.6%	7%	$P<.001$
G3/4 neutropenia	45.7%	35.2%	$P<.01$
Worse with CD			
Hand-foot syndrome, PPE	2.2%	12%	$P<.001$
G3/4 thrombocytopenia	6.2%	15.9%	$P<.001$
≥G2 mucositis	7.0%	13.9%	$P<.001$
≥G2 nausea	24.2%	35.2%	$P<.001$
≥G2 vomiting	15.6%	22.5%	$P<.001$

CA125, cancer antigen 125; CI, confidence interval; D/C, discontinue; G, grade; HR, hazard ratio; PFS, progression-free survival; PLD, pegylated liposomal doxorubicin; PPE, palmar-plantar erythrodysesthesia; RECIST, Response Evaluation Criteria in Solid Tumors.

- ○ Toxicities of CD included a greater degree of mucositis, nausea, vomiting, and PPE. These side effects were generally short term and manageable.
- ○ The addition of PLD to carboplatin appears to reduce the risk of hypersensitivity reactions (HSR) to carboplatin. The rate of HSR with carboplatin retreatment alone is 23% (Alberts et al. 2008a). The mechanism for this reduced effect is unknown.
- This trial was designed to be a noninferiority trial but actually demonstrated superiority of CD over CP. Testing for superiority in the setting on noninferiority is considered acceptable.
- PFS is considered a valid endpoint for recurrent platinum-sensitive ovarian cancer (du Bois et al. 2005b; Bast et al. 2007). PFS reflects tumor shrinkage and disease stabilization effects and is not confounded by the impact of subsequent treatment as the OS endpoint can be.
- Aside from treatment arm, other covariates that predicted improved PFS included therapy-free interval >12 months (HR, 0.56; 95% CI, 0.48-0.65), lack of measurable disease, and CA125 <100.

- Possible explanations for improved PFS with carboplatin and PLD:
  - Carboplatin appears to enhance the activity of PLD. CD has superior OS to carboplatin alone in platinum-sensitive ovarian cancer in a small randomized controlled trial (26 vs 18 months, $P=.02$) (Alberts et al. 2008a).
  - Duration of therapy was longer with CD (21 vs 16 weeks) because the interval between cycles was longer (4 vs 3 weeks) and because of lower toxicity-related treatment discontinuations. The time from end of treatment to progression was almost similar between arms (6.7 months for CD, 5.9 months for CP).

OCEANS (Aghajanian, JCO 2012)

REFERENCE

- Aghajanian C, et al. OCEANS: a randomized, double-blind, placebo-controlled phase III trial of chemotherapy with or without bevacizumab in patients with platinum-sensitive recurrent epithelial ovarian, primary peritoneal, or fallopian tube cancer. *J Clin Oncol.* 2012;30(17):2039-2045. PMID: 22529265. (Aghajanian et al. 2012)

TRIAL SPONSOR

- Genentech, South San Francisco, CA

RATIONALE FOR TRIAL

- Patients with platinum-sensitive recurrent ovarian cancer (relapse ≥6 months from initial platinum-based therapy) are usually retreated with platinum-based chemotherapy (Parmar et al. 2003; Pfisterer et al. 2006a; Pujade-Lauraine et al. 2010).
- The combination of gemcitabine and carboplatin (GC) was approved for use in platinum-sensitive ovarian cancer in 2004 in Europe and in 2006 in the United States based on an intergroup (AGO-OVAR/NCIC-CTG/EORTC) phase III study (Pfisterer et al. 2006a). Compared to carboplatin alone, the combination of gemcitabine with carboplatin improved progression-free survival from 5.8 months to 8.6 months (HR, 0.72; 95% CI, 0.58-0.90; $P=.0031$) (Pfisterer et al. 2006a).
- Bevacizumab is a monoclonal antibody targeting vascular endothelial growth factor (VEGF-A) and has demonstrated activity in phase II studies in recurrent ovarian cancer.

- GOG 170D treated 62 patients who had received 1 to 2 prior regimens (platinum sensitive or platinum resistant) with single-agent bevacizumab at 15 mg/kg every 3 weeks and showed an objective response rate of 21% and a median duration of response of 10.3 months. Forty percent of patients were progression free at 6 months (Burger et al. 2007).
- In a single-arm study evaluating bevacizumab with metronomic cyclophosphamide, 70 patients who had received 1 to 3 prior regimens (platinum sensitive or platinum resistant) demonstrated a 24% objective response rate and 56% of patients were progression free at 6 months (Garcia et al. 2008). Four patients (5.7%) had a gastrointestinal (GI) perforation or fistula.
- Forty-four patients with platinum-refractory or platinum-resistant ovarian cancer, recurrence after 2 to 3 prior regimens, and progression during or within 3 months of topotecan or pegylated liposomal doxorubicin showed a response rate of 15.9%, and 27.8% of patients were progression free at 6 months (Cannistra et al. 2007). While single-agent bevacizumab was active in this heavily pretreated population, there were 5 GI perforations (11%), leading to early closure of this study.
- Based on data demonstrating efficacy of bevacizumab in recurrent ovarian cancer, OCEANS (Ovarian Cancer Study Comparing Efficacy and Safety of Chemotherapy and Anti-Angiogenic Therapy in Platinum-Sensitive Recurrent Disease) was designed as a randomized, double-blind, phase III trial to compare GC to GC + bevacizumab in patients with platinum-sensitive ovarian cancer.

PATIENT POPULATION
- N = 484 randomized.
- Enrollment from April 2007 to January 2010.

Inclusion Criteria
- Recurrent ovarian cancer with disease progression ≥6 months after completion of front-line platinum-based chemotherapy.
- Measurable disease according to RECIST version 1.0 (Therasse et al. 2000).
- ECOG status of 0 or 1 (Oken et al. 1982).
- Life expectancy of at least 12 weeks.
- Adequate bone marrow, coagulation, renal, and hepatic function.

Exclusion Criteria
- Prior chemotherapy for recurrent ovarian cancer.
- Prior treatment with bevacizumab or other VEGF pathway-targeted therapy.
- Other malignancies within 5 years (unless low risk of recurrence).
- History of abdominal fistula, GI perforation, or intra-abdominal abscess.
- Clinical signs or symptoms of GI obstruction.
- Requirement for parenteral hydration or nutrition.
- Nonhealing wound, ulcer, or bone fracture.
- Bleeding diatheses or significant coagulopathy.
- Known central nervous system (CNS) disease (except for treated brain metastases).
- Clinically significant cardiovascular disease.
- Major surgical procedure within 28 days of enrollment or anticipated surgery during course of study.

TREATMENT DETAILS
- Dosing matched to AGO-OVAR-NCIC CTG-EORTC trial (Pfisterer et al. 2006).

Arm 1: Gemcitabine + Carboplatin + Placebo (GC + PL).
- Gemcitabine 1000 mg/m^2 on days 1 and 8.
- Carboplatin area under the curve 4 mg/mL/min on day 1 based on the Calvert formula.
- Placebo on day 1 or each cycle, administered before GC.
- Cycles repeated every 21 days.

Arm 2: Gemcitabine + Carboplatin + Bevacizumab (GC + BV).
- Gemcitabine 1000 mg/m^2 on days 1 and 8.
- Carboplatin area under the curve 4 mg/mL/min on day 1 based on the Calvert formula.
- Bevacizumab 15 mg/kg IV on day 1 or each cycle, administered before GC.
- Cycles repeated every 21 days.

Additional Treatment Details
- Patients received 6 cycles but were allowed to receive up to 10 cycles if continued response was seen.

- After completion of GC, placebo or bevacizumab was continued until progressive disease or unacceptable toxicity.

Treatment Modifications
- Day 1 treatment held if ANC <1500, hemoglobin <8.5, or platelets <100,000 within 24 hours of scheduled treatment.
- Cycles could be delayed for a maximum of 3 weeks until minimum values achieved.
- Day 8 gemcitabine dose modifications were made per the package insert.
- Bevacizumab or placebo could be held for toxicity for a maximum of 6 weeks. Beyond 6 weeks, bevacizumab was discontinued.
- If a component of therapy was discontinued for toxicity, the other components could still be administered per protocol.

ASSESSMENTS
- CT scan every 9 weeks from day 1 of cycle 1, regardless of treatment delay or discontinuation. Radiologic evaluation was done according to RECIST 1.0.
- Progression could be determined clinically but not by CA125 elevation alone.
- Toxicity was graded according to the CTCAE version 3.0.
- Patients were observed for adverse events for 30 days after treatment discontinuation and survival every 3 months until death.

ENDPOINTS
- PFS, as determined by investigators (primary endpoint).
- Overall response rate.
- Overall survival.
- Duration of response.

STATISTICAL CONSIDERATIONS

Stratification Factors
- Time from last platinum treatment to recurrence (6-12 months, >12 months).
- Cytoreductive surgery for recurrence (yes, no).

Sample Size
- Approximately 317 progression events were required to detect a PFS HR of 0.73 in favor of the bevacizumab arm with a 2-sided α of .05 and 80% power.

Statistical Tests

- Kaplan-Meier test (Kaplan and Meier 1958) was used to estimate the median PFS and duration of response (DOR) for each treatment group.
- The Brookmeyer-Crowley method (Brookmeyer and Crowley 1982) was used to construct 95% confidence intervals for median values.
- The Cox regression model was used to estimate the stratified HR.
- A 2-sided stratified log-rank test was used to compare between groups..
- The Cochran-Mantel-Haenszel test was used to compare response rates.
- Efficacy analyses were performed on the intent-to-treat population.
- Safety analyses were performed on all patients who received at least 1 partial dose of any part of protocol treatment.
- Study was blinded, but patients could be unblinded at time of progression at the request of the investigator.

Additional Statistical Considerations

- Trial was initiated as a phase II study with extensive safety reviews focused on GI toxicity.
- After approximately 20 patients were accrued to each arm and no perforations were reported after >10 weeks of follow-up, the trial was converted to a phase III trial.

CONCLUSION OF TRIAL

- Gemcitabine, carboplatin (GC) + bevacizumab administered until progression extends progression-free survival compared to GC in patients with platinum-sensitive recurrent ovarian cancer.

COMMENTS

- This is the first randomized phase III study to demonstrate a positive outcome for the addition of a biologic therapy to standard chemotherapy in platinum-sensitive recurrent ovarian cancer.
  - Improvement in PFS.
  - Improvement in ORR.
  - Improvement in DOR.
  - No difference in OS, but data are immature at the time of publication.
  - No new safety concerns, no reports of GI perforation during treatment.
- Subgroup analyses all supported the primary analysis. PFS was superior with bevacizumab for subcategories of age, ECOG performance status, platinum-free interval, and cytoreductive surgery status.

Table 5.8 Results of OCEANS

Treatment arm	GC+PL N=242	GC+BV N=242	Statistics
Patient characteristics			
Median age (range)	61 (28-86)	60 (38-87)	
Time from prior chemotherapy			
6-12 months	42%	41%	
≥12 months	58%	59%	
Serous	83.5%	78.1%	
Endometrioid	6.6.%	5.4%	
Mucinous	0.4%	1.2%	
Clear cell	2.5%	3.7%	
Other	7.0%	11.6%	
Second cytoreduction			
Yes	10%	12%	
No	90%	88%	
Treatment delivery			
Median No. of chemotherapies (range)	6 (1-10)	6 (1-10)	
Median No. of PL or BV (range)	10 (1-36)	12 (1-43)	
Treatment D/C, progression	66.1%	43.0%	
Treatment D/C, HTN	0%	3.6%	
Treatment D/C, proteinuria	0%	2.4%	
Subsequent cancer therapy	88%	84%	
Subsequent bevacizumab	31%	15%	
Efficacy			
Median PFS	8.4 months	12.4 months	HR 0.48 (95% CI, 0.38-0.61)
Overall RR	57.4%	78.5%	$P<.0001$
Duration of response	7.4 months	10.4 months	HR 0.53 (95% CI, 0.41-0.70)
Median OS (immature data)	35.2 months	33.3 months	
Toxicity			
Serious adverse events	24.9%	34.8%	
G3-5 toxicity	82.4%	89.5%	
≥G3 hypertension	0.4%	17.4%	
≥G3 proteinuria	0.9%	8.5%	
RPLS	0%	1.2%	

BV, bevacizumab; CI, confidence interval; D/C, discontinue; GC+BV, gemcitabine and carboplatin+bevacizumab; GC+PL, gemcitabine and carboplatin+placebo; HR, hazard ratio; HTN, hypertension; OS, overall survival; PFS, progression-free survival; PL, placebo; RPLS, reversible posterior leukoencephalopathy syndrome; RR, response rate.

- The overall response rate was 21% higher in the BV arm. The majority of responses were partial responses.
- There was no difference in overall survival, but the data are immature at the time of publication. There was a high degree of data censoring beyond 18 months, and the median OS was longer than expected in both arms.
- Toxicity comments.
  - Proteinuria tended to develop after more extended bevacizumab treatment and was monitored using urine protein-to-creatinine ratio measurements. The median time to development of grade 3 or higher proteinuria was 26.5 months.
  - Three cases of reversible posterior leukoencephalopathy syndrome were reported in the bevacizumab arm: 2 cases were confirmed by magnetic resonance imaging.
  - No GI perforations occurred during study treatment or within the 30-day safety period. Two GI perforations occurred in the bevacizumab arm after the safety period, both at 69 days after study drug discontinuation. Patient 1 received 34 cycles of bevacizumab and developed small bowel obstruction and gastric ulcer perforation at 69 days. Patient 2 received 39 cycles of bevacizumab and developed intestinal perforation at 69 days after study drug discontinuation and after receipt of 1 dose of pegylated liposomal doxorubicin off study.
  - The rates of neutropenia and febrile neutropenia were similar in both arms.
- As ovarian cancer becomes a chronic illness, treatments that prolong PFS and time without cytotoxic chemotherapy are clinically relevant.
- Limitations of OCEANS:
  - Lack of quality-of-life data.
  - Lack of specimen collection for biomarker analysis.
- Strengths of OCEANS:
  - Robustness of primary endpoint with strict adherence to RECIST-defined progression and its supportive independent review committee (IRC) analysis and the schedule of assessments.
  - The 4-month improved PFS is well above the frequency of radiologic assessments (every 9 weeks) (Panageas et al. 2007; Dancey et al. 2009).
- Platinum-based doublets are accepted as the best treatment option for platinum-sensitive recurrent ovarian cancer (ROC) based on ICON4,

AGO-OVAR-NCIC CTG-EORTC, and CALYPSO (Caelyx in Platinum Sensitive Ovarian Patients) trials (Parmar et al. 2003; Pfisterer et al. 2006a; Pujade-Lauraine et al. 2010). Data from OCEANS suggest that the addition of bevacizumab to the GC doublet improves outcomes.
- ICON4 and CALYPSO differ from OCEANS based on inclusion of nonmeasurable and CA125-evaluable disease, allowed length of cytotoxic chemotherapy, assessment modalities, assessment intervals and method to determine progression. These factors influence survival.

AURELIA (Pujade-Lauraine, JCO 2014)

REFERENCE

- Pujade-Lauraine E, et al. Bevacizumab combined with chemotherapy for platinum-resistant recurrent ovarian cancer: The AURELIA open-label randomized phase III trial. *J Clin Oncol.* 2014;32(13):1302-1308. PMID: 24637997. (Pujade-Lauraine et al. 2014)

TRIAL SPONSOR

- Written on behalf of the European Network of Gynaecological Oncological Trial Groups (ENGOT)–Gynecologic Cancer Intergroup (GCIG) investigators
- Sponsored by F. Hoffmann-La Roche (Basel, Switzerland), which also provided third-party writing assistance

RATIONALE FOR TRIAL

- Approximately 25% of patients with advanced ovarian cancer have first relapse within 6 months of primary platinum-based chemotherapy and are classified as having platinum-resistant disease. Almost all patients with recurrent ovarian cancer eventually develop platinum resistance.
- The most active single agents for platinum-resistant disease are PLD, paclitaxel, and topotecan (Gordon et al. 2001; Buda et al. 2004; Mutch et al. 2007; Vergote et al. 2009).
- Median overall survival is approximately 12 months for platinum-resistant ovarian cancer (Naumann and Coleman 2011).
- Combined chemotherapy appears to increase toxicity without improving efficacy (Buda et al. 2004; Sehouli et al. 2008; Lortholary et al. 2012).

- An alternative treatment strategy is to combine single-agent chemotherapy with a biologic therapy.
- Bevacizumab.
  - Is a monoclonal antibody that targets all isoforms of VEGF-A.
  - Has activity in platinum-resistant ovarian cancer as a monotherapy (Burger et al. 2007; Cannistra et al. 2007) and combined with chemotherapy (Garcia et al. 2008; McGonigle et al. 2011).
- AURELIA (Avastin Use in Platinum-Resistant Epithelial Ovarian Cancer) is a randomized trial evaluating the combination of bevacizumab and chemotherapy in platinum-resistant ovarian cancer.

PATIENT POPULATION
- N=361 enrolled.
- Enrolled between October 2009 and April 2011.
- Histologically confirmed epithelial ovarian, fallopian tube, or primary peritoneal cancer.
- Measurable disease by RECIST version 1.0 or assessable by GCIG CA-125 response criteria.
- Progression within 6 months of completing ≥4 cycles of platinum-based therapy.

Inclusion Criteria
- Age ≥18 years.
- ECOG performance status ≤2.
- Adequate liver, renal, and bone marrow function.

Exclusion Criteria.
- Strict exclusion criteria were defined to reduce the risk of GI perforation, which was a concern in patients with heavily pretreated ovarian cancer (Cannistra et al. 2007).
- More than 2 prior anticancer regimens.
- Refractory disease (progression during previous platinum-containing therapy).
- Risk factors for bowel complications.
  - History of bowel obstruction (including subocclusive disease) related to disease.
  - History of abdominal fistula.
  - History of GI perforation.
  - History of intra-abdominal abscess.

- Evidence of rectosigmoid involvement by pelvic examination.
  - Bowel involvement seen on computed tomography.
  - Clinical symptoms of bowel obstruction.
- Prior radiotherapy to the pelvis or abdomen.
- Surgery (including open biopsy) within 4 weeks of study therapy (within 24 hours if a minor surgical procedure).
- Anticipated need for major surgery during study treatment.
- Current or recent treatment with another investigational drug within 30 days of first study dose.
- Untreated CNS symptoms or symptomatic CNS metastasis.
- History or evidence of thrombotic or hemorrhagic disorders within 6 months before first study treatment.
- Uncontrolled hypertension.
- Active clinically significant cardiovascular disease.
- Nonhealing wound, ulcer, or bone fracture.

TREATMENT DETAILS

Standard Chemotherapy Selection

- Investigator choice of single-agent chemotherapy with appropriate premedications.
  - Paclitaxel 80 mg/m^2 IV on days 1, 8, 15, and 22 every 4 weeks.
  - PLD 40 mg/m^2 IV on day 1 every 4 weeks.
  - Topotecan 4 mg/m^2 IV on days 1, 8, and 15 every 4 weeks.
  - Topotecan 1.25 mg/m^2 IV on days 1 to 5 every 3 weeks.
- After chemotherapy regimen was selected, patients were randomized to chemotherapy vs chemotherapy plus bevacizumab.
- Chemotherapy and bevacizumab were continued until disease progression, unacceptable toxicity, or withdrawal of consent.
- Investigator selection of chemotherapy was evenly distributed due to capping of the cohorts.
  - PLD, n = 126, complete accrual in October 2010.
  - Paclitaxel, n = 115, complete accrual in April 2011.
  - Topotecan, n = 120, complete accrual in April 2011.

Arm 1: Chemotherapy Alone (CT)

Arm 2: Chemotherapy Plus Bevacizumab (BEV-CT)

- Bevacizumab 10 mg/kg every 2 weeks or
- Bevacizumab 15 mg/kg every 3 weeks for patients receiving topotecan every 3 weeks.

Drug Discontinuation
- For patients receiving BEV-CT, if 1 agent was discontinued for toxicity, the other could be continued as a single agent.
- Bevacizumab was discontinued for any grade GI perforation.

Dose Reductions.
- Bevacizumab dose reductions were not allowed.
- Chemotherapy dose modification guidelines were according to standard clinical practice.

Crossovers
- Patients assigned to CT could cross over to single-agent bevacizumab 15 mg/kg every 3 weeks on clear evidence for progression after a careful risk-benefit assessment.
- Patients assigned to BEV-CT received standard-of-care treatment without bevacizumab at progression.

ASSESSMENTS
- Imaging studies.
  - At baseline and every 8 weeks (or every 9 weeks for patients receiving topotecan every 3 weeks), using the same technique. Computed tomography and magnetic resonance imaging (in case of contrast allergy) were the preferred imaging modalities.
  - Reponses were confirmed by computed tomography scan at least 4 weeks after the first response.
- Follow-up: patients were observed for survival for ≥12 months.
- Safety: assessed before each cycle and within 30 days of completing treatment.
- Adverse events: graded according to the NCI CTCAE (version 3.0).

ENDPOINTS
- Investigator-assessed PFS by RECIST—defined as the interval between randomization and first radiologically documented disease progression or death (primary endpoint).
- ORR by RECIST (version 1.0) alone, GCIG CA-125 criteria alone, or both criteria combined.
- OS.
- Safety.
- Tolerability.
- Quality of life.

STATISTICAL CONSIDERATIONS.

Stratification Factors
- Selected chemotherapy (PLD vs paclitaxel vs topotecan).
- Prior antiangiogenic therapy (yes vs no).
- Platinum-free interval (<3 months vs 3-6 months).

Sample Size
- Initially, a sample size of 300 patients was planned so that 228 progression events would provide 80% power with a 1-sided log-rank test at an α of .05, assuming a hazard ratio of 0.72 corresponding to a median PFS of 4.0 months with CT vs 5.56 months with BEV-CT.
- The sample size was increased to 332 patients to provide 80% power to detect a PFS HR of 0.70 with a 2-sided log-rank test with an α of 0.05 after 247 events, assuming a median PFS of 4.0 months with CT and 5.7 months with BEV-CT.
- The independent data monitoring committee (IDMC) recommended the sample size be increased to ≥360 patients with a primary analysis planned after 290 PFS events based on an HR of 0.72 and 80% power.

Statistical Tests
- Unstratified 2-sided log-rank test used to compare PFS between the 2 treatment arms.
- Stratified 2-sided log-rank test was used for the post hoc analysis.
- Exploratory analyses of safety and efficacy were prespecified for the subgroup of patients with ascites at baseline.
- Post hoc analyses were performed to determine the proportion of patients undergoing paracentesis during study therapy.

CONCLUSION OF TRIAL
- In patients with platinum-resistant ovarian cancer, the addition of bevacizumab to chemotherapy significantly improves PFS and ORR. OS is not improved, and no new safety signals for bevacizumab have been observed. This should be considered a standard treatment option for platinum-resistant ovarian cancer.

COMMENTS
- This is the first randomized phase III trial to demonstrate a PFS advantage with combined therapy compared to single-agent therapy.
  - The benefit to PFS was seen across all subgroup analyses.

Table 5.9 Results of AURELIA

Treatment arm	Chemotherapy alone N = 182	Chemotherapy plus bevacizumab N = 179	Statistics
Patient characteristics			
Median age (range)	61 (25-84)	62 (25-80)	
<3 months, prior chemotherapy	25%	28%	
Two prior chemotherapies	43%	40%	
Prior antiangiogenic	8%	7%	
Serous/adenocarcinoma	84%	87%	
Endometrioid	5%	5%	
Clear cell	7%	2%	
Grade 1	5%	6%	
Grade 2	26%	30%	
Grade 3	58%	53%	
Unknown grade	11%	12%	
Measurable disease	79%	80%	
Ascites	30%	33%	
Treatment delivery			
Median duration	3 cycles (range 1-17)	6 cycles (range 1-24)	
Efficacy			
Median PFS	3.4 months	6.7 months	HR 0.48 (95% CI, 0.38-0.60)
ORR	12.6%	30.9%	$P<.001$
ORR, RECIST alone	11.8%	27.3%	$P=.001$
ORR, GCIG CA125 alone	11.6%	31.8%	$P<.001$
Median OS	13.3 months	16.6 months	HR 0.85 (95% CI, 0.66, 1.08)
Required paracentesis	17%	2%	
Toxicity			
AE, special interest	40.3%	57.0%	
≥G2 hypertension	7%	20%	
≥G2 proteinuria	0%	2%	
≥G2 GI perforation	0%	2%	
≥G2 fistula, abscess	0%	2%	
Arterial thrombosis	0%	2%	
Venous thrombosis	4%	3%	

AE, adverse event; CA125, cancer antigen 125; CI, confidence interval; GCIG, Gynecologic Cancer InterGroup; HR, hazard ratio; ORR, overall response rate; OS, overall survival; PFS, progression-free survival; RECIST, Response Evaluation Criteria in Solid Tumors.

- Chemotherapy exposure was greater in the BEV-CT arm, reflecting the longer PFS.
- The trial was not powered to detect a difference in OS, and crossover to bevacizumab was allowed.
  - At the time of data cutoff for OS analysis, 40% of patients in the CT arm had crossed over to receive bevacizumab after progression on CT alone.
- The addition of bevacizumab appears to improve the control of ascites.
- The 2.2% rate of GI perforation is lower than previously reported (Cannistra et al. 2007; Simpkins et al. 2007).
  - Strict exclusion criteria were used to ensure high-risk patients were not enrolled.
- Safety of bevacizumab.
  - Higher rates of grade ≥2 hypertension and proteinuria.
  - No new safety signals.
  - The higher cumulative incidence of peripheral neuropathy and HFS in the bevacizumab-containing arm likely reflects the longer chemotherapy exposure and longer PFS.
- The AURELIA results add to the literature demonstrating improved PFS with the addition of bevacizumab to chemotherapy.
  - GOG 218 (Burger et al. 2011).
  - ICON7 (Perren et al. 2011).
  - OCEANS (Aghajanian et al. 2012).
- The utility of bevacizumab use after relapse and front-line bevacizumab containing therapy is unknown.
  - In AURELIA, only 7% of patients received prior antiangiogenic therapy, so no conclusions can be drawn from this study.
  - In colorectal cancer, survival is improved with second-line bevacizumab use (Bennouna et al. 2013).
- Criticisms of trial.
  - Potential for bias as PFS was determined by investigators.
  - No third arm with bevacizumab alone.
- Patient-reported outcomes are described in an accompanying article (Stockler et al. 2014).

Abbreviations

AACR	American Association for Cancer Research
ACTION	Adjuvant ChemoTherapy in Ovarian Neoplasm Trial
AGO	Arbeitsgemeinschaft Gynakologische Onkologie
AGO-OVAR	Arbeitsgemeinscharft Gynakologische Onkologie Studieengrupp Ovarialkarzinom
ALP	Alkaline phosphatase
ALT	Alanine aminotransferase
ANC	Absolute neutrophil count
ANZGOG	Australia New Zealand Gynaecological Oncology Group
ASCO	American Society of Clinical Oncology
AST	Aspartate aminotransferase
AUC	Area under the curve
AURELIA	Avastin Use in Platinum-Resistant Epithelial Ovarian Cancer
BEV	Bevacizumab
BSA	Bovine serum albumin
BUN	Blood urea nitrogen
CA125	Cancer Antigen 125
CALYPSO	Caelyx in Platinum Sensitive Ovarian Patients
CAP	Cyclophosphamide (C), doxorubicin/Adriamycin (A), cisplatin (P)
CBC	Complete blood count
CD	Carboplatin and pegylated liposomal doxorubicin
CEA	Carcinoembryonic antigen
CI	Confidence interval
CNS	Central nervous system
CP	Cyclophosphamide (C), cisplatin (P)

CR	Complete response
CTCAE	Common Toxicity Criteria for Adverse Events
CT scan	Computed tomography scan
DCR	Disease control rate
D5W	5% dextrose in water
DOR	Duration of response
ECG	Electrocardiogram
ECHO	Echocardiogram
ECOG	Eastern Cooperative Oncology Group
EDTA	Ethylenediaminetetraacetic acid
ENGOT	European Network of Gynaecological Oncological Trial Groups
EORTC	European Organization for Research and Treatment of Cancer
FACT-O	Functional Assessment of Cancer Therapy—Ovarian
FDA	Food and Drug Administration
FIGO	International Federation of Gynecology and Obstetrics
FLIC	Functional Living Index–Cancer
GC	Gemcitabine and carboplatin
GCIG	Gynecologic Cancer InterGroup
G-CSF	Granulocyte colony-stimulating factor
GEICO	Grupo Espanol de Investigacion en Cancer de Ovario
GFR	Glomerular filtration rate
GI	Gastrointestinal
GICOG	Gruppo Interregionale Collaborativo in Oncologico Ginecologia
GINECO	Groupe d'Investigateurs Nationaux pour l'Etude des Cancers Ovariens
GM-CSF	Granulocyte macrophage colony-stimulating factor
GOG	Gynecologic Oncology Group
HFS	Hand-foot syndrome
HR	Hazard ratio
HSR	Hypersensitivity reaction
ICON	International Collaborative Ovarian Neoplasm
IDMC	Independent Data Monitoring Committee
IL-6	Interleukin 6
IP	Intraperitoneal
IRC	Independent review committee
IRFMN	Instituto Mario Negri, Milan, Italy
ITG	Integrated Therapeutics Group

Abbreviations

IV	Intravenous
JGOG	Japanese Gynecologic Oncology Group
LMP	Low malignant potential
LVEF	Left ventricular ejection fraction
MaNGO	Mario Negri Gynecologic Oncology
MITO	Multicentre Italian Trials in Ovarian Cancer
MRC CTU	Clinical Trials Unit of the Medical Research Council
MRI	Magnetic resonance imaging
MTD	Maximum tolerated dose
NCCTG	North Central Cancer Treatment Group
NCI	National Cancer Institute
NCIC	National Cancer Institute of Canada
NCI-C-CTG	National Cancer Institute of Canada Clinical Trials Group
NMR	Nuclear magnetic resonance
NOCOVA	Nordic Gynecological Cancer Study Group
NS	Not significant
NSGO	Nordic Society for Gynecologic Oncology
OCEANS	Ovarian Cancer Study Comparing Efficacy and Safety of Chemotherapy and Anti-Angiogenic Therapy in Platinum-Sensitive Recurrent Disease
ORR	Overall response rate
OS	Overall survival
pCR	Pathologic complete response
PD	Progressive disease
PFS	Progression-free survival
PLD	Pegylated liposomal doxorubicin
PPE	Palmar-plantar erythrodysesthesia
PR	Partial response
PS	Papillary serous
PT	Paclitaxel plus cisplatin
QLQ	Quality-of-life questionnaires
QOL	Quality of life
RCOG	Royal College of Obstetricians and Gynaecologists
RECIST	Response Evaluation Criteria in Solid Tumors
RFS	Recurrence-free survival
ROC	Recurrent ovarian cancer
RR	Response rate

SAAK	Swiss Group for Clinical Cancer Research
SD	Stable disease
SWOG	Southwest Oncology Group
TC	Paclitaxel plus carboplatin
ULN	Upper limit of normal
VEGF	Vascular endothelial growth factor
WHO	World Health Organization

References

Aaronson NK, Ahmedzai S, Bergman B, et al. (1993). The European Organization for Research and Treatment of Cancer QLQ-C30: a quality-of-life instrument for use in international clinical trials in oncology. *J Natl Cancer Inst.* 85(5):365-376.

Aghajanian C, Blank SV, Goff BA, et al. (2012). OCEANS: a randomized, double-blind, placebo-controlled phase III trial of chemotherapy with or without bevacizumab in patients with platinum-sensitive recurrent epithelial ovarian, primary peritoneal, or fallopian tube cancer. *J Clin Oncol.* 30(17):2039-2045.

A'Hern RP, Gore ME (1995). Impact of doxorubicin on survival in advanced ovarian cancer. *J Clin Oncol.* 13(3):726-732.

Alberts DS, Green S, Hannigan EV, et al. (1992). Improved therapeutic index of carboplatin plus cyclophosphamide versus cisplatin plus cyclophosphamide: final report by the Southwest Oncology Group of a phase III randomized trial in stages III and IV ovarian cancer. *J Clin Oncol.* 10(5):706-717.

Alberts DS, Liu PY, Hannigan EV, et al. (1996). Intraperitoneal cisplatin plus intravenous cyclophosphamide versus intravenous cisplatin plus intravenous cyclophosphamide for stage III ovarian cancer. *N Engl J Med.* 335(26):1950-1955.

Alberts DS, Liu PY, Wilczynski SP, et al.; Southwest Oncology Group (2008a). Randomized trial of pegylated liposomal doxorubicin (PLD) plus carboplatin versus carboplatin in platinum-sensitive (PS) patients with recurrent epithelial ovarian or peritoneal carcinoma after failure of initial platinum-based chemotherapy (Southwest Oncology Group Protocol S0200). *Gynecol Oncol.* 108(1):90-94.

Alberts DS, Markman M, Armstrong D, Rothenberg ML, Muggia F, Howell SB (2002). Intraperitoneal therapy for stage III ovarian cancer: a therapy whose time has come! *J Clin Oncol.* 20(19):3944-3946.

Alberts DS, Marth C, Alvarez RD, et al.; Consortium GCT (2008b). Randomized phase 3 trial of interferon gamma-1b plus standard carboplatin/paclitaxel versus carboplatin/paclitaxel alone for first-line treatment of advanced ovarian and primary peritoneal carcinomas: results from a prospectively designed analysis of progression-free survival. *Gynecol Oncol.* 109(2):174-181.

Ando M, Minami H, Ando Y, et al. (2000). Multi-institutional validation study of carboplatin dosing formula using adjusted serum creatinine level. *Clin Cancer Res.* 6(12):4733-4738.

Ang C, Chan KK, Bryant A, Naik R, Dickinson HO (2011). Ultra-radical (extensive) surgery versus standard surgery for the primary cytoreduction of advanced epithelial ovarian cancer. *Cochrane Database Syst Rev.* 4:CD007697.

Armstrong D, Rowinsky E, Donehower R, et al. (1995). A phase II trial of topotecan as salvage therapy in epithelial ovarian cancer. *Proc Am Soc Clin Oncol.* 14:A769 (abstr).

Armstrong DK, Bundy B, Wenzel L, et al.; Gynecologic Oncology Group (2006). Intraperitoneal cisplatin and paclitaxel in ovarian cancer. *N Engl J Med.* 354(1):34-43.

Bagri A, Berry L, Gunter B, et al. (2010). Effects of anti-VEGF treatment duration on tumor growth, tumor regrowth, and treatment efficacy. *Clin Cancer Res.* 16(15):3887-3900.

Bajetta E, Di Leo A, Biganzoli L, et al. (1996). Phase II study of vinorelbine in patients with pretreated advanced ovarian cancer: activity in platinum-resistant disease. *J Clin Oncol.* 14(9):2546-2551.

Baker TR, Piver MS, Hempling RE (1993). The addition of etoposide and ifosfamide to cisplatin as second line therapy in ovarian carcinoma. *Eur J Gynaecol Oncol.* 14(1):18-22.

Basen-Engquist K, Bodurka-Bevers D, Fitzgerald MA, et al. (2001). Reliability and validity of the functional assessment of cancer therapy-ovarian. *J Clin Oncol.* 19(6):1809-1817.

Bast RC, Thigpen JT, Arbuck SG, et al. (2007). Clinical trial endpoints in ovarian cancer: report of an FDA/ASCO/AACR Public Workshop. *Gynecol Oncol.* 107(2):173-176.

Bell J, Brady MF, Young RC, et al.; Gynecologic Oncology Group (2006). Randomized phase III trial of three versus six cycles of adjuvant carboplatin and paclitaxel in early stage epithelial ovarian carcinoma: a Gynecologic Oncology Group study. *Gynecol Oncol.* 102(3):432-439.

Benedet JL, Bender H, Jones H III, Ngan HY, Pecorelli S (2000). FIGO staging classifications and clinical practice guidelines in the management of gynecologic cancers. FIGO Committee on Gynecologic Oncology. *Int J Gynaecol Obstet.* 70(2):209-262.

Bennouna J, Sastre J, Arnold D, et al.; Investigators MLS (2013). Continuation of bevacizumab after first progression in metastatic colorectal cancer (ML18147): a randomised phase 3 trial. *Lancet Oncol.* 14(1):29-37.

Bertelsen K, Grenman S, Rustin GJ (1999). How long should first-line chemotherapy continue? *Ann Oncol.* 10(suppl 1):17-20.

Bertelsen K, Jakobsen A, Andersen JE, et al. (1987). A randomized study of cyclophosphamide and cis-platinum with or without doxorubicin in advanced ovarian carcinoma. *Gynecol Oncol.* 28(2):161-169.

Bertelsen K, Jakobsen A, Stroyer J, et al. (1993). A prospective randomized comparison of 6 and 12 cycles of cyclophosphamide, adriamycin, and cisplatin in advanced epithelial ovarian cancer: a Danish Ovarian Study Group trial (DACOVA). *Gynecol Oncol.* 49(1):30-36.

Bjorkholm E, Pettersson F, Einhorn N, Krebs I, Nilsson B, Tjernberg B (1982). Long-term follow-up and prognostic factors in ovarian carcinoma: the radiumhemmet series 1958 to 1973. *Acta Radiol Oncol.* 21(6):413-419.

Bolis G, Colombo N, Pecorelli S, et al. (1995). Adjuvant treatment for early epithelial ovarian cancer: results of two randomised clinical trials comparing cisplatin to no further treatment or chromic phosphate (32P). G.I.C.O.G.: Gruppo Interregionale Collaborativo in Ginecologia Oncologica. *Ann Oncol.* 6(9):887-893.

Bolis G, Scarfone G, Giardina G, et al.; Associazione per la Ricerca in Ginecologia Oncologia Study Group (2001). Carboplatin alone vs carboplatin plus epidoxorubicin as second-line therapy for cisplatin- or carboplatin-sensitive ovarian cancer. *Gynecol Oncol.* 81(1):3-9.

Bookman MA, Brady MF, McGuire WP, et al. (2009). Evaluation of new platinum-based treatment regimens in advanced-stage ovarian cancer: a phase III trial of the Gynecologic Cancer Intergroup. *J Clin Oncol.* 27(9):1419-1425. [Erratum, *J Clin Oncol.* 2009;1427:2305]

Bookman MA, Malmstrom H, Bolis G, et al. (1998). Topotecan for the treatment of advanced epithelial ovarian cancer: an open-label phase II study in patients treated after prior chemotherapy that contained cisplatin or carboplatin and paclitaxel. *J Clin Oncol.* 16(10):3345-3352.

Bookman MA, McGuire WP III, Kilpatrick D, et al. (1996). Carboplatin and paclitaxel in ovarian carcinoma: a phase I study of the Gynecologic Oncology Group. *J Clin Oncol.* 14(6):1895-1902.

Brewer CA, Blessing JA, Nagourney RA, Morgan M, Hanjani P (2006). Cisplatin plus gemcitabine in platinum-refractory ovarian or primary peritoneal cancer: a phase II study of the Gynecologic Oncology Group. *Gynecol Oncol.* 103(2):446-450.

Bristow RE, Chi DS (2006). Platinum-based neoadjuvant chemotherapy and interval surgical cytoreduction for advanced ovarian cancer: a meta-analysis. *Gynecol Oncol*. 103(3):1070-1076.

Bristow RE, Tomacruz RS, Armstrong DK, Trimble EL, Montz FJ (2002). Survival effect of maximal cytoreductive surgery for advanced ovarian carcinoma during the platinum era: a meta-analysis. *J Clin Oncol*. 20(5):1248-1259.

Brookmeyer R, Crowley J (1982). A confidence interval for the median survival time. *Biometrics*. 1:29-41.

Browder T, Butterfield CE, Kraling BM, et al. (2000). Antiangiogenic scheduling of chemotherapy improves efficacy against experimental drug-resistant cancer. *Cancer Res*. 60(7):1878-1886.

Buda A, Floriani I, Rossi R, et al. (2004). Randomised controlled trial comparing single agent paclitaxel vs epidoxorubicin plus paclitaxel in patients with advanced ovarian cancer in early progression after platinum-based chemotherapy: an Italian Collaborative Study from the Mario Negri Institute, Milan, G.O.N.O. (Gruppo Oncologico Nord Ovest) group and I.O.R. (Istituto Oncologico Romagnolo) group. *Br J Cancer*. 90(11):2112-2117.

Burger RA, Brady MF, Bookman MA, et al.; Gynecologic Oncology Group (2011). Incorporation of bevacizumab in the primary treatment of ovarian cancer. *N Engl J Med*. 365(26):2473-2483.

Burger RA, Sill MW, Monk BJ, Greer BE, Sorosky JI (2007). Phase II trial of bevacizumab in persistent or recurrent epithelial ovarian cancer or primary peritoneal cancer: a Gynecologic Oncology Group Study. *J Clin Oncol*. 25(33):5165-5171.

Buyse M (1993). Interim analyses, stopping rules and data monitoring in clinical trials in Europe. *Stat Med*. 12(5-6):509-520.

Calvert AH, Newell DR, Gumbrell LA, et al. (1989). Carboplatin dosage: prospective evaluation of a simple formula based on renal function. *J Clin Oncol*. 7(11):1748-1756.

Cannistra SA (1993). Cancer of the ovary. *N Engl J Med*. 329(21):1550-1559.

Cannistra SA, Matulonis UA, Penson RT, et al. (2007). Phase II study of bevacizumab in patients with platinum-resistant ovarian cancer or peritoneal serous cancer. *J Clin Oncol*. 25(33):5180-5186. [Erratum, *J Clin Oncol*. 2008;5126:1773.

Carter NJ, Keam SJ (2007). Trabectedin : a review of its use in the management of soft tissue sarcoma and ovarian cancer. *Drugs*. 67(15):2257-2276.

Chan JK, Tian C, Fleming GF, et al. (2010). The potential benefit of 6 vs. 3 cycles of chemotherapy in subsets of women with early-stage high-risk epithelial ovarian cancer: an exploratory analysis of a Gynecologic Oncology Group study. *Gynecol Oncol*. 116(3):301-306.

References

Chemotherapy in advanced ovarian cancer: an overview of randomised clinical trials. Advanced Ovarian Cancer Trialists Group. (1991). *BMJ.* 303(6807):884-893.

Chiara S, Conte P, Franzone P, et al. (1994). High-risk early-stage ovarian cancer: randomized clinical trial comparing cisplatin plus cyclophosphamide versus whole abdominal radiotherapy. *Am J Clin Oncol.* 17(1):72-76.

Claret L, Girard P, Hoff PM, et al. (2009). Model-based prediction of phase III overall survival in colorectal cancer on the basis of phase II tumor dynamics. *J Clin Oncol.* 27(25):4103-4108.

Cockroft DW, Gault MH (1976). Prediction of creatinine clearance from serum creatinine. *Nephron.* 16(1):31-41.

Colombo N, Guthrie D, Chiari S, et al.; International Collaborative Ovarian Neoplasm c (2003). International Collaborative Ovarian Neoplasm trial 1: a randomized trial of adjuvant chemotherapy in women with early-stage ovarian cancer. *J Natl Cancer Inst.* 95(2):125-132.

Connelly E, Markman M, Kennedy A, et al. (1996). Paclitaxel delivered as a 3-hr infusion with cisplatin in patients with gynecologic cancers: unexpected incidence of neurotoxicity. *Gynecol Oncol.* 62(2):166-168.

Cox DR (1972). Regression models and life tables. *J R Stat Soc B.* 34:187-202.

Crawford SC, Vasey PA, Paul J, Hay A, Davis JA, Kaye SB (2005). Does aggressive surgery only benefit patients with less advanced ovarian cancer? Results from an international comparison within the SCOTROC-1 Trial. *J Clin Oncol.* 23(34):8802-8811. [Erratum, *J Clin Oncol.* 2006;8824:1224]

Creemers GJ, Bolis G, Gore M, et al. (1996). Topotecan, an active drug in the second-line treatment of epithelial ovarian cancer: results of a large European phase II study. *J Clin Oncol.* 14(12):3056-3061.

Cull A, Howat S, Greimel E, et al.; Group EQoL and Scottish Gynaecological Cancer Trials Group (2001). Development of a European Organization for Research and Treatment of Cancer questionnaire module to assess the quality of life of ovarian cancer patients in clinical trials: a progress report. *Eur J Cancer.* 37(1):47-53.

Cyclophosphamide plus cisplatin versus cyclophosphamide, doxorubicin, and cisplatin chemotherapy of ovarian carcinoma: a meta-analysis. The Ovarian Cancer Meta-Analysis Project. (1991). *J Clin Oncol.* 9(9):1668-1674.

D'Agostino G, Amant F, Berteloot P, Scambia G, Vergote I (2003). Phase II study of gemcitabine in recurrent platinum-and paclitaxel-resistant ovarian cancer. *Gynecol Oncol.* 88(3):266-269.

Dancey JE, Dodd LE, Ford R, et al. (2009). Recommendations for the assessment of progression in randomised cancer treatment trials. *Eur J Cancer.* 45(2):281-289.

De Placido S, Scambia G, Di Vagno G, et al. (2004). Topotecan compared with no therapy after response to surgery and carboplatin/paclitaxel in patients with ovarian cancer: Multicenter Italian Trials in Ovarian Cancer (MITO-1) randomized study. *J Clin Oncol.* 22(13):2635-2642.

Decker DG, Fleming TR, Malkasian GD Jr, Webb MJ, Jeffries JA, Edmonson JH (1982). Cyclophosphamide plus cis-platinum in combination: treatment program for stage III or IV ovarian carcinoma. *Obstet Gynecol.* 60(4): 481-487.

Dembo AJ, Bush RS, Beale FA, et al. (1979). Ovarian carcinoma: improved survival following abdominopelvic irradiation in patients with a completed pelvic operation. *Am J Obstet Gynecol.* 134(7):793-800.

Dent SF, Klaassen D, Pater JL, Zee B, Whitehead M (2000). Second primary malignancies following the treatment of early stage ovarian cancer: update of a study by the National Cancer Institute of Canada—Clinical Trials Group (NCIC-CTG). *Ann Oncol.* 11(1):65-68.

Dizon DS, Hensley ML, Poynor EA, et al. (2002). Retrospective analysis of carboplatin and paclitaxel as initial second-line therapy for recurrent epithelial ovarian carcinoma: application toward a dynamic disease state model of ovarian cancer. *J Clin Oncol.* 20(5):1238-1247.

Donald S, Verschoyle RD, Greaves P, et al. (2003). Complete protection by high-dose dexamethasone against the hepatotoxicity of the novel antitumor drug yondelis (ET-743) in the rat. *Cancer Res.* 63(18):5902-5908.

du Bois A, Belau A, Wagner U, et al.; Arbeitsgemeinschaft Gynaekologische Onkologie Ovarian Cancer Study G (2005a). A phase II study of paclitaxel, carboplatin, and gemcitabine in previously untreated patients with epithelial ovarian cancer FIGO stage IC-IV (AGO-OVAR protocol OVAR-8). *Gynecol Oncol.* 96(2):444-451.

du Bois A, Burges A, Meier W, et al.; Arbeitsgemeinschaft Gynaekologische Onkologie Studiengruppe Ovarialkarzinom (2006a). Pegylated liposomal doxorubicin and carboplatin in advanced gynecologic tumors: a prospective phase I/II study of the Arbeitsgemeinschaft Gynaekologische Onkologie Studiengruppe Ovarialkarzinom (AGO-OVAR). *Ann Oncol.* 17(1):93-96.

du Bois A, Herrstedt J, Hardy-Bessard AC, et al. (2010). Phase III trial of carboplatin plus paclitaxel with or without gemcitabine in first-line treatment of epithelial ovarian cancer. *J Clin Oncol.* 28(27):4162-4169.

du Bois A, Luck HJ, Bauknecht T, et al. (1997). Phase I/II study of the combination of carboplatin and paclitaxel as first-line chemotherapy in patients with advanced epithelial ovarian cancer. *Ann Oncol.* 8(4):355-361.

du Bois A, Luck HJ, Meier W, et al.; Arbeitsgemeinschaft Gynakologische Onkologie Ovarian Cancer Study Group (2003). A randomized clinical trial of cisplatin/paclitaxel versus carboplatin/paclitaxel as first-line treatment of ovarian cancer. *J Natl Cancer Inst.* 95(17):1320-1329.

du Bois A, Luck HJ, Pfisterer J, et al. (2001). Second-line carboplatin and gemcitabine in platinum sensitive ovarian cancer—a dose-finding study by the Arbeitsgemeinschaft Gynakologische Onkologie (AGO) Ovarian Cancer Study Group. *Ann Oncol.* 12(8):1115-1120.

du Bois A, Meier W, Luck HJ, et al. (2002). Chemotherapy versus hormonal treatment in platinum- and paclitaxel-refractory ovarian cancer: a randomised trial of the German Arbeitsgemeinschaft Gynaekologische Onkologie (AGO) Study Group Ovarian Cancer. *Ann Oncol.* 13(2):251-257.

du Bois A, Pfisterer J, Burchardi N, et al.; Arbeitsgemeinschaft Gynaekologische Onkologie Studiengruppe Ovarialkarzinom and Kommission Uterus (2007). Combination therapy with pegylated liposomal doxorubicin and carboplatin in gynecologic malignancies: a prospective phase II study of the Arbeitsgemeinschaft Gynaekologische Onkologie Studiengruppe Ovarialkarzinom (AGO-OVAR) and Kommission Uterus (AGO-K-Ut). *Gynecol Oncol.* 107(3):518-525.

du Bois A, Quinn M, Thigpen T, et al. (2005b). 2004 consensus statements on the management of ovarian cancer: final document of the 3rd International Gynecologic Cancer Intergroup Ovarian Cancer Consensus Conference (GCIG OCCC 2004). *Ann Oncol.* 16(suppl 8):viii7-viii12.

du Bois A, Reuss A, Pujade-Lauraine E, Harter P, Ray-Coquard I, Pfisterer J (2009). Role of surgical outcome as prognostic factor in advanced epithelial ovarian cancer: a combined exploratory analysis of 3 prospectively randomized phase 3 multicenter trials: by the Arbeitsgemeinschaft Gynaekologische Onkologie Studiengruppe Ovarialkarzinom (AGO-OVAR) and the Groupe d'Investigateurs Nationaux Pour les Etudes des Cancers de l'Ovaire (GINECO). *Cancer.* 115(6):1234-1244.

du Bois A, Weber B, Rochon J, et al.; Arbeitsgemeinschaft Gynaekologische Onkologie Ovarian Cancer Study Group, Ovarian Cancer Study Group and Groupe d'Investigateurs Nationaux pour l'Etude des Cancers Ovariens (2006b). Addition of epirubicin as a third drug to carboplatin-paclitaxel in first-line treatment of advanced ovarian cancer: a prospectively randomized gynecologic cancer intergroup trial by the Arbeitsgemeinschaft Gynaekologische Onkologie Ovarian Cancer Study Group and the Groupe d'Investigateurs Nationaux pour l'Etude des Cancers Ovariens. *J Clin Oncol.* 24(7):1127-1135.

Dvorak HF, Nagy JA, Dvorak JT, Dvorak AM (1988). Identification and characterization of the blood vessels of solid tumors that are leaky to circulating macromolecules. *Am J Pathol.* 133(1):95-109.

Einhorn LH, Williams SD, Loehrer PJ, et al. (1989). Evaluation of optimal duration of chemotherapy in favorable-prognosis disseminated germ cell tumors: a Southeastern Cancer Study Group protocol. *J Clin Oncol.* 7(3):387-391.

Einzig AI, Wiernik PH, Sasloff J, Runowicz CD, Goldberg GL (1992). Phase II study and long-term follow-up of patients treated with taxol for advanced ovarian adenocarcinoma. *J Clin Oncol*. 10(11):1748-1753.

Eisenhauer EA, ten Bokkel Huinink WW, Swenerton KD, et al. (1994). European-Canadian randomized trial of paclitaxel in relapsed ovarian cancer: high-dose versus low-dose and long versus short infusion. *J Clin Oncol*. 12(12): 2654-2666.

Eisenhauer EA, Vermorken JB, van Glabbeke M (1997). Predictors of response to subsequent chemotherapy in platinum pretreated ovarian cancer: a multivariate analysis of 704 patients [see comments]. *Ann Oncol*. 8(10):963-968.

Eksborg S, Stendahl U, Lonroth U (1986). Comparative pharmacokinetic study of adriamycin and 4'epi-adriamycin after their simultaneous intravenous administration. *Eur J Clin Pharmacol*. 30(5):629-631.

Eskens FA, Sleijfer S (2008). The use of bevacizumab in colorectal, lung, breast, renal and ovarian cancer: where does it fit? *Eur J Cancer*. 44(16): 2350-2356.

Fanning J, Bennett TZ, Hilgers RD (1992). Meta-analysis of cisplatin, doxorubicin, and cyclophosphamide versus cisplatin and cyclophosphamide chemotherapy of ovarian carcinoma. *Obstet Gynecol*. 80(6):954-960.

Fayers PM (2001). Interpreting quality of life data: population-based reference data for the EORTC QLQ-C30. *Eur J Cancer*. 37(11):1331-1334.

Ferrandina G, Ludovisi M, Lorusso D, et al. (2008). Phase III trial of gemcitabine compared with pegylated liposomal doxorubicin in progressive or recurrent ovarian cancer. *J Clin Oncol*. 26(6):890-896.

Ferrandina G, Paris I, Ludovisi M, et al. (2005). Gemcitabine and liposomal doxorubicin in the salvage treatment of ovarian cancer: updated results and long-term survival. *Gynecol Oncol*. 98(2):267-273.

Ferrero JM, Weber B, Geay JF, et al. (2007). Second-line chemotherapy with pegylated liposomal doxorubicin and carboplatin is highly effective in patients with advanced ovarian cancer in late relapse: a GINECO phase II trial. *Ann Oncol*. 18(2):263-268.

Folkman J (1971). Tumor angiogenesis: therapeutic implications. *N Engl J Med*. 285(21):1182-1186.

Francis P, Rowinsky E, Schneider J, Hakes T, Hoskins W, Markman M (1995). Phase I feasibility and pharmacologic study of weekly intraperitoneal paclitaxel: a Gynecologic Oncology Group pilot study. *J Clin Oncol*. 13(12): 2961-2967.

Freedman LS (1982). Tables of the number of patients required in clinical trials using the logrank test. *Stat Med*. 1(2):121-129.

Friedlander M, Buck M, Wyld D, et al. (2007). Phase II study of carboplatin followed bysequential gemcitabine and paclitaxel as first-line treatment for advanced ovarian cancer. *Int J Gynecol Cancer.* 17(2):350-358.

Friedlander M, Millward MJ, Bell D, et al. (1998). A phase II study of gemcitabine in platinum pre-treated patients with advanced epithelial ovarian cancer. *Ann Oncol.* 9(12):1343-1345.

Fyles AW, Thomas GM, Pintilie M, Ackerman I, Levin W (1998). A randomized study of two doses of abdominopelvic radiation therapy for patients with optimally debulked stage I, II, and III ovarian cancer. *Int J Radiat Oncol Biol Phys.* 41(3):543-549.

Gabizon AA, Muggia FM (1997). Initial clinical evaluation of pegylated-liposomal doxorubicin in solid tumors. In: Woodle MC, Storm G, eds. *Long Circulating Liposomes: Old Drugs, New Therapeutics.* Austin, TX: Landes Bioscience: 165-174.

Garcia AA, Hirte H, Fleming G, et al. (2008). Phase II clinical trial of bevacizumab and low-dose metronomic oral cyclophosphamide in recurrent ovarian cancer: a trial of the California, Chicago, and Princess Margaret Hospital phase II consortia. *J Clin Oncol.* 26(1):76-82.

Gaynor JJ, Fever EJ, Tan CC, et al. (1993). On the use of cause-specific failure and conditional failure probabilities: examples from clinical oncology data. *J Am Stat Assn.* 88:400-409.

Gelber RD, Cole BF, Gelber S, Goldhirsch A (1995). Comparing treatments using quality-adjusted survival: the Q-TWIST method. *Am Statist.* 49:161-169.

Gelman R, Gelber R, Henderson IC, Coleman CN, Harris JR (1990). Improved methodology for analyzing local and distant recurrence. *J Clin Oncol.* 8(3):548-555.

George SL, Desu MM (1974). Planning the size and duration of a clinical trial studying the time to some critical event. *J Chronic Dis.* 27(1):15-24.

Ghersi D, Parmar MK, Stewart LA, Marsoni S, Williams CJ (1992). Early ovarian cancer and the icon trials. *Eur J Cancer.* 28A(6-7):1297.

Goel R, Cleary SM, Horton C, et al. (1989). Effect of sodium thiosulfate on the pharmacokinetics and toxicity of cisplatin. *J Natl Cancer Inst.* 81(20):1552-1560.

Goff BA, Thompson T, Greer BE, Jacobs A, Storer B; Puget Sound Oncology Consortium (2003). Treatment of recurrent platinum resistant ovarian or peritoneal cancer with gemcitabine and doxorubicin: a phase I/II trial of the Puget Sound Oncology Consortium (PSOC 1602). *Am J Obstet Gynecol.* 188(6):1556-1562, discussion 1562-1564.

Goldie JH, Coldman AJ (1979). A mathematic model for relating the drug sensitivity of tumors to their spontaneous mutation rate. *Cancer Treat Rep.* 63(11-12):1727-1733.

Goncalves A, Braud AC, Viret F, et al. (2003). Phase I study of pegylated liposomal doxorubicin (Caelyx) in combination with carboplatin in patients with advanced solid tumors. *Anticancer Res.* 23(4):3543-3548.

Gonzalez-Martin AJ, Calvo E, Bover I, et al. (2005). Randomized phase II trial of carboplatin versus paclitaxel and carboplatin in platinum-sensitive recurrent advanced ovarian carcinoma: a GEICO (Grupo Espanol de Investigacion en Cancer de Ovario) study. *Ann Oncol.* 16(5):749-755.

Gordon AN, Fleagle JT, Guthrie D, Parkin DE, Gore ME, Lacave AJ (2001). Recurrent epithelial ovarian carcinoma: a randomized phase III study of pegylated liposomal doxorubicin versus topotecan. *J Clin Oncol.* 19(14):3312-3322.

Gordon AN, Granai CO, Rose PG, et al. (2000). Phase II study of liposomal doxorubicin in platinum- and paclitaxel-refractory epithelial ovarian cancer. *J Clin Oncol.* 18(17):3093-3100.

Gordon AN, Tonda M, Sun S, Rackoff W; Doxil Study 30-49 Investigators (2004). Long-term survival advantage for women treated with pegylated liposomal doxorubicin compared with topotecan in a phase 3 randomized study of recurrent and refractory epithelial ovarian cancer. *Gynecol Oncol.* 95(1):1-8.

Gore M, Mainwaring P, A'Hern R, et al. (1998). Randomized trial of dose-intensity with single-agent carboplatin in patients with epithelial ovarian cancer. London Gynaecological Oncology Group. *J Clin Oncol.* 16(7):2426-2434.

Gore M, Oza A, Rustin G, et al. (2002). A randomised trial of oral versus intravenous topotecan in patients with relapsed epithelial ovarian cancer. *Eur J Cancer.* 38(1):57-63.

Gore ME, Fryatt I, Wiltshaw E, Dawson T (1990). Treatment of relapsed carcinoma of the ovary with cisplatin or carboplatin following initial treatment with these compounds. *Gynecol Oncol.* 36(2):207-211.

Grambsch PM, Therneau TM (1994). Proportional hazards tests and diagnostics based on weighted residuals. *Biometrika.* 81:515-526.

Green S, Weiss GR (1992). Southwest Oncology Group standard response criteria, endpoint definitions and toxicity criteria. *Invest New Drugs.* 10(4):239-253.

Greene MH, Boice JD Jr, Greer BE, Blessing JA, Dembo AJ (1982). Acute nonlymphocytic leukemia after therapy with alkylating agents for ovarian cancer: a study of five randomized clinical trials. *N Engl J Med.* 307(23):1416-1421.

Greene RF, Collins JM, Jenkins JF, Speyer JL, Myers CE (1983). Plasma pharmacokinetics of adriamycin and adriamycinol: implications for the design of in vitro experiments and treatment protocols. *Cancer Res.* 43(7):3417-3421.

Greer BE, Bundy BN, Ozols RF, et al. (2005). Implications of second-look laparotomy in the context of optimally resected stage III ovarian cancer: a nonrandomized comparison using an explanatory analysis: a Gynecologic Oncology Group study. *Gynecol Oncol.* 99(1):71-79.

Greggi S, Salerno MG, D'Agostino G, et al. (2001). Topotecan and gemcitabine in platinum/paclitaxel-resistant ovarian cancer. *Oncology.* 60(1):19-23.

Greimel E, Bottomley A, Cull A, et al.; EORTC Quality of Life Group and the Quality of Life Unit (2003). An international field study of the reliability and validity of a disease-specific questionnaire module (the QLQ-OV28) in assessing the quality of life of patients with ovarian cancer. *Eur J Cancer.* 39(10):1402-1408.

Griffiths CT (1975). Surgical resection of tumor bulk in the primary treatment of ovarian carcinoma. *Natl Cancer Inst Monogr.* 42:101-104.

Gronroos M, Nieminen U, Kauppila A, Kauppila O, Saksela E, Vayrynen M (1984). A prospective, randomized, national trial for treatment of ovarian cancer: the role of chemotherapy and external irradiation. *Eur J Obstet Gynecol Reprod Biol.* 17(1):33-42.

Gupta SK, John S, Naik R, et al. (2005). A multicenter phase II study of gemcitabine, paclitaxel, and cisplatin in chemonaive advanced ovarian cancer. *Gynecol Oncol.* 98(1):134-140.

Hacker NF, Berek JS, Lagasse LD, Nieberg RK, Elashoff RM (1983). Primary cytoreductive surgery for epithelial ovarian cancer. *Obstet Gynecol.* 61(4):413-420.

Hakes TB, Chalas E, Hoskins WJ, et al. (1992). Randomized prospective trial of 5 versus 10 cycles of cyclophosphamide, doxorubicin, and cisplatin in advanced ovarian carcinoma. *Gynecol Oncol.* 45(3):284-289.

Harrison ML, Gore ME, Spriggs D, et al. (2007). Duration of second or greater complete clinical remission in ovarian cancer: exploring potential endpoints for clinical trials. *Gynecol Oncol.* 106(3):469-475.

Heintz AP, Odicino F, Maisonneuve P, et al. (2006). Carcinoma of the ovary. FIGO 26th Annual Report on the Results of Treatment in Gynecological Cancer. *Int J Gynaecol Obstet.* 95(suppl 1):S161-S192.

Helewa ME, Krepart GV, Lotocki R (1986). Staging laparotomy in early epithelial ovarian carcinoma. *Am J Obstet Gynecol.* 154(2):282-286.

Hensley ML, Correa DD, Thaler H, et al. (2006). Phase I/II study of weekly paclitaxel plus carboplatin and gemcitabine as first-line treatment of advanced-stage ovarian cancer: pathologic complete response and longitudinal assessment of impact on cognitive functioning. *Gynecol Oncol.* 102(2):270-277.

Hertzberg RP, Caranfa MJ, Hecht SM (1989). On the mechanism of topoisomerase I inhibition by camptothecin: evidence for binding to an enzyme-DNA complex. *Biochemistry.* 28(11):4629-4638.

Hoskins P, Eisenhauer E, Beare S, et al. (1998). Randomized phase II study of two schedules of topotecan in previously treated patients with ovarian cancer: a National Cancer Institute of Canada Clinical Trials Group study. *J Clin Oncol.* 16(6):2233-2237.

Hoskins P, Eisenhauer E, Vergote I, et al. (2000). Phase II feasibility study of sequential couplets of cisplatin/topotecan followed by paclitaxel/cisplatin as primary treatment for advanced epithelial ovarian cancer: a National Cancer Institute of Canada Clinical Trials Group Study. *J Clin Oncol.* 18(24):4038-4044.

Hoskins P, Vergote I, Cervantes A, et al. (2010). Advanced ovarian cancer: phase III randomized study of sequential cisplatin-topotecan and carboplatin-paclitaxel vs carboplatin-paclitaxel. *J Natl Cancer Inst.* 102(20):1547-1556.

Hoskins PJ (2009). Triple cytotoxic therapy for advanced ovarian cancer: a failed application, not a failed strategy. *J Clin Oncol.* 27(9):1355-1358.

Hoskins PJ, Swenerton KD (1994). Oral etoposide is active against platinum-resistant epithelial ovarian cancer. *J Clin Oncol.* 12(1):60-63.

Hoskins WJ, Bundy BN, Thigpen JT, Omura GA (1992). The influence of cytoreductive surgery on recurrence-free interval and survival in small-volume stage III epithelial ovarian cancer: a Gynecologic Oncology Group study. *Gynecol Oncol.* 47(2):159-166.

Hou JY, Kelly MG, Yu H, et al. (2007). Neoadjuvant chemotherapy lessens surgical morbidity in advanced ovarian cancer and leads to improved survival in stage IV disease. *Gynecol Oncol.* 105(1):211-217.

Houghton PJ, Cheshire PJ, Myers L, Stewart CF, Synold TW, Houghton JA (1992). Evaluation of 9-dimethylaminomethyl-10-hydroxycamptothecin against xenografts derived from adult and childhood solid tumors. *Cancer Chemother Pharmacol.* 31(3):229-239.

Howell SB, Pfeifle CL, Wung WE, et al. (1982). Intraperitoneal cisplatin with systemic thiosulfate protection. *Ann Intern Med.* 97(6):845-851.

Howell SB, Zimm S, Markman M, et al. (1987). Long-term survival of advanced refractory ovarian carcinoma patients with small-volume disease treated with intraperitoneal chemotherapy. *J Clin Oncol.* 5(10):1607-1612.

Hreshchyshyn MM, Park RC, Blessing JA, et al. (1980). The role of adjuvant therapy in stage I ovarian cancer. *Am J Obstet Gynecol.* 138(2):139-145.

Hsiang YH, Lihou MG, Liu LF (1989). Arrest of replication forks by drug-stabilized topoisomerase I-DNA cleavable complexes as a mechanism of cell killing by camptothecin. *Cancer Res.* 49(18):5077-5082.

Hurwitz H, Fehrenbacher L, Novotny W, et al. (2004). Bevacizumab plus irinotecan, fluorouracil, and leucovorin for metastatic colorectal cancer. *N Engl J Med.* 350(23):2335-2342.

International Collaborative Ovarian Neoplasm Group (1998). ICON2: randomised trial of single-agent carboplatin against three-drug combination of CAP (cyclophosphamide, doxorubicin, and cisplatin) in women with ovarian cancer. ICON Collaborators. International Collaborative Ovarian Neoplasm Study. *Lancet.* 352(9140):1571-1576.

International Collaborative Ovarian Neoplasm Group (2002). Paclitaxel plus carboplatin versus standard chemotherapy with either single-agent carboplatin or cyclophosphamide, doxorubicin, and cisplatin in women with ovarian cancer: the ICON3 randomised trial. *Lancet.* 360(9332):505-515.

Jacob JH, Gershenson DM, Morris M, Copeland LJ, Burke TW, Wharton JT (1991). Neoadjuvant chemotherapy and interval debulking for advanced epithelial ovarian cancer. *Gynecol Oncol.* 42(2):146-150.

Jain RK (1987). Transport of molecules across tumor vasculature. *Cancer Metastasis Rev.* 6(4):559-593.

Jakobsen A, Bertelsen K, Andersen JE, et al. (1997). Dose-effect study of carboplatin in ovarian cancer: a Danish Ovarian Cancer Group study. *J Clin Oncol.* 15(1):193-198.

Jelliffe RW (1973). Letter: creatinine clearance: bedside estimate. *Ann Intern Med.* 79(4):604-605.

Jordan MA, Wendell K, Gardiner S, Derry WB, Copp H, Wilson L (1996). Mitotic block induced in HeLa cells by low concentrations of paclitaxel (Taxol) results in abnormal mitotic exit and apoptotic cell death. *Cancer Res.* 56(4):816-825.

Kang S, Nam BH (2009). Does neoadjuvant chemotherapy increase optimal cytoreduction rate in advanced ovarian cancer? Meta-analysis of 21 studies. *Ann Surg Oncol.* 16(8):2315-2320.

Kaplan EL, Meier P (1958). Non-parametric estimation from incomplete observations. *J Am Stat Assoc.* 53:457-481.

Katsumata N, Yasuda M, Isonishi S, et al.; Japanese Gynecologic Oncology Group (2013). Long-term results of dose-dense paclitaxel and carboplatin versus conventional paclitaxel and carboplatin for treatment of advanced epithelial ovarian, fallopian tube, or primary peritoneal cancer (JGOG 3016): a randomised, controlled, open-label trial. *Lancet Oncol.* 14(10):1020-1026.

Katsumata N, Yasuda M, Takahashi F, et al.; Japanese Gynecologic Oncology Group (2009). Dose-dense paclitaxel once a week in combination with carboplatin every 3 weeks for advanced ovarian cancer: a phase 3, open-label, randomised controlled trial. *Lancet.* 374(9698):1331-1338.

Kehoe S, Hook J, Nankivell M, et al. (2015). Primary chemotherapy versus primary surgery for newly diagnosed advanced ovarian cancer (CHORUS): an open-label, randomised, controlled, non-inferiority trial. *Lancet.* 386(9990):249-257.

Kirmani S, Lucas WE, Kim S, et al. (1991). A phase II trial of intraperitoneal cisplatin and etoposide as salvage treatment for minimal residual ovarian carcinoma. *J Clin Oncol.* 9(4):649-657.

Klaassen D, Shelley W, Starreveld A, et al. (1988). Early stage ovarian cancer: a randomized clinical trial comparing whole abdominal radiotherapy, melphalan, and intraperitoneal chromic phosphate: a National Cancer Institute of Canada Clinical Trials Group report. *J Clin Oncol.* 6(8):1254-1263.

Klauber N, Parangi S, Flynn E, Hamel E, D'Amato RJ (1997). Inhibition of angiogenesis and breast cancer in mice by the microtubule inhibitors 2-methoxyestradiol and taxol. *Cancer Res.* 57(1):81-86.

Krafft W, Morack G, Flach W, et al. (1980). The therapy of the early ovarian cancer (T1/T2 M0 N0) (author's transl) [in German]. *Arch Geschwulstforsch.* 50(7):664-671.

Krasner CN, McMeekin DS, Chan S, et al. (2007). A phase II study of trabectedin single agent in patients with recurrent ovarian cancer previously treated with platinum-based regimens. *Br J Cancer.* 97(12):1618-1624.

Kruskal WH, Wallis WA (1952). Use of ranks in one criterion variance analysis. *J Am Stat Assn.* 47:583-621.

Kudelka AP, Tresukosol D, Edwards CL, et al. (1996). Phase II study of intravenous topotecan as a 5-day infusion for refractory epithelial ovarian carcinoma. *J Clin Oncol.* 14(5):1552-1557.

Kurman RJ, Shih Ie M (2008). Pathogenesis of ovarian cancer: lessons from morphology and molecular biology and their clinical implications. *Int J Gynecol Pathol.* 27(2):151-160.

Lachlin JM, Foulkes MA (1986). Evauation of sample size and power for analyses of survival with allowance for non-uniform patient entry, losses to follow-up, noncompliance and stratification. *Biometrics.* 42:507-519.

Lambert HE, Rustin GJ, Gregory WM, Nelstrop AE (1997). A randomized trial of five versus eight courses of cisplatin or carboplatin in advanced epithelial ovarian carcinoma. A North Thames Ovary Group Study. *Ann Oncol.* 8(4): 327-333.

Le T, Adolph A, Krepart GV, Lotocki R, Heywood MS (2002). The benefits of comprehensive surgical staging in the management of early-stage epithelial ovarian carcinoma. *Gynecol Oncol.* 85(2):351-355.

Levey AS, Coresh J, Greene T, et al.; Chronic Kidney Disease Epidemiology Collaboration (2006). Using standardized serum creatinine values in the modification of diet in renal disease study equation for estimating glomerular filtration rate. *Ann Intern Med.* 145(4):247-254.

Levin L, Hryniuk WM (1987). Dose intensity analysis of chemotherapy regimens in ovarian carcinoma. *J Clin Oncol.* 5(5):756-767.

References

Lokich J, Anderson N (1998). Carboplatin versus cisplatin in solid tumors: an analysis of the literature. *Ann Oncol.* 9(1):13-21.

Lopes NM, Adams EG, Pitts TW, Bhuyan BK (1993). Cell kill kinetics and cell cycle effects of taxol on human and hamster ovarian cell lines. *Cancer Chemother Pharmacol.* 32(3):235-242.

Lopez AM, Wallace L, Dorr RT, Koff M, Hersh EM, Alberts DS (1999). Topical DMSO treatment for pegylated liposomal doxorubicin-induced palmar-plantar erythrodysesthesia. *Cancer Chemother Pharmacol.* 44(4):303-306.

Lortholary A, Largillier R, Weber B, et al. (2012). Weekly paclitaxel as a single agent or in combination with carboplatin or weekly topotecan in patients with resistant ovarian cancer: the CARTAXHY randomized phase II trial from Groupe d'Investigateurs Nationaux pour l'Etude des Cancers Ovariens (GINECO). *Ann Oncol.* 23(2):346-352.

Los G, Mutsaers PH, van der Vijgh WJ, Baldew GS, de Graaf PW, McVie JG (1989). Direct diffusion of cis-diamminedichloroplatinum(II) in intraperitoneal rat tumors after intraperitoneal chemotherapy: a comparison with systemic chemotherapy. *Cancer Res.* 49(12):3380-3384.

Lund B, Hansen OP, Theilade K, Hansen M, Neijt JP (1994). Phase II study of gemcitabine (2',2'-difluorodeoxycytidine) in previously treated ovarian cancer patients. *J Natl Cancer Inst.* 86(20):1530-1533.

Lund B, Neijt JP (1996). Gemcitabine in cisplatin-resistant ovarian cancer. *Semin Oncol.* 23(5)(suppl 10):72-76.

Mannel RS, Brady MF, Kohn EC, et al. (2011). A randomized phase III trial of IV carboplatin and paclitaxel × 3 courses followed by observation versus weekly maintenance low-dose paclitaxel in patients with early-stage ovarian carcinoma: a Gynecologic Oncology Group Study. *Gynecol Oncol.* 122(1):89-94.

Mantel N (1966). Evaluation of survival data and two new rank order statistics arising in its consideration. *Cancer Chemother Rep.* 50(3):163-170.

Mantel N, Haenszel W (1959). Statistical aspects of the analysis of data from retrospective studies of disease. *J Natl Cancer Inst.* 22(4):719-748.

Markman M (1998). Intraperitoneal therapy of ovarian cancer. *Semin Oncol.* 25(3):356-360.

Markman M, Berek JS, Blessing JA, McGuire WP, Bell J, Homesley HD (1992). Characteristics of patients with small-volume residual ovarian cancer unresponsive to cisplatin-based ip chemotherapy: lessons learned from a Gynecologic Oncology Group phase II trial of ip cisplatin and recombinant alpha-interferon. *Gynecol Oncol.* 45(1):3-8.

Markman M, Bundy BN, Alberts DS, et al. (2001). Phase III trial of standard-dose intravenous cisplatin plus paclitaxel versus moderately high-dose carboplatin followed by intravenous paclitaxel and intraperitoneal cisplatin in small-volume stage III ovarian carcinoma: an intergroup study of the Gynecologic Oncology Group, Southwestern Oncology Group, and Eastern Cooperative Oncology Group. *J Clin Oncol.* 19(4):1001-1007.

Markman M, Hakes T, Barakat R, Curtin J, Almadrones L, Hoskins W (1996). Follow-up of Memorial Sloan-Kettering Cancer Center patients treated on National Cancer Institute Treatment Referral Center protocol 9103: paclitaxel in refractory ovarian cancer. *J Clin Oncol.* 14(3):796-799.

Markman M, Kennedy A, Webster K, Peterson G, Kulp B, Belinson J (2000). Phase 2 trial of liposomal doxorubicin (40 mg/m(2)) in platinum/paclitaxel-refractory ovarian and fallopian tube cancers and primary carcinoma of the peritoneum. *Gynecol Oncol.* 78(3, pt 1):369-372.

Markman M, Liu PY, Wilczynski S, et al.; Southwest Oncology Group and Gynecologic Oncology Group (2003a). Phase III randomized trial of 12 versus 3 months of maintenance paclitaxel in patients with advanced ovarian cancer after complete response to platinum and paclitaxel-based chemotherapy: a Southwest Oncology Group and Gynecologic Oncology Group trial. *J Clin Oncol.* 21(13):2460-2465.

Markman M, Rothman R, Hakes T, et al. (1991). Second-line platinum therapy in patients with ovarian cancer previously treated with cisplatin. *J Clin Oncol.* 9(3):389-393.

Markman M, Webster K, Zanotti K, Kulp B, Peterson G, Belinson J (2003b). Phase 2 trial of single-agent gemcitabine in platinum-paclitaxel refractory ovarian cancer. *Gynecol Oncol.* 90(3):593-596.

Marth C, Hiebl S, Oberaigner W, Winter R, Leodolter S, Sevelda P (2009). Influence of department volume on survival for ovarian cancer: results from a prospective quality assurance program of the Austrian Association for Gynecologic Oncology. *Int J Gynecol Cancer.* 19(1):94-102.

Matsuo S, Imai E, Horio M, et al. (2009). Revised equations for estimated GFR from serum creatinine in Japan. *Am J Kidney Dis.* 53(6):982-992.

McGonigle KF, Muntz HG, Vuky J, et al. (2011). Combined weekly topotecan and biweekly bevacizumab in women with platinum-resistant ovarian, peritoneal, or fallopian tube cancer: results of a phase 2 study. *Cancer.* 117(16):3731-3740.

McGuire WP, Blessing JA, Bookman MA, Lentz SS, Dunton CJ (2000). Topotecan has substantial antitumor activity as first-line salvage therapy in platinum-sensitive epithelial ovarian carcinoma: a Gynecologic Oncology Group Study. *J Clin Oncol.* 18(5):1062-1067.

McGuire WP, Hoskins WJ, Brady MF, et al. (1995). Assessment of dose-intensive therapy in suboptimally debulked ovarian cancer: a Gynecologic Oncology Group study. *J Clin Oncol.* 13(7):1589-1599.

References

McGuire WP, Hoskins WJ, Brady MF, et al. (1996). Cyclophosphamide and cisplatin compared with paclitaxel and cisplatin in patients with stage III and stage IV ovarian cancer. *N Engl J Med.* 334(1):1-6.

McGuire WP, Rowinsky EK, Rosenshein NB, et al. (1989). Taxol: a unique antineoplastic agent with significant activity in advanced ovarian epithelial neoplasms. *Ann Intern Med.* 111(4):273-279.

Meco D, Colombo T, Ubezio P, et al. (2003). Effective combination of ET-743 and doxorubicin in sarcoma: preclinical studies. *Cancer Chemother Pharmacol.* 52(2):131-138.

Mehta C, Petal N (1983). A network algorithm for performing Fisher's exact test in $r \times c$ contingency tables. *J Am Stat Assoc.* 78:427-434.

Miller AB, Hoogstraten B, Staquet M, Winkler A (1981). Reporting results of cancer treatment. *Cancer.* 47(1):207-214.

Monk BJ, Herzog TJ, Kaye SB, et al. (2010). Trabectedin plus pegylated liposomal doxorubicin in recurrent ovarian cancer. *J Clin Oncol.* 28(19):3107-3114.

Morice P, Wicart-Poque F, Rey A, et al. (2001). Results of conservative treatment in epithelial ovarian carcinoma. *Cancer.* 92(9):2412-2418.

Muggia FM, Braly PS, Brady MF, et al. (2000). Phase III randomized study of cisplatin versus paclitaxel versus cisplatin and paclitaxel in patients with suboptimal stage III or IV ovarian cancer: a Gynecologic Oncology Group study. *J Clin Oncol.* 18(1):106-115.

Muggia FM, Hainsworth JD, Jeffers S, et al. (1997). Phase II study of liposomal doxorubicin in refractory ovarian cancer: antitumor activity and toxicity modification by liposomal encapsulation. *J Clin Oncol.* 15(3):987-993.

Mutch DG, Orlando M, Goss T, et al. (2007). Randomized phase III trial of gemcitabine compared with pegylated liposomal doxorubicin in patients with platinum-resistant ovarian cancer. *J Clin Oncol.* 25(19):2811-2818.

Naumann RW, Coleman RL (2011). Management strategies for recurrent platinum-resistant ovarian cancer. *Drugs.* 71(11):1397-1412.

Neijt JP, Engelholm SA, Tuxen MK, et al. (2000). Exploratory phase III study of paclitaxel and cisplatin versus paclitaxel and carboplatin in advanced ovarian cancer. *J Clin Oncol.* 18(17):3084-3092.

Neijt JP, Engelholm SA, Witteveen PO, et al. (1997). Paclitaxel (175 mg/m2 over 3 hours) with cisplatin or carboplatin in previously untreated ovarian cancer: an interim analysis. *Semin Oncol.* 24(5)(suppl 15):S15-36-S15-39.

Neijt JP, ten Bokkel Huinink WW, van der Burg ME, et al. (1984). Randomised trial comparing two combination chemotherapy regimens (Hexa-CAF vs CHAP-5) in advanced ovarian carcinoma. *Lancet.* 2(8403):594-600.

Neijt JP, ten Bokkel Huinink WW, van der Burg ME, et al. (1987). Randomized trial comparing two combination chemotherapy regimens (CHAP-5 v CP) in advanced ovarian carcinoma. *J Clin Oncol.* 5(8):1157-1168.

Neijt JP, ten Bokkel Huinink WW, van der Burg ME, et al. (1991). Long-term survival in ovarian cancer: mature data from the Netherlands Joint Study Group for Ovarian Cancer. *Eur J Cancer.* 27(11):1367-1372.

NIH consensus conference. Ovarian cancer. Screening, treatment, and follow-up. NIH Consensus Development Panel on Ovarian Cancer. (1995). *JAMA.* 273(6):491-497.

Norton L (2001). Theoretical concepts and the emerging role of taxanes in adjuvant therapy. *Oncologist.* 6(suppl 3):30-35.

O'Brien ME, Wigler N, Inbar M, et al.; Group CBCS (2004). Reduced cardiotoxicity and comparable efficacy in a phase III trial of pegylated liposomal doxorubicin HCl (CAELYX/Doxil) versus conventional doxorubicin for first-line treatment of metastatic breast cancer. *Ann Oncol.* 15(3):440-449.

O'Brien PC, Fleming TR (1979). A multiple testing procedure for clinical trials. *Biometrics.* 35(3):549-556.

Oken MM, Creech RH, Tormey DC, et al. (1982). Toxicity and response criteria of the Eastern Cooperative Oncology Group. *Am J Clin Oncol.* 5(6):649-655.

O'Malley CD, Cress RD, Campleman SL, Leiserowitz GS (2003). Survival of Californian women with epithelial ovarian cancer, 1994-1996: a population-based study. *Gynecol Oncol.* 91(3):608-615.

Omura G, Blessing JA, Ehrlich CE, et al. (1986). A randomized trial of cyclophosphamide and doxorubicin with or without cisplatin in advanced ovarian carcinoma: a Gynecologic Oncology Group Study. *Cancer.* 57(9):1725-1730.

Omura GA, Bundy BN, Berek JS, Curry S, Delgado G, Mortel R (1989). Randomized trial of cyclophosphamide plus cisplatin with or without doxorubicin in ovarian carcinoma: a Gynecologic Oncology Group Study. *J Clin Oncol.* 7(4):457-465.

Omura GA, Morrow CP, Blessing JA, et al. (1983). A randomized comparison of melphalan versus melphalan plus hexamethylmelamine versus adriamycin plus cyclophosphamide in ovarian carcinoma. *Cancer.* 51(5):783-789.

Osoba D, Rodrigues G, Myles J, Zee B, Pater J (1998). Interpreting the significance of changes in health-related quality-of-life scores. *J Clin Oncol.* 16(1):139-144.

Oudard S, Thierry A, Jorgensen TJ, Rahman A (1991). Sensitization of multidrug-resistant colon cancer cells to doxorubicin encapsulated in liposomes. *Cancer Chemother Pharmacol.* 28(4):259-265.

Oza AM, Cook AD, Pfisterer J, et al.; ICON7 trial investigators (2015). Standard chemotherapy with or without bevacizumab for women with newly diagnosed ovarian cancer (ICON7): overall survival results of a phase 3 randomised trial. *Lancet Oncol.* 16(8):928-936.

Ozols RF (1994). Treatment of ovarian cancer: current status. *Semin Oncol.* 21(2) (suppl 2):1-9; quiz 10, 58.

Ozols RF, Bundy BN, Greer BE, et al.; Gynecologic Oncology Group (2003). Phase III trial of carboplatin and paclitaxel compared with cisplatin and paclitaxel in patients with optimally resected stage III ovarian cancer: a Gynecologic Oncology Group study. *J Clin Oncol.* 21(17):3194-3200.

Panageas KS, Ben-Porat L, Dickler MN, Chapman PB, Schrag D (2007). When you look matters: the effect of assessment schedule on progression-free survival. *J Natl Cancer Inst.* 99(6):428-432.

Parmar MK, Ledermann JA, Colombo N, et al.; ICON and Collaborators AGO (2003). Paclitaxel plus platinum-based chemotherapy versus conventional platinum-based chemotherapy in women with relapsed ovarian cancer: the ICON4/AGO-OVAR-2.2 trial. *Lancet.* 361(9375):2099-2106.

Pectasides D, Fountzilas G, Aravantinos G, et al. (2006). Advanced stage clear-cell epithelial ovarian cancer: the Hellenic Cooperative Oncology Group experience. *Gynecol Oncol.* 102(2):285-291.

Pepe MS, Mori M (1993). Kaplan-Meier, marginal or conditional probability curves in summarizing competing risks failure time data? *Stat Med.* 12(8): 737-751.

Perren TJ, Swart AM, Pfisterer J, et al.; ICON7 trial investigators (2011). A phase 3 trial of bevacizumab in ovarian cancer. *N Engl J Med.* 365(26):2484-2496.

Peto R, Peto J (1972). Asymptomatically efficient rank invariant procedures. *J R Stat Soc A.* 135:185-207.

Pfisterer J, Plante M, Vergote I, et al. (2006a). Gemcitabine plus carboplatin compared with carboplatin in patients with platinum-sensitive recurrent ovarian cancer: an intergroup trial of the AGO-OVAR, the NCIC CTG, and the EORTC GCG. *J Clin Oncol.* 24(29):4699-4707.

Pfisterer J, Weber B, Reuss A, et al. (2006b). Randomized phase III trial of topotecan following carboplatin and paclitaxel in first-line treatment of advanced ovarian cancer: a gynecologic cancer intergroup trial of the AGO-OVAR and GINECO. *J Natl Cancer Inst.* 98(15):1036-1045.

Piccart MJ, Bertelsen K, James K, et al. (2000). Randomized intergroup trial of cisplatin-paclitaxel versus cisplatin-cyclophosphamide in women with advanced epithelial ovarian cancer: three-year results. *J Natl Cancer Inst.* 92(9): 699-708.

Piccart MJ, Green JA, Lacave AJ, et al. (2000). Oxaliplatin or paclitaxel in patients with platinum-pretreated advanced ovarian cancer: a randomized phase II study of the European Organization for Research and Treatment of Cancer Gynecology Group. *J Clin Oncol.* 18(6):1193-1202.

Pignata S, De Placido S, Biamonte R, et al. (2006). Residual neurotoxicity in ovarian cancer patients in clinical remission after first-line chemotherapy with carboplatin and paclitaxel: the Multicenter Italian Trial in Ovarian cancer (MITO-4) retrospective study. *BMC Cancer.* 6:5.

Pignata S, Scambia G, Ferrandina G, et al. (2011). Carboplatin plus paclitaxel versus carboplatin plus pegylated liposomal doxorubicin as first-line treatment for patients with ovarian cancer: the MITO-2 randomized phase III trial. *J Clin Oncol.* 29(27):3628-3635.

Pignata S, Scambia G, Katsaros D, et al.; Multicentre Italian Trials in Ovarian cancer (MITO-7), Groupe d'Investigateurs Nationaux pour l'Etude des Cancers Ovariens et du sein (GINECO), Mario Negri Gynecologic Oncology (MaNGO), European Network of Gynaecological Oncological Trial Groups (ENGOT-OV-10) and Gynecologic Cancer InterGroup (GCIG) Investigators (2014). Carboplatin plus paclitaxel once a week versus every 3 weeks in patients with advanced ovarian cancer (MITO-7): a randomised, multicentre, open-label, phase 3 trial. *Lancet Oncol.* 15(4):396-405.

Pignata S, Scambia G, Savarese A, et al. (2009). Carboplatin and pegylated liposomal doxorubicin for advanced ovarian cancer: preliminary activity results of the MITO-2 phase III trial. *Oncology.* 76(1):49-54.

Piver MS (1982). Optimal surgical therapy in stage I and II ovarian malignancies. *Int J Radiat Oncol Biol Phys.* 8(2):247-249.

Piver MS, Barlow JJ, Lele SB (1978). Incidence of subclinical metastasis in stage I and II ovarian carcinoma. *Obstet Gynecol.* 52(1):100-104.

Polterauer S, Vergote I, Concin N, et al. (2012). Prognostic value of residual tumor size in patients with epithelial ovarian cancer FIGO stages IIA-IV: analysis of the OVCAD data. *Int J Gynecol Cancer.* 22(3):380-385.

Polychemotherapy for early breast cancer: an overview of the randomised trials. Early Breast Cancer Trialists' Collaborative Group. (1998). *Lancet.* 352(9132):930-942.

Potter ME, Partridge EE, Hatch KD, Soong SJ, Austin JM, Shingleton HM (1991). Primary surgical therapy of ovarian cancer: how much and when. *Gynecol Oncol.* 40(3):195-200.

Prefontaine M, Gelfand AT, Donovan JT, Powell JL (1994). Reproducibility of tumor measurements in ovarian cancer: a study of interobserver variability. *Gynecol Oncol.* 55(1):87-90.

Pujade-Lauraine E, Hilpert F, Weber B, et al. (2014). Bevacizumab combined with chemotherapy for platinum-resistant recurrent ovarian cancer: the AURELIA open-label randomized phase III trial. *J Clin Oncol.* 32(13):1302-1308.

Pujade-Lauraine E, Wagner U, Aavall-Lundqvist E, et al. (2010). Pegylated liposomal doxorubicin and carboplatin compared with paclitaxel and carboplatin for patients with platinum-sensitive ovarian cancer in late relapse. *J Clin Oncol.* 28(20):3323-3329.

Raspagliesi F, Zanaboni F, Vecchione F, et al. (2004). Gemcitabine combined with oxaliplatin (GEMOX) as second-line chemotherapy in patients with advanced ovarian cancer refractory or resistant to platinum and taxane. *Oncology.* 67(5-6):376-381.

Redman CW, Mould J, Warwick J, et al. (1993). The West Midlands epithelial ovarian cancer adjuvant therapy trial. *Clin Oncol (R Coll Radiol).* 5(1):1-5.

Reimer RR, Hoover R, Fraumeni JF Jr, Young RC (1977). Acute leukemia after alkylating-agent therapy of ovarian cancer. *N Engl J Med.* 297(4):177-181.

Reynolds T (1999). Why randomized surgical oncology trials are so scarce. *J Natl Cancer Inst.* 91(14):1182-1183.

Richardson GS, Scully RE, Nikrui N, Nelson JH Jr. (1985). Common epithelial cancer of the ovary (2). *N Engl J Med.* 312(7):415-424.

Rose PG (2005). Gemcitabine reverses platinum resistance in platinum-resistant ovarian and peritoneal carcinoma. *Int J Gynecol Cancer.* 15(suppl 1):18-22.

Rose PG, Blessing JA, Mayer AR, Homesley HD (1998a). Prolonged oral etoposide as second-line therapy for platinum-resistant and platinum-sensitive ovarian carcinoma: a Gynecologic Oncology Group study. *J Clin Oncol.* 16(2):405-410.

Rose PG, Fusco N, Fluellen L, Rodriguez M (1998b). Second-line therapy with paclitaxel and carboplatin for recurrent disease following first-line therapy with paclitaxel and platinum in ovarian or peritoneal carcinoma. *J Clin Oncol.* 16(4):1494-1497.

Rose PG, Mossbruger K, Fusco N, Smrekar M, Eaton S, Rodriguez M (2003). Gemcitabine reverses cisplatin resistance: demonstration of activity in platinum- and multidrug-resistant ovarian and peritoneal carcinoma. *Gynecol Oncol.* 88(1):17-21.

Rose PG, Nerenstone S, Brady MF, et al.; Gynecologic Oncology Group (2004). Secondary surgical cytoreduction for advanced ovarian carcinoma. *N Engl J Med.* 351(24):2489-2497.

Rose PG, Smrekar M, Fusco N (2005). A phase II trial of weekly paclitaxel and every 3 weeks of carboplatin in potentially platinum-sensitive ovarian and peritoneal carcinoma. *Gynecol Oncol.* 96(2):296-300.

Rosenberg P, Andersson H, Boman K, et al. (2002). Randomized trial of single agent paclitaxel given weekly versus every three weeks and with peroral versus intravenous steroid premedication to patients with ovarian cancer previously treated with platinum. *Acta Oncol.* 41(5):418-424.

Rowinsky EK, Donehower RC (1995). Paclitaxel (taxol). *N Engl J Med.* 332(15): 1004-1014.

Rowinsky EK, Gilbert MR, McGuire WP, et al. (1991a). Sequences of taxol and cisplatin: a phase I and pharmacologic study. *J Clin Oncol.* 9(9):1692-1703.

Rowinsky EK, Grochow LB, Hendricks CB, et al. (1992). Phase I and pharmacologic study of topotecan: a novel topoisomerase I inhibitor. *J Clin Oncol.* 10(4):647-656.

Rowinsky EK, McGuire WP, Guarnieri T, Fisherman JS, Christian MC, Donehower RC (1991b). Cardiac disturbances during the administration of taxol. *J Clin Oncol.* 9(9):1704-1712.

Royston P, Parmar MK (2002). Flexible parametric proportional-hazards and proportional-odds models for censored survival data, with application to prognostic modelling and estimation of treatment effects. *Stat Med.* 21(15):2175-2197.

Rubin SC, Randall TC, Armstrong KA, Chi DS, Hoskins WJ (1999). Ten-year follow-up of ovarian cancer patients after second-look laparotomy with negative findings. *Obstet Gynecol.* 93(1):21-24.

Rustin GJ, Marples M, Nelstrop AE, Mahmoudi M, Meyer T (2001). Use of CA-125 to define progression of ovarian cancer in patients with persistently elevated levels. *J Clin Oncol.* 19(20):4054-4057.

Rustin GJ, Quinn M, Thigpen T, et al. (2004). Re: New guidelines to evaluate the response to treatment in solid tumors (ovarian cancer). *J Natl Cancer Inst.* 96(6):487-488.

Rustin GJ, Timmers P, Nelstrop A, et al. (2006). Comparison of CA-125 and standard definitions of progression of ovarian cancer in the intergroup trial of cisplatin and paclitaxel versus cisplatin and cyclophosphamide. *J Clin Oncol.* 24(1):45-51.

Saltz L, Sirott M, Young C, et al. (1993). Phase I clinical and pharmacology study of topotecan given daily for 5 consecutive days to patients with advanced solid tumors, with attempt at dose intensification using recombinant granulocyte colony-stimulating factor. *J Natl Cancer Inst.* 85(18):1499-1507.

Schemper M, Smith TL (1996). A note on quantifying follow-up in studies of failure time. *Control Clin Trials.* 17(4):343-346.

Schneider JG (1994). Intraperitoneal chemotherapy. *Obstet Gynecol Clin North Am.* 21(1):195-212.

Schoenfeld D (1981). The asymptotic properties of nonparemetric tests for comapring survival distributions. *Biometrika.* 68(1):316-319.

Schrag D, Earle C, Xu F, et al. (2006). Associations between hospital and surgeon procedure volumes and patient outcomes after ovarian cancer resection. *J Natl Cancer Inst.* 98(3):163-171.

Schueler JA, Trimbos JB, Hermans J, Fleuren GJ (1998). The yield of surgical staging in presumed early stage ovarian cancer: benefits or doubts? *Int J Gynecol Cancer.* 95:125-132.

Scully RE (1977). Ovarian tumors: a review. *Am J Pathol.* 87(3):686-720.

Sehouli J, Stengel D, Mustea A, et al.; Ovarian Cancer Study Group of the Nord-Ostdeutsche Gesellschaft fur Gynakologische Onkologie (2008). Weekly paclitaxel and carboplatin (PC-W) for patients with primary advanced ovarian cancer: results of a multicenter phase-II study of the NOGGO. *Cancer Chemother Pharmacol.* 61(2):243-250.

Sehouli J, Stengel D, Oskay-Oezcelik G, et al. (2008). Nonplatinum topotecan combinations versus topotecan alone for recurrent ovarian cancer: results of a phase III study of the North-Eastern German Society of Gynecological Oncology Ovarian Cancer Study Group. *J Clin Oncol.* 26(19):3176-3182.

Sessa C, De Braud F, Perotti A, et al. (2005). Trabectedin for women with ovarian carcinoma after treatment with platinum and taxanes fails. *J Clin Oncol.* 23(9):1867-1874.

Sevelda P, Gitsch E, Dittrich C, et al. (1987). Therapeutic and prognostic results of a prospective multicenter ovarian cancer study of FIGO stages I and II [in German]. *Geburtshilfe Frauenheilkd.* 47(3):179-185.

Shapiro F, Schneider J, Markman M, et al. (1997). High-intensity intravenous cyclophosphamide and cisplatin, interim surgical debulking, and intraperitoneal cisplatin in advanced ovarian carcinoma: a pilot trial with ten-year follow-up. *Gynecol Oncol.* 67(1):39-45.

Shapiro JD, Millward MJ, Rischin D, et al. (1996). Activity of gemcitabine in patients with advanced ovarian cancer: responses seen following platinum and paclitaxel. *Gynecol Oncol.* 63(1):89-93.

Sigurdsson K, Johnsson JE, Trope C (1982). Carcinoma of the ovary, stages I and II: a prospective randomized study of the effects of postoperative chemotherapy and radiotherapy. *Ann Chir Gynaecol.* 71(6):321-329.

Simon R (1986). Confidence intervals for reporting results of clinical trials. *Ann Intern Med.* 105(3):429-435.

Simpkins F, Belinson JL, Rose PG (2007). Avoiding bevacizumab related gastrointestinal toxicity for recurrent ovarian cancer by careful patient screening. *Gynecol Oncol.* 107(1):118-123.

Skipper HE (1974). Thoughts on cancer chemotherapy and combination modality therapy (1974). *JAMA.* 230(7):1033-1035.

Smith JP, Rutledge FN, Delclos L (1975). Postoperative treatment of early cancer of the ovary: a random trial between postoperative irradiation and chemotherapy. *Natl Cancer Inst Monogr.* 42:149-153.

Smith MA, Ungerleider RS, Korn EL, Rubinstein L, Simon R (1997). Role of independent data-monitoring committees in randomized clinical trials sponsored by the National Cancer Institute. *J Clin Oncol.* 15(7):2736-2743.

Smith TJ, Khatcheressian J, Lyman GH, et al. (2006). 2006 update of recommendations for the use of white blood cell growth factors: an evidence-based clinical practice guideline. *J Clin Oncol.* 24(19):3187-3205.

Soper JT, Johnson P, Johnson V, Berchuck A, Clarke-Pearson DL (1992). Comprehensive restaging laparotomy in women with apparent early ovarian carcinoma. *Obstet Gynecol.* 80(6):949-953.

Stockler MR, Hilpert F, Friedlander M, et al. (2014). Patient-reported outcome results from the open-label phase III AURELIA trial evaluating bevacizumab-containing therapy for platinum-resistant ovarian cancer. *J Clin Oncol.* 32(13): 1309-1316.

Stuart GC, Kitchener H, Bacon M, et al. (2011). 2010 Gynecologic Cancer Inter-Group (GCIG) consensus statement on clinical trials in ovarian cancer: report from the Fourth Ovarian Cancer Consensus Conference. *Int J Gynecol Cancer.* 21(4):750-755.

Sugiyama T, Kamura T, Kigawa J, et al. (2000). Clinical characteristics of clear cell carcinoma of the ovary: a distinct histologic type with poor prognosis and resistance to platinum-based chemotherapy. *Cancer.* 88(11):2584-2589.

Sutton GP, Blessing JA, Homesley HD, Berman ML, Malfetano J (1989). Phase II trial of ifosfamide and mesna in advanced ovarian carcinoma: a Gynecologic Oncology Group Study. *J Clin Oncol.* 7(11):1672-1676.

Swenerton K, Jeffrey J, Stuart G, et al. (1992). Cisplatin-cyclophosphamide versus carboplatin-cyclophosphamide in advanced ovarian cancer: a randomized phase III study of the National Cancer Institute of Canada Clinical Trials Group. *J Clin Oncol.* 10(5):718-726.

Swisher EM, Mutch DG, Rader JS, Elbendary A, Herzog TJ (1997). Topotecan in platinum- and paclitaxel-resistant ovarian cancer. *Gynecol Oncol.* 66(3):480-486.

Takahashi N, Li WW, Banerjee D, Scotto KW, Bertino JR (2001). Sequence-dependent enhancement of cytotoxicity produced by ecteinascidin 743 (ET-743) with doxorubicin or paclitaxel in soft tissue sarcoma cells. *Clin Cancer Res.* 7(10):3251-3257.

Takano M, Sugiyama T, Yaegashi N, et al. (2007). Progression-free survival and overall survival of patients with clear cell carcinoma of the ovary treated with paclitaxel-carboplatin or irinotecan-cisplatin: retrospective analysis. *Int J Clin Oncol.* 12(4):256-260.

Temple R (2006). Hy's law: predicting serious hepatotoxicity. *Pharmacoepidemiol Drug Saf.* 15(4):241-243.

References

ten Bokkel Huinink W, Gore M, Carmichael J, et al. (1997). Topotecan versus paclitaxel for the treatment of recurrent epithelial ovarian cancer. *J Clin Oncol.* 15(6):2183-2193.

ten Bokkel Huinink W, Lane SR, Ross GA; International Topotecan Study Group (2004). Long-term survival in a phase III, randomised study of topotecan versus paclitaxel in advanced epithelial ovarian carcinoma. *Ann Oncol.* 15(1): 100-103.

Tewari D, Monk BJ, Hunter M, Falkner CA, Burger RA (2004). Gemcitabine and cisplatin chemotherapy is an active combination in the treatment of platinum-resistant ovarian and peritoneal carcinoma. *Invest New Drugs.* 22(4):475-480.

Theodoulou M, Hudis C (2004). Cardiac profiles of liposomal anthracyclines: greater cardiac safety versus conventional doxorubicin? *Cancer.* 100(10):2052-2063.

Therasse P, Arbuck SG, Eisenhauer EA, et al. (2000). New guidelines to evaluate the response to treatment in solid tumors. European Organization for Research and Treatment of Cancer, National Cancer Institute of the United States, National Cancer Institute of Canada. *J Natl Cancer Inst.* 92(3):205-216.

Thierry AR, Dritschilo A, Rahman A (1992). Effect of liposomes on P-glycoprotein function in multidrug resistant cells. *Biochem Biophys Res Commun.* 187(2): 1098-1105.

Thigpen JT, Blessing JA, Ball H, Hummel SJ, Barrett RJ (1994). Phase II trial of paclitaxel in patients with progressive ovarian carcinoma after platinum-based chemotherapy: a Gynecologic Oncology Group study. *J Clin Oncol.* 12(9): 1748-1753.

Travis LB, Curtis RE, Boice JD Jr, Platz CE, Hankey BF, Fraumeni JF Jr. (1996). Second malignant neoplasms among long-term survivors of ovarian cancer. *Cancer Res.* 56(7):1564-1570.

Travis LB, Holowaty EJ, Bergfeldt K, et al. (1999). Risk of leukemia after platinum-based chemotherapy for ovarian cancer. *N Engl J Med.* 340(5):351-357.

Trimbos B, Timmers P, Pecorelli S, et al. (2010). Surgical staging and treatment of early ovarian cancer: long-term analysis from a randomized trial. *J Natl Cancer Inst.* 102(13):982-987.

Trimbos JB (1991). Treatment of early ovarian cancer. *Eur J Cancer.* 27(10): 1196-1198.

Trimbos JB, Parmar M, Vergote I, et al. (2003a). International Collaborative Ovarian Neoplasm trial 1 and Adjuvant ChemoTherapy In Ovarian Neoplasm trial: two parallel randomized phase III trials of adjuvant chemotherapy in patients with early-stage ovarian carcinoma. *J Natl Cancer Inst.* 95(2):105-112.

Trimbos JB, Vergote I, Bolis G, et al. (2003b). Impact of adjuvant chemotherapy and surgical staging in early-stage ovarian carcinoma: European Organisation for Research and Treatment of Cancer-Adjuvant ChemoTherapy in Ovarian Neoplasm trial. *J Natl Cancer Inst.* 95(2):113-125.

Trope C, Kaern J, Hogberg T, et al. (2000). Randomized study on adjuvant chemotherapy in stage I high-risk ovarian cancer with evaluation of DNA-ploidy as prognostic instrument. *Ann Oncol.* 11(3):281-288.

Trotti A, Byhardt R, Stetz J, et al. (2000). Common toxicity criteria: version 2.0: an improved reference for grading the acute effects of cancer treatment: impact on radiotherapy. *Int J Radiat Oncol Biol Phys.* 47(1):13-47.

Uziely B, Jeffers S, Isacson R, et al. (1995). Liposomal doxorubicin: antitumor activity and unique toxicities during two complementary phase I studies. *J Clin Oncol.* 13(7):1777-1785.

Vail DM, Chun R, Thamm DH, Garrett LD, Cooley AJ, Obradovich JE (1998). Efficacy of pyridoxine to ameliorate the cutaneous toxicity associated with doxorubicin containing pegylated (Stealth) liposomes: a randomized, double-blind clinical trial using a canine model. *Clin Cancer Res.* 4(6):1567-1571.

van der Burg ME, Hoff AM, van Lent M, Rodenburg CJ, van Putten WL, Stoter G (1991). Carboplatin and cyclophosphamide salvage therapy for ovarian cancer patients relapsing after cisplatin combination chemotherapy. *Eur J Cancer.* 27(3):248-250.

van der Burg ME, van Lent M, Buyse M, et al. (1995). The effect of debulking surgery after induction chemotherapy on the prognosis in advanced epithelial ovarian cancer. Gynecological Cancer Cooperative Group of the European Organization for Research and Treatment of Cancer. *N Engl J Med.* 332(10):629-634.

van Warmerdam LJ, Huizing MT, Giaccone G, et al. (1997). Clinical pharmacology of carboplatin administered in combination with paclitaxel. *Semin Oncol.* 24(1)(suppl 2):S2-97-S92-104.

Vasey PA, Jayson GC, Gordon A, et al.; Scottish Gynaecological Cancer Trials Group (2004). Phase III randomized trial of docetaxel-carboplatin versus paclitaxel-carboplatin as first-line chemotherapy for ovarian carcinoma. *J Natl Cancer Inst.* 96(22):1682-1691.

Vergote I, De Brabanter J, Fyles A, et al. (2001). Prognostic importance of degree of differentiation and cyst rupture in stage I invasive epithelial ovarian carcinoma. *Lancet.* 357(9251):176-182.

Vergote I, De Wever I, Tjalma W, Van Gramberen M, Decloedt J, van Dam P (1998). Neoadjuvant chemotherapy or primary debulking surgery in advanced ovarian carcinoma: a retrospective analysis of 285 patients. *Gynecol Oncol.* 71(3): 431-436.

Vergote I, Finkler N, del Campo J, et al. (2009). Phase 3 randomised study of canfosfamide (Telcyta, TLK286) versus pegylated liposomal doxorubicin or topotecan as third-line therapy in patients with platinum-refractory or -resistant ovarian cancer. *Eur J Cancer.* 45(13):2324-2332.

Vergote I, Himmelmann A, Frankendal B, Scheistroen M, Vlachos K, Trope C (1992). Hexamethylmelamine as second-line therapy in platin-resistant ovarian cancer. *Gynecol Oncol.* 47(3):282-286.

Vergote I, Rustin GJ, Eisenhauer EA, et al. (2000). Re: new guidelines to evaluate the response to treatment in solid tumors [ovarian cancer]. Gynecologic Cancer Intergroup. *J Natl Cancer Inst.* 92(18):1534-1535.

Vergote I, Trope CG, Amant F, et al. (2010). Neoadjuvant chemotherapy or primary surgery in stage IIIC or IV ovarian cancer. *N Engl J Med.* 363(10): 943-953.

Vergote IB, Vergote-De Vos LN, Abeler VM, et al. (1992). Randomized trial comparing cisplatin with radioactive phosphorus or whole-abdomen irradiation as adjuvant treatment of ovarian cancer. *Cancer.* 69(3):741-749.

Vermorken JB, Ten Bokkel Huinink WW, Eisenhauer EA, et al. (1993). Advanced ovarian cancer: carboplatin versus cisplatin. *Ann Oncol.* 4(suppl 4):41-48.

Vernooij F, Heintz AP, Witteveen PO, van der Heiden-van der Loo M, Coebergh JW, van der Graaf Y (2008). Specialized care and survival of ovarian cancer patients in the Netherlands: nationwide cohort study. *J Natl Cancer Inst.* 100(6):399-406.

Verweij J, Lund B, Beijnen J, et al. (1993). Phase I and pharmacokinetics study of topotecan, a new topoisomerase I inhibitor. *Ann Oncol.* 4(8):673-678.

Vogl SE, Pagano M, Kaplan BH, Greenwald E, Arseneau J, Bennett B (1983). Cisplatin based combination chemotherapy for advanced ovarian cancer: high overall response rate with curative potential only in women with small tumor burdens. *Cancer.* 51(11):2024-2030.

von Mehren M, Schilder RJ, Cheng JD, et al. (2008). A phase I study of the safety and pharmacokinetics of trabectedin in combination with pegylated liposomal doxorubicin in patients with advanced malignancies. *Ann Oncol.* 19(10): 1802-1809.

von Minckwitz G, Puglisi F, Cortes J, et al. (2014). Bevacizumab plus chemotherapy versus chemotherapy alone as second-line treatment for patients with HER2-negative locally recurrent or metastatic breast cancer after first-line treatment with bevacizumab plus chemotherapy (TANIA): an open-label, randomised phase 3 trial. *Lancet Oncol.* 15(11):1269-1278.

Walton L, Ellenberg SS, Major F Jr, Miller A, Park R, Young RC (1987). Results of second-look laparotomy in patients with early-stage ovarian carcinoma. *Obstet Gynecol.* 70(5):770-773.

West RJ, Zweig SF (1997). Meta-analysis of chemotherapy regimens for ovarian carcinoma: a reassessment of cisplatin, cyclophosphamide and doxorubicin versus cisplatin and cyclophosphamide. *Eur J Gynaecol Oncol*. 18(5):343-348.

Wils J, Blijham G, Naus A, et al. (1986). Primary or delayed debulking surgery and chemotherapy consisting of cisplatin, doxorubicin, and cyclophosphamide in stage III-IV epithelial ovarian carcinoma. *J Clin Oncol*. 4(7):1068-1073.

Winter WE III, Maxwell GL, Tian C, et al.; Gynecologic Oncology Group Study (2007). Prognostic factors for stage III epithelial ovarian cancer: a Gynecologic Oncology Group Study. *J Clin Oncol*. 25(24):3621-3627.

Winter WE III, Maxwell GL, Tian C, et al.; Gynecologic Oncology Group (2008). Tumor residual after surgical cytoreduction in prediction of clinical outcome in stage IV epithelial ovarian cancer: a Gynecologic Oncology Group Study. *J Clin Oncol*. 26(1):83-89.

Yedema CA, Kenemans P, Wobbes T, et al. (1992). Use of serum tumor markers in the differential diagnosis between ovarian and colorectal adenocarcinomas. *Tumour Biol*. 13(1-2):18-26.

Yoshida S, Furukawa N, Haruta S, et al. (2009). Theoretical model of treatment strategies for clear cell carcinoma of the ovary: focus on perspectives. *Cancer Treat Rev*. 35(7):608-615.

Young RC, Brady MF, Nieberg RK, et al. (2003). Adjuvant treatment for early ovarian cancer: a randomized phase III trial of intraperitoneal 32P or intravenous cyclophosphamide and cisplatin—a gynecologic oncology group study. *J Clin Oncol*. 21(23):4350-4355.

Young RC, Decker DG, Wharton JT, et al. (1983). Staging laparotomy in early ovarian cancer. *JAMA*. 250(22):3072-3076.

Young RC, Walton LA, Ellenberg SS, et al. (1990). Adjuvant therapy in stage I and stage II epithelial ovarian cancer: results of two prospective randomized trials. *N Engl J Med*. 322(15):1021-1027.

Zanetta G, Chiari S, Rota S, et al. (1997). Conservative surgery for stage I ovarian carcinoma in women of childbearing age. *Br J Obstet Gynaecol*. 104(9):1030-1035.

Zanotti KM, Belinson JL, Kennedy AW, Webster KD, Markman M (2000). Treatment of relapsed carcinoma of the ovary with single-agent paclitaxel following exposure to paclitaxel and platinum employed as initial therapy. *Gynecol Oncol*. 79(2):211-215.

Zhang L, Conejo-Garcia JR, Katsaros D, et al. (2003). Intratumoral T cells, recurrence, and survival in epithelial ovarian cancer. *N Engl J Med*. 348(3):203-213.

Zia MI, Siu LL, Pond GR, Chen EX (2005). Comparison of outcomes of phase II studies and subsequent randomized control studies using identical chemotherapeutic regimens. *J Clin Oncol*. 23(28):6982-6991.

Index

"t" following page number indicates table.

abdominal pain. *See* toxicity, abdominal pain
absolute neutrophil count (ANC): GOG 157, 39; GOG 132, 72
ACTION trial (Trimbos 2003b, Trimbos 2010), 1, 19, 23, 24–32, 43, 193, 197
Adjuvant ChemoTherapy in Ovarian Neoplasm Trial. *See* ACTION trial
Adriamycin. *See* doxorubicin
Adriamycin + cyclophosphamide. *See* cyclophosphamide + doxorubicin/ Adriamycin (CA)
Adriamycin + cyclophosphamide + platinum. *See* cyclophosphamide + doxorubicin/ Adriamycin + platinum (CAP)
advanced-stage ovarian cancer, CA125 normalization: OV16, 143t; paclitaxel + carboplatin (TC), 143t
advanced-stage ovarian cancer, negative second look: cyclophosphamide + cisplatin (CP), 56t; cyclophosphamide + doxorubicin + cisplatin (CAP), 52t; cyclophosphamide + cisplatin (CP), 52t; GOG 52, 52t; GOG 97, 56t; measurable, 56t; non-measurable, 56t
advanced-stage ovarian cancer, overall survival: AGO/OVAR-3, 104t; AGO-OVAR9, 136t; carboplatin, 69t, 94t; carboplatin + pegylated liposomal doxorubicin (C-PLD), 130t; CHORUS, 183–185, 185t; cisplatin, 73t; clear cell histology, 125t, 149t; cyclophosphamide + cisplatin (CP), 56t, 61t, 65t, 84t; cyclophosphamide + doxorubicin (CA), 49t; cyclophosphamide + doxorubicin + cisplatin (CAP), 49t, 52t, 69t; cyclophosphamide + cisplatin (CP), 52t; Danish Netherlands Trial, 78t; dose-dense paclitaxel + carboplatin, 124t; EORTC 55971, 177t; EORTC-GCG 55865, 167t; GOG 47, 49t; GOG 52, 52t; GOG 97, 56t; GOG 104, 65t; GOG 111, 61t; GOG 114, 89t; GOG 132, 73t; GOG 152, 172t; GOG 158, 98t; GOG 172, 113t; GOG 182/ICON5, 118t; GOG 218, 155t; high-risk group, 149t; ICON2, 69t; ICON3, 94t; ICON7, 149t; interval debulking surgery, 167t, 172t; intraperitoneal cisplatin-based chemotherapy, 65t, 89t, 113t; JGOG 3016, 124t; low-grade serous histology, 149t; measurable disease, 49t, 65t, 113t; MITO-2, 130t; mucinous histology, 125t; neoadjuvant chemotherapy, 177t, 185t; no interval debulking surgery, 167t, 172t; non-measurable disease, 49t; no visible residual disease, 113t; optimal, 124; optimal stage III, 189; OV-10, 84t; OV16, 143t; paclitaxel, 73t; paclitaxel + carboplatin (TC), 78t, 94t, 98t, 104t, 124t, 130t, 136t, 143t, 149t, 155t; paclitaxel + carboplatin + bevacizumab (PCB), 149t,

295

advanced-stage ovarian cancer, overall survival (*cont.*)
  155t; paclitaxel + cisplatin (TP), 61t, 73t, 78t, 84t, 89t, 98t, 104t, 113t; primary debulking, 177t, 185t; serous histology, 125t; stage IV, 189; suboptimal, 124t; suboptimal stage III, 189
advanced-stage ovarian cancer, pathologic complete response: cisplatin, 73t; cyclophosphamide + cisplatin (CP), 65t, 84t; GOG 104, 65t; GOG 132, 73t; GOG 158, 98t; GOG 172, 113t; intraperitoneal cisplatin-based chemotherapy, 65t, 113t; OV-10, 84t; paclitaxel, 73t; paclitaxel + carboplatin (TC), 98t; paclitaxel + cisplatin (TP), 73t, 84t, 98t, 113t
advanced-stage ovarian cancer, progression-free interval: carboplatin, 69t; cyclophosphamide + doxorubicin (CA), 49t; cyclophosphamide + doxorubicin + cisplatin (CAP), 49t, 52t, 69t; cyclophosphamide + cisplatin (CP), 52t, 84t; GOG 47, 49t; GOG 52, 52t; ICON2, 69t; OV-10, 84t; paclitaxel + cisplatin (TP), 84t
advanced-stage ovarian cancer, progression-free survival: AGO/OVAR-3, 104t; AGO-OVAR9, 136t; carboplatin, 94t; carboplatin + pegylated liposomal doxorubicin (C-PLD), 130t; CHORUS, 185t; cisplatin, 73t; clear cell histology, 125t; cyclophosphamide + cisplatin (CP), 56t, 61t; docetaxel + carboplatin, 108t; dose-dense paclitaxel + carboplatin, 124t; EORTC 55971, 177t; EORTC-GCG 55865, 167t; GOG 97, 56t; GOG 111, 61t; GOG 114, 89t; GOG 132, 73t; GOG 152, 172t; GOG 158, 98t; GOG 172, 113t; GOG 178/SWOG 9701, 190t; GOG 182/ICON5, 118t; GOG 218, 155t; high-risk group, 149t; ICON3, 94t; ICON7, 149t; interval debulking surgery, 167t, 172t; intraperitoneal cisplatin-based chemotherapy, 89t, 113t; JGOG 3016, 124t; maintenance paclitaxel, 190t; measurable disease, 113t; MITO-2, 130t; MITO-7, 160t; mucinous histology, 125t; neoadjuvant chemotherapy, 177t, 185t; no interval debulking surgery, 167t, 172t; no visible residual disease, 113t; optimal, 124t; OV16, 143t; paclitaxel, 73t; paclitaxel + carboplatin (TC), 94t, 98t, 104t, 108t, 124t, 130t, 136t, 143t, 149t, 155t, 160t; paclitaxel + carboplatin + bevacizumab (PCB), 149t, 155t; paclitaxel + cisplatin (TP), 61t, 73t, 89t, 98t, 104t, 113t; primary debulking surgery, 177t, 185t; SCOTROC, 108t; serous histology, 124t; suboptimal, 124t; weekly paclitaxel + carboplatin, 160t
advanced-stage ovarian cancer, RECIST response: AGO/OVAR-3, 104t; cisplatin, 73t; cyclophosphamide + cisplatin (CP), 56t, 61t; cyclophosphamide + doxorubicin (CA), 49t; cyclophosphamide + doxorubicin + cisplatin (CAP), 49t; Danish Netherlands Trial, 78t; GOG 47, 49t; GOG 97, 56t; GOG 111, 61t; GOG 132, 73t; OV16, 143t; paclitaxel, 73t; paclitaxel + carboplatin (TC), 78t, 104t, 143t; paclitaxel + cisplatin (TP), 61t, 73t, 78t, 104t
advanced-stage ovarian cancer, response duration: cyclophosphamide + doxorubicin (CA), 49t; cyclophosphamide + doxorubicin + cisplatin (CAP), 49t; GOG 47, 49t
advanced-stage ovarian cancer, response rate: AGO-OVAR9, 136t; carboplatin + pegylated liposomal doxorubicin (C-PLD), 130t; cyclophosphamide + cisplatin (CP), 61t, 84t; Danish Netherlands Trial, 78t; docetaxel + carboplatin, 108t; dose-dense paclitaxel + carboplatin, 124t; GOG 111, 61t; ICON7, 149t; JGOG 3016, 124t; MITO-2, 130t; MITO-7, 160t; OV-10, 84t; OV16, 143t; paclitaxel + carboplatin (TC), 78t, 108t, 124t, 130t, 136t, 143t, 149t, 160t; paclitaxel + carboplatin + bevacizumab (PCB), 149t; paclitaxel + cisplatin (TP), 61t, 78t, 84t; SCOTROC, 108t; weekly paclitaxel + carboplatin, 160t
age, prognostic factor, 52, 64
AGO. *See* Arbeitsgemeinschaft Gynakologische Onkologie
AGO-OVAR-3 (du Bois 2003), 46, 91, 99, 100–105, 223
AGO-OVAR-9 (du Bois, 2010), 46, 132–137

Index

AGO-OVAR/NCIC/EORTC (Pfisterer 2006a), 115, 133, 200, 222–228, 242, 243, 249, 251, 255–256
alkylating agent and risk of leukomegenesis, 48
allergic reaction. *See* toxicity, allergic reaction
alopecia. *See* toxicity, alopecia
altretamine, FDA approval, 235
ALZA Corp, 207
analysis of covariance, CHORUS, 183
analysis of variance: AGO-OVAR/NCIC/ EORTC trial, 227; Doxil Study 30–49, 212
anaphylaxis. *See* toxicity, anaphylaxis
anemia. *See* toxicity, anemia
angiogenesis, 145, 151
anorexia. *See* toxicity, anorexia
antibiotics, SCOTROC, 107
antiemetic regimens: AGO-OVAR-3, 102; CALYPSO, 245; GICOG trials, 11; SCOTROC, 107
ANZGOG. *See* Australia and New Zealand Gynecologic Oncology Group
Arbeitsgemeinschaft Gynakologische Onkologie (AGO), 100, 132, 145, 217, 222, 243
area under the curve (AUC): Calvert formula, 33, 68, 76, 87, 91, 96, 101, 107, 120–121, 128, 133, 158, 195, 218, 244; pegylated liposomal doxorubicin, 208
arterial thrombosis. *See* toxicity, arterial thrombosis
arthralgia. *See* toxicity, arthralgia
ascertainment bias, 37
ascites: AURELIA, 260, 262; prognostic significance, 17
Asian ethnicity, survival differences, 125
assessable disease: AGO-OVAR/NCIC/ EORTC trial, 223; Doxil Study 30–49, 209; gemcitabine versus PLD trial, 230; unidimensional, 209
assessment methods: ACTION, 21; GOG 47, 48; ICON1, 21
assessment schedule: AGO-OVAR-3, 102–103; AGO-OVAR9, 134; AGO-OVAR/NCIC/EORTC trial, 224; AURELIA, 259; CALYPSO, 245; CHORUS, 181; Danish Netherlands Trial, 77; Doxil Study 30–49, 211; EORTC 55971, 175; EORTC-GCG 55865, 165; gemcitabine versus PLD trial, 230; GICOG trials, 12; GOG 52, 51; GOG 97, 55; GOG 111, 59; GOG 114, 88; GOG 132, 72; GOG 152, 170; GOG 157, 40; GOG 158, 97; GOG 172, 111; GOG 175, 196; GOG 178/SWOG 9701, 188–189; GOG 218, 153; ICON1, 34, 37; ICON2, 68; ICON3, 92; ICON4/AGO-OVAR 2.2, 219; ICON7, 146; JGOG 3016, 122; MITO-2, 128, 129; MITO-7, 159; OCEANS, 252, 255; OV-10, 83; OV16, 140, 141; OVA-301, 238; SCOTROC, 107–109
atrioventricular block, 60
AURELIA (Pujade-Lauraine 2014), 200, 256–262
Australia and New Zealand Gynecologic Oncology Group, 114, 145, 243
autologous bone marrow rescue, 57
Aventis Pharmaceuticals, 105

barium enema: EORTC 55971, 174; GICOG trials, 11; GOG 7601, 3; GOG 7602, 6; OV16, 138
benzodiazepines, 11
bevacizumab: activity in ovarian cancer, 145, 151, 249, 257, 262; activity in platinum-resistant recurrent ovarian cancer, 257, 260; activity in platinum-sensitive recurrent ovarian cancer, 253; angiogenesis, 151; arterial thrombosis, 153; benefit with increased disease severity, 150; BOOST trial, 150; bowel perforation, 150, 153; breast cancer, 150, 151; coagulopathy, 153; colon cancer, 150, 151, 262; combined with carboplatin and gemcitabine, 251; combined with metronomic cyclophosphamide, 250; combined with paclitaxel weekly, 258; combined with pegylated liposomal doxorubicin, 258; combined with topotecan, 258; convergence of survival curves, 156; cost-effectiveness, 151; dose adjustment for weight change, 153; dose duration, 156; dose modifications, 252; dose selection, 156; durable benefit, 150; duration of response, 250; exclusion criteria, 251, 257–258; fistula, 250;

bevacizumab (*cont.*)
gastrointestinal perforation, 250, 255, 257–258, 262; GOG 218, 151–157; hypersensitivity, 153; ICON7, 145–151; hypertension, 150, 153; intestinal obstruction, 153; maintenance therapy, 146, 152, 157, 252; monoclonal antibody, 145, 151, 249, 257; phase II results, 249; proteinuria, 255; regrowth of tumor, 156; response rate, 250, 255; reversible posterior leukoencephalopathy syndrome, 153, 255; proteinuria, 153; timing from surgery, 251; timing of maximum impact, 148; venous thrombosis, 153; wound healing, 146, 153, 251

bilirubin. *See* toxicity, bilirubin

biologic progression-free interval, ICON7, 147

biomarkers, ICON7, 151

bleeding. *See* toxicity, bleeding

Blyth-Still-Casella method, AGO-OVAR9, 135

bone marrow function: AGO-OVAR-3, 101; AGO-OVAR9, 133; AGO-OVAR/NCIC/EORTC trial, 223; Danish Netherlands Trial, 75; Doxil Study 30–49, 209; GOG 97, 54; GOG 111, 58; GOG 114, 87; GOG 132, 71; GOG 152, 169; GOG 158, 96; GOG 175, 196; GOG 182/ICON5, 115; JGOG 3016, 120; MITO-7, 158; OV-10, 81; OV16, 138; OVA-301, 236; topotecan versus paclitaxel study, 202

borderline ovarian tumors: inclusion in trial, 5, 9; indolent course, 5

bowel obstruction. *See* toxicity bowel obstruction

bowel perforation. *See* gastrointestinal perforation

bowel resection, CHORUS, 181

bradyarrhythmias, 60

Breslow tests for significance, Danish Netherlands Trial, 77

Bristol-Meyers Squibb, 75

Brookmeyer-Crowley method, OCEANS, 253

CA. *See* cyclophosphamide+doxorubicin/Adriamycin

CA125: assessable disease, 230, 244; AURELIA, 257, 259; CALYPSO, 244, 245; criteria for disease progression, 122, 141, 171; CHORUS, 181, 182; Danish Netherlands Trial, 77, 79; Doxil Study 30–49, 209; EORTC-GCG 55865, 165; GCIG criteria, 153, 244, 245, 257, 259; gemcitabine versus PLD trial, 229, 230; GICOG, 12; GOG 97, 55; GOG 104, 63; GOG 132, 72; GOG 152, 170; GOG 172, 111; GOG 175, 196; GOG 178/SWOG 9701, 187; GOG 182/ICON5, 117; GOG 218, 153; ICON4/AGO-OVAR 2.2, 218, 219; ICON7, 148; JGOG 3016, 122; MITO-7, 159; normalization as endpoint, 144; OCEANS, 252; OV-10, 83; OV16, 140; OV16, 141; prognostic factor, 233, 248; Rustin method, 107, 153–154, 230; SCOTROC, 107–109; sign of progressive disease, 79; surrogate for outcome, 83, 144

CA125 normalization in advanced-stage ovarian cancer. *See* advanced-stage ovarian cancer, CA125 normalization

CA125 progression in recurrent ovarian cancer. *See* recurrent ovarian cancer, progression by CA125

CA125 response in recurrent ovarian cancer. *See* recurrent ovarian cancer, response by CA125 criteria

CA125 to CEA ratio: CHORUS, 179; EORTC 55971, 174; JGOG 3016, 120; OV16, 138

Calvert formula: AGO-OVAR-3, 101; AGO-OVAR9, 133; CALYPSO, 244; Danish Netherlands Trial, 76; GOG 114, 87; GOG 158, 96; GOG 175, 195; ICON1, 33; ICON2, 68; ICON3, 91; ICON4/AGO-OVAR 2.2, 218; JGOG 3016, 120, 121; MITO-2, 128; MITO-7, 158; SCOTROC, 107

CALYPSO (Pujade-Lauraine 2010), 200, 242–249, 249, 255–256

cancer-specific survival, definition, 29

cancer-specific survival in high-risk early-stage ovarian cancer. *See* early-stage ovarian cancer, high-risk, cancer-specific survival

CAP. *See* cyclophosphamide+doxorubicin/Adriamycin+platinum (CAP)

carboplatin: ACTION, 21, 27; AGO-OVAR/NCIC/EORTC trial, 223; AUC 2, 158;

Index

AUC 4, 224; AUC 5, 33, 68, 76, 107, 128, 115, 128, 133, 139, 146, 223, 244, 251; AUC 6, 99, 101, 116, 120, 121, 152, 158, 195; AUC 7, 107; AUC 7.5, 39, 96, 99; AUC 9, 86, 90; Calvert formula, 76, 91, 96, 101, 107, 120, 121, 128, 134, 158, 195, 218, 224, 244, 251; Cockcroft-Gault formula, 68, 128, 139, 158, 219, 244; combination regimens, 33; dose, 99; dose reduction, 224; dose reduction for GFR method, 68; early-stage ovarian cancer, 20, 25, 33; equivalence to CAP, 68; equivalence to cisplatin, 66, 91, 95, 103; FDA approval, 235; first-line treatment, 95; hypersensitivity reaction, 246, 248; ICON1, 21; ICON2, 68, 91; ICON3, 91, 100; ICON4/AGO-OVAR 2.2, 218; inferior to cisplatin, 75; Jelliffe method, 87, 96, 101, 121, 134, 195, 224; less toxicity than cisplatin, 67, 75, 99, 100, 103, 105; maximum tolerated dose, 101; neurotoxicity, 99; platinum-sensitive ovarian cancer, 222, 243; preferred agent in early-stage ovarian cancer, 24, 37; progression-free survival, 225; recommendation against upfront use, 96; SCOTROC, 107; substitution for cisplatin, 82; toxicity, 95; use in United Kingdom, 67; weekly administration, 161
carboplatin+docetaxel. *See* docetaxel+carboplatin
carboplatin+gemcitabine: AGO-OVAR/NCIC/EORTC trial, 222–228, 242, 243; approval in Europe, 249; approval in United States, 249; combined with bevacizumab, 251; dose reduction, 224; OCEANS, 251; platinum-sensitive ovarian cancer, 227; progression-free survival, 225, 249; response rate, 223
carboplatin+paclitaxel. *See* paclitaxel+carboplatin (TC)
carboplatin+pegylated liposomal doxorubicin (PLD): alternative front-line therapy, 131; CALYPSO, 244, 249; duration of therapy, 249; MITO-2, 126–132; overall survival, 244, 249; platinum-sensitive ovarian cancer, 249; progression-free survival, 244; response rate, 243–244; superior to carboplatin alone, 249; toxicity profile, 131

cardiac function: Doxil Study 30–49, 209; OVA-301, 236, 238
cardiac ischemia. *See* toxicity, cardiac ischemia
cardiac toxicity. *See* toxicity, cardiac
central nervous system bleeding. *See* toxicity, central nervous system bleeding
chemical tumor debulking, 86
chemoresistance: early-stage ovarian cancer, 42; influence on survival, 137; time to treatment failure, 137
chemotherapy, superiority of combination regimens, 66
chest radiography: Doxil Study 30–49, 211; GICOG trials, 11, 12; GOG 152, 170; GOG 178/SWOG 9701, 187; GOG 7601, 3; GOG 7602, 6
Chi-square test: ACTION, 29; CALYPSO, 246; ICON1/ACTION, 21, 23; ICON3, 92; ICON4/AGO-OVAR 2.2, 220; JGOG 3016, 123; MITO-2, 131; OV10, 83; test for interaction, 92; test for trend, 92
chlorambucil, GOG 97, 55
chlorpheniramine, 106
CHORUS (Kehoe 2015), 162, 178–185
chromic phosphate (^{32}P). *See* intraperitoneal ^{32}P
cimetidine, 39, 76, 88, 96, 102, 106, 196
cisplatin: ACTION, 21, 26; dose adjustment, 71; dosing, 11, 33, 71; efficacy, 47; equivalence to carboplatin, 66, 91; equivalence to PC (paclitaxel+cisplatin), 74; FDA approval, 235; GICOG trials, 11; GOG 132, 70; higher dose in GOG 132, 71; ICON4/AGO-OVAR 2.2, 219; immediate versus delayed treatment, 13–14; intraperitoneal, 63, 86, 88; renal monitoring, 48, 51; superiority of, 12, 20, 48; toxicity, 99
cisplatin+cyclophosphamide. *See* cyclophosphamide+cisplatin (CP)
cisplatin+cyclophosphamide+doxorubicin/Adriamycin. *See* cyclophosphamide+doxorubicin/Adriamycin+platinum (CAP)
cisplatin+doxorubicin/Adriamycin+cyclophosphamide. *See* cyclophosphamide+doxorubicin/Adriamycin+platinum (CAP)

cisplatin+paclitaxel. *See* paclitaxel+ cisplatin (TP)
clear cell histology: no benefit with dose-dense paclitaxel administration, 123; poor response to chemotherapy, 199; prognostic factor, 2, 17; response rate to chemotherapy, 44–45; worse outcomes, 5, 9, 52
clemastine, 102
clinical response rate, GOG 97, 57
clinical trials limitations, 235
coagulopathy: bevacizumab, 153; GOG 218, 153
Cochran-Mantel-Haenszel: Doxil Study 30–49, 212; OCEANS, 253; OV16, 142
Cockcroft-Gault formula: CALYPSO, 244; ICON2, 68; ICON4/AGO-OVAR 2.2, 219; MITO-2, 128; MITO-7, 158; OV16, 139
Colonoscopy: EORTC 55971, 174; OV16, 138
combination chemotherapy, recurrent ovarian cancer, 215
Common Terminology Criteria for Adverse Events (CTCAE): AGO-OVAR9, 134; AGO-OVAR/NCIC/EORTC trial, 225; AURELIA, 259; CALYPSO, 245; CHORUS, 182; Doxil Study 30–49, 211; gemcitabine versus PLD trial, 230; GOG 152, 170; GOG 182/ICON5, 115; GOG 218, 153; MITO-2, 129; MITO-7, 159; OCEANS, 252; OVA-301, 238; SCOTROC, 107; topotecan versus paclitaxel trial, 204
competing risks: GOG 157, 40; GOG 95, 17
complete pathologic response in advanced-stage ovarian cancer. *See* advanced-stage ovarian cancer, pathologic complete response
complete response (CR): Doxil Study 30–49, 211; GOG 47, 48; EORTC-GCG 55865, 165; topotecan versus paclitaxel trial, 203
computed tomography (CT) scan: AGO-OVAR-3, 103; AURELIA, 259; CALYPSO, 245; CHORUS, 181; Danish Netherlands Trial, 77; Doxil Study 30–49, 209, 211; EORTC 55971, 175; EORTC-GCG 55865, 165; gemcitabine versus PLD trial, 230; GICOG trials, 11, 12; GOG 132, 72; GOG 152, 170; GOG 178/SWOG 9701, 187; GOG 218, 153; GOG 7601, 3; GOG 7602, 6; ICON7, 147; JGOG 3016, 122; MITO-2, 129; MITO-7, 159; OCEANS, 252; OV-10, 83; OV16, 140; SCOTROC, 107–109; topotecan versus paclitaxel study, 202
confidence limits, Simon method, 5, 7
congestive heart failure. *See* toxicity, congestive heart failure
constipation. *See* toxicity, constipation
cost effectiveness: bevacizumab, 151; endpoint, 83; ICON7, 151
covariance matrix, GOG 172, 112
covariance parameters, GOG 172, 112
Cox proportional hazards regression: ACTION, 27; AGO-OVAR9, 135; AGO-OVAR/NCIC/EORTC trial, 227; CALYPSO, 246; CHORUS, 183; Danish Netherlands Trial, 77; EORTC 55971, 176; EORTC-GCG 55865, 165; gemcitabine versus PLD trial, 231; GICOG trials, 12; GOG 52, 52; GOG 104, 64; GOG 114, 88; GOG 158, 97; GOG 172, 112; GOG 178/SWOG 9701, 191; GOG 218, 154; GOG 7601, 4; GOG 7602, 7; ICON2, 68; ICON7, 148; MITO-2, 131; OCEANS, 253; OV-10, 83; OVA-301, 239; topotecan versus paclitaxel trial, 206
C-reactive protein, 79
creatine phosphokinase, OVA-301, 236
creatinine: parameters to discontinue chemotherapy, 11; parameters to hold chemotherapy, 11
creatinine clearance: Danish Netherlands Trial, 76; ICON2, 68; MITO-2, 128; parameters to discontinue chemotherapy, 11; parameters to hold chemotherapy, 11
Cremophor EL, 76
crossover: AURELIA, 259, 262; gemcitabine versus PLD trial, 230; GOG 111, 62, 85; GOG 132, 74; GOG 178/SWOG 9701, 194; GOG 218, 157; ICON1, 37; ICON3, 95; OV-10, 85
CTCAE. *See* Common Terminology Criteria for Adverse Events
CT scan. *See* computed tomography scan
cumulative incidence, 12

cutaneous toxicity. *See* toxicity, skin
cyclophosphamide: alkylating agent, 48; dose modifications, 59; hemorrhagic cystitis, 55; maintenance therapy in GOG 47, 47, 48; metronomic, 250
cyclophosphamide+cisplatin (CP): disease control rate with, 57, 58; dose modifications, 82; EORTC-GCG 55865, 164; equivalence to cyclophosphamide+ doxorubicin/Adriamycin+platinum (CAP), 100; GOG 52, 51, 100; GOG 95, 9, 15, 16; GOG 97, 53; GOG 104, 63; GOG 111, 58, 80, 100; GOG 114 arm discontinued, 87; inferiority compared to paclitaxel+cisplatin (TP) regimen, 60, 74, 83, 90; inferiority compared to single-agent platinum, 95; intensive intravenous dosing, 54; intraperitoneal dosing, 63; OV-10, 80, 81, 100; possible antagonistic effect, 74; standard intravenous dosing, 54; standard of care, 57, 201; superiority of, 17; toxicity of, 56
cyclophosphamide+doxorubicin/Adriamycin (CA): GOG 47, 47; subsequent treatment with cisplatin, 49–50
cyclophosphamide+doxorubicin/Adriamycin+platinum (CAP): first line treatment, 95; GOG 47, 47, 48, 100; GOG 52, 51; ICON1, 21, 33; ICON2, 36, 67, 91; ICON3, 92, 100; lower cyclophosphamide dose than in CA regimen, 52; superiority over cyclophosphamide+ doxorubicin, 48, 50, 100; superiority over cyclophosphamide+cisplatin, 66–67; toxicity, 70; use in Italy, 67
cystectomy (bladder), CHORUS, 181
cytoreductive surgery: drug-resistant clones, 163; EORTC-GCG 55865, 162–168; rationale, 163; tumor growth rate, 163

Danish Netherlands trial (Neijt 2000), 46, 75–79, 91, 99, 105
death due to treatment. *See* toxicity, death due to treatment
delay in treatment: AGO-OVAR-3, 102; AGO-OVAR/NCIC/EORTC trial, 224; CALYPSO, 245; gemcitabine versus PLD trial, 230; GOG 104, 63; GOG 111, 59; GOG 132, 72; GOG 157, 39; GOG 158, 96–97; GOG 172, 111; GOG 175, 196; GOG 178/SWOG 9701, 188; GOG 182/ ICON5, 117; JGOG, 121; MITO-2, 128; OCEANS, 252; OV16, 139; OVA-301, 241; SCOTROC, 107
dermatologic toxicity. *See* toxicity, skin
dexamethasone, 11, 39, 59, 76, 81, 88, 96, 102, 106, 196, 203, 237
diaphragm stripping, CHORUS, 181
diarrhea. *See* toxicity, diarrhea
diphenhydramine, 39, 59, 76, 81, 88, 96, 106, 196
disease control rate in recurrent ovarian cancer. *See* recurrent ovarian cancer, disease-control rate
disease-free survival in high-risk early-stage ovarian cancer. *See* early-stage ovarian cancer, high-risk, disease-free survival
disease-free survival in low-risk early-stage ovarian cancer. *See* early-stage ovarian cancer, low-risk, disease-free survival
disease-free survival in stage I ovarian cancer. *See* stage I ovarian cancer, disease-free survival
docetaxel: activity in ovarian cancer, 105; combination with carboplatin, 105, 106, 109; dexamethasone treatment, 106; dose, 106; dose discontinuation, 107; dose reduction, 106, 107; hypersensitivity reaction, 107; substitution for paclitaxel, 152
docetaxel+carboplatin, 105–109
dose-dense paclitaxel: antiangiogenic effect, 123; hematologic toxicity, 123; improved survival, 123; rationale, 123
dose escalation: GOG 47, 48; GOG 52, 51; topotecan versus paclitaxel trial, 203
dose intensity: GOG 97, 54; GOG 114, 88; GOG 157, 39; no impact on outcome, 57, 126; topotecan versus paclitaxel trial, 203
dose reduction: AGO-OVAR-3, 102; AGO-OVAR9, 133, 134; AGO-OVAR/ NCIC/EORTC trial, 224; AURELIA, 259; CALYPSO, 245; Danish Netherlands Trial, 76; Doxil Study 30–49, 210, 214t; gemcitabine versus PLD trial, 230; GOG 47, 47–48; GOG 52, 51; GOG 97,

dose reduction (*cont.*)
  54; GOG 157, 39; GOG 158, 96; GOG 172, 111; GOG 175, 196; GOG 178/ SWOG 9701, 188; GOG 182/ICON5, 117; JGOG 3016, 121; MITO-2, 128; MITO-7, 158; OV16, 139, 140; OVA-301, 237; pegylated liposomal doxorubicin, 210; SCOTROC, 106–107; topotecan, 210; topotecan versus paclitaxel trial, 203, 207
Doxil study 30–49 (Gordon 2001, Gordon 2004), 115, 200, 207–217, 234, 242, 243, 256
doxorubicin (Adriamycin): alopecia, 127; cardiac toxicity, 127; congestive heart failure, 48, 51; cumulative dose, 48, 51; dose-limiting toxicity, 127; first-line treatment, 126; gastrointestinal toxicity, 127; improved survival, 126, 132; lack of treatment benefit, 50, 52; myelosuppression, 127; toxicity, 48, 208
doxorubicin + cyclophosphamide. *See* cyclophosphamide + doxorubicin/ Adriamycin (CA)
doxorubicin + cyclophosphamide + platinum. *See* cyclophosphamide + doxorubicin/ Adriamycin + platinum (CAP)
duration of chemotherapy, 38
duration of response in recurrent ovarian cancer. *See* recurrent ovarian cancer, duration of response
dyspnea. *See* toxicity, dyspnea

early-stage ovarian cancer: GOG 7601, 1–5; prevalence, 37; recurrence risk, 17, 25, 32, 37, 38, 42, 43, 194
early-stage ovarian cancer, high-risk: GCIG consensus recommendations, 194; GICOG trials, 9–15; GOG 7602, 5–9; recurrence risk, 7, 17, 36; survival, 7, 36
early-stage ovarian cancer, high-risk, cancer-specific survival: ACTION, 29t, 31t; grade 3 tumors, 31t; no further therapy, 29t, 31t; non-optimally staged, 29t, 31t; optimally staged, 29t, 31t; platinum-based chemotherapy, 29t, 31t
early-stage ovarian cancer, high-risk, disease-free survival: cisplatin, 14t; GICOG trial 2, 14t; GOG 157, 42; intraperitoneal ^{32}P, 14t
early-stage ovarian cancer, high-risk, overall survival: ACTION, 28t; by histology, 45t; carboplatin + paclitaxel, 41t; cisplatin, 14t; cyclophosphamide + cisplatin (CP), 18t; GICOG trial 2, 14t; GOG 95, 18t; GOG 157, 41t; GOG 175, 198t; GOG 7602, 8t; ICON1, 35t; ICON1/ACTION, 22t; intraperitoneal ^{32}P, 8t, 14t, 18t; maintenance chemotherapy, 198t; melphalan, 8t; no further therapy, 22t, 28t, 35t; non-optimally staged, 28t; non-serous histology, 45t; optimally staged, 28t; paclitaxel + carboplatin (TC), 41t; platinum-based chemotherapy, 22t, 28t, 35t; serous histology, 45t
early-stage ovarian cancer, high-risk, recurrence-free survival: ACTION, 28t, 29t, 31t; by ascites, 45t; by cytology, 45t; by grade, 45t; by histology, 45t; by performance status, 45t; by stage, 45t; by tumor rupture, 45t; GOG 157, 45t; grade 3 tumors, 31t; ICON1, 35t; ICON1/ ACTION, 22t; no further therapy, 22t, 28t, 29t, 31t, 35t; non-optimally staged, 28t, 29t, 31t; non-serous histology, 45t; optimally staged, 28t, 29t, 31t; platinum-based chemotherapy, 22t, 28t, 29t, 31t, 35t; serous histology, 45t
early-stage ovarian cancer, high-risk, recurrence rate: ACTION, 28t, 29t; carboplatin + paclitaxel, 41t; complete staging, 41t; cyclophosphamide + cisplatin (CP), 18t; GOG 95, 18t; GOG 157, 41t; GOG 158, 100; GOG 175, 198t; intraperitoneal ^{32}P, 18t; maintenance chemotherapy, 198t; no further therapy, 28t, 29t; paclitaxel + carboplatin (TC), 41t; platinum-based chemotherapy, 28t, 29t; stage I, 42; stage II, 42; stage III, 100
early-stage ovarian cancer, low-risk: cisplatin in, 15; definition, 5, 10; GICOG trials, 9–15; GOG 7601, 1–5, 25; no further treatment, 5, 10, 25
early-stage ovarian cancer, low-risk, disease-free survival: cisplatin, 13t; GICOG trial 1, 13t; GOG 7601, 4t; melphalan, 4t; no further treatment, 4t, 13t
early-stage ovarian cancer, low-risk, overall survival: cisplatin, 13t; GICOG trial 1, 13t; no further treatment, 13t

Index

early termination of trial: federal mandate, 192; GOG 178/SWOG 9701, 189–190, 191, 192
Eastern Cooperative Oncology Group (ECOG), 86
echocardiogram, 211
ECOG. *See* Eastern Cooperative Oncology Group
Ecteinascidia turbinata, 235
electrocardiography: CALYPSO, 245; GOG 152, 170
Eli Lilly & Co, 228
endpoints: adverse events, 122, 141, 175; biologic progression-free interval, 147; CA125 as surrogate for outcome, 83, 144, 182; CA125 normalization at three cycles, 144; clinical response rate, 83, 171; complications, 117; cost-effectiveness, 83; cumulative dose delivery, 117; disease control rate, 231; dose intensity, 117; duration of response, 204, 212, 225, 239, 252; endorsed by AACR, 235; endorsed by ASCO, 235; endorsed by FDA, 235; endorsed by GCIG, 157; FACT-O/TOI score, 159; five-year survival, 68; health economics, 147; laboratory results, 147; negative second look, 53; non-standardized, 235; objective response rate, 159; overall response rate, 239, 252, 259; overall survival, 12, 21, 27, 34, 55, 60, 68, 72, 83, 88, 92, 97, 103, 109, 112, 117, 122, 129, 134, 141, 147, 159, 165, 171, 175, 182, 189, 196, 212, 219, 225, 228, 231, 238, 252, 259; pathologic response rate, 63, 90; performance status, 147; progression-free interval, 53, 55, 68, 153; progression-free survival, 60, 72, 77, 83, 88, 92, 97, 103, 109, 112, 117, 122, 129, 135, 141, 147, 153, 159, 165, 171, 175, 182, 189, 219, 225, 231, 238, 246, 252, 259; proportion without progression, 103; quality of life, 83, 103, 109, 112, 129, 135, 147, 175, 182, 219, 225, 239, 259; recurrence-free survival, 21, 27, 34; recurrence rate, 40, 196; relapse-free survival, 12; response rate, 48, 55, 72, 122, 137, 204, 212; response to treatment, 103, 135, 147, 225; safety, 212, 239, 259; surrogate, 235; survival, 2, 7, 53, 63, 68, 137, 204; time at risk of recurrence, 40; time to progression, 212; time to recurrence, 196, 204; time to response, 204, 212; time to treatment failure, 137; tolerability, 259; toxicity, 103, 117, 129, 135, 147, 159, 212, 225; translational research, 147; treatment activity, 129
ENGOT. *See* European Network of Gynaecological Oncological Trial Group
EORTC. *See* European Organization of Research and Treatment in Cancer
EORTC 55971 (Vergote 2010), 162, 174–178, 182
EORTC-GCG 55865 (van der Burg 1995), 162, 162–168, 168, 171, 173
epogen, 136t
erythropoietin, 145t, 214t
ethylenediaminetetraacetic acid (EDTA) clearance, Danish Netherlands Trial, 76
etoposide: lack of cross-resistance to platinum and taxanes, 208; response rates, 215; second-line therapy, 201
European Network of Gynaecological Oncological Trial Group (ENGOT), 157, 256
European Organization of Research and Treatment in Cancer (EORTC), 19, 24, 80, 138, 163, 174, 222, 243
exact linear rank test, MITO-2, 131

fatigue. *See* toxicity, fatigue
febrile neutropenia. *See* toxicity, febrile neutropenia
fever. *See* toxicity, fever
F. Hoffmann-La Roche, 256
filgrastim, GOG 157, 39
fine needle aspiration, EORTC 55971, 174
Fisher's exact test: gemcitabine versus PLD trial, 231; GOG 104, 64; GOG 218, 154; JGOG 3016, 123; MITO-2, 131; OV-10, 83; OV16, 142
fistula. *See* toxicity, fistula
flexible parametric survival models, ICON7, 148
Food and Drug Administration, approval of pegylated liposomal doxorubicin, 208
Freedman's method for sample size calculation, gemcitabine versus PLD trial, 231
Functional Assessment of Cancer Therapy—Gynecologic Oncology Group—Ntx, MITO-7, 159

Functional Assessment of Cancer Therapy—Ovarian (FACT-O) questionnaire: GOG 172, 111; GOG 218, 153, 154; MITO-7, 159, 160t; primary endpoint, 159

Functional Living Index—Cancer (FLIC), GOG 97, 55

gastrointestinal perforation. *See* toxicity, gastrointestinal perforation

gastrointestinal toxicity. *See* toxicity, gastrointestinal

gastroscopy: EORTC 55971, 174; OV16, 138

GCIG. *See* Gynecologic Cancer Intergroup

GCIG criteria for CA125 response, 153, 244, 245, 257, 259

GEICO. *See* Grupo de Investigacion de Cancer De Ovario

gemcitabine: combination regimens, 223–224, 229, 251; combined with paclitaxel and carboplatin, 116–117, 132–137; dose modifications, 252; dose reduction, 224; dosing, 230; FDA approval, 235; front-line chemotherapy, 116–117, 132–137; gemcitabine versus PLD trial, 228–234; fatigue, 137; hematologic toxicity, 137; lack of cross-resistance to platinum and taxanes, 208; nucleoside analogue, 223; phase II studies, 229; platinum-resistant ovarian cancer, 229; recurrent ovarian cancer, 115, 132, 133, 223, 243; response rates, 215

gemcitabine+carboplatin. *See* carboplatin+gemcitabine

Gemcitabine versus PLD trial (Mutch 2007), 132, 200, 228–234, 256

Gemzar. *See* gemcitabine

Genentech, 249

genitourinary toxicity. *See* toxicity, genitourinary

GICOG trials (Bolis 1995), 1, 9–15, 19, 20, 24, 25, 32, 36, 38, 193, 197

GINECO. *See* Group d'Investigateurs Nationaux pour l'Etude des Cancers Ovariens

global deterioration of health, GOG 218, 154

global test of heterogeneity, GICOG trials, 12

glomerular filtration rate (GFR): 24-hour urine collection, 218; edetic acid, 107; equivalent to creatinine clearance, 87; GOG 114, 87; ICON1, 33; ICON2, 68; nuclear renogram, 139; peroxidase-antiperoxidase method can result in excessive dosing, 125; radioisotope method, 218; SCOTROC, 107

GOG. *See* Gynecologic Oncology Group

GOG 47 (Omura 1986), 46, 46–50, 50, 100

GOG 52 (Omura 1989), 46, 50–53, 100

GOG 95 (Young, 2003), 1, 15–19, 38, 193, 197

GOG 97 (McGuire 1995), 46, 52–57

GOG 104 (Alberts 1996), 46, 62–66, 90, 110, 189

GOG 111 (McGuire 1996), 38, 46, 57–62, 66, 70, 74, 80, 83, 85, 87, 90, 91, 95, 100, 105, 189, 191, 194, 201, 208

GOG 114 (Markman 2001), 46, 86–90, 110

GOG 132 (Muggia 2000), 46, 70–74, 91, 95, 189, 191

GOG 152 (Rose 2004), 162, 168–173, 175

GOG 157 (Bell 2006, Chan 2007), 1, 37–45, 193, 194, 197, 199

GOG 158 (Ozols 2003), 46, 91, 95–100, 194

GOG 172 (Armstrong 2006), 46, 90, 109–114

GOG 175 (Mannel 2011), 186, 193–199

GOG 178/SWOG 9701 (Markman 2003), 186, 186–193, 194, 195

GOG 182/ICON5 (Bookman 2009), 46, 100, 114–119, 120, 137, 142

GOG 218 (Burger 2011), 46, 150, 151–157, 262

GOG 7601 (Young 1990), 1, 1–5, 15, 20, 23, 25, 36, 37, 193

GOG 7602 (Young 1990), 1, 5–9, 32, 38, 42, 193, 197

grade, prognostic factor, 2, 30, 52

Grambsch-Therneau test, CHORUS, 183

granulocyte colony-stimulating factors (G-CSFs): AGO-OVAR-3, 102; AGO-OVAR9, 134, 136t; Doxil Study 30–49, 210, 214t; gemcitabine versus PLD trial, 230; GOG 132, 72; GOG 152, 169; GOG 158, 96–97; GOG 172, 111; GOG 175, 196; GOG 178/SWOG 9701, 188; GOG 182/ICON5, 117; GOG 218, 152; JGOG 3016, 121; OV-10, 82; OV16,

Index

145t; OVA-301, 237, 240t; SCOTROC, 107; topotecan versus paclitaxel trial, 203, 206t, 207.
granulocyte count, prognostic impact, 79
granulocyte macrophage colony-stimulating factors (GM-CSFs), AGO-OVAR9, 134
granulocyte toxicity. *See* toxicity, granulocyte
Group d'Investigateurs Nationaux pour l'Etude des Cancers Ovariens (GINECO), 127, 132, 145, 243
Grupo de Investigacion de Cancer De Ovario (GEICO), 138, 145
Gynecologic Cancer Intergroup (GCIG), 132, 138, 141, 145, 157, 256
Gynecologic Oncology Group (GOG), 1, 5, 15, 37, 46, 50, 53, 57, 62, 70, 86, 95, 110, 114, 151, 168, 187, 193

hand-foot syndrome. *See* toxicity, palmar-plantar erythrodysesthesia (PPE)
hazard functions, ICON7, 148
hazard ratio, pooled, 23
hearing loss. *See* toxicity, ototoxicity
heart block. *See* toxicity, heart block
hematologic function. *See* bone marrow function
hematologic parameters to treat: AGO-OVAR9, 134; dose-dense paclitaxel, 121; JGOG 3016, 121; MITO-2, 128; OV16, 139
hematologic toxicity. *See* toxicity, hematologic
hemoglobin, prognostic impact, 79
hemorrhagic cystitis. *See* toxicity, hemorrhagic cystitis
hepatic function: AGO-OVAR-3, 101; AGO-OVAR9, 133; Danish Netherlands Trial, 76; Doxil Study 30–49, 209; GOG 97, 54; GOG 111, 58, GOG 114, 87; GOG 132, 71; GOG 152, 169; GOG 158, 96; GOG 182/ICON5, 115; JGOG 3016, 120; OV-10, 81; OVA-301, 236; topotecan versus paclitaxel study, 202
hepatic toxicity. *See* toxicity, hepatic
heterogeneity: statistical, 24, 42, 131; tumors, 44
hexamethylmelamine: response rates, 215; second-line therapy, 201
high-dose chemotherapy with stem cell support, treatment option for recurrent ovarian cancer, 215
histamine H1 antagonist, 203
histamine H2 antagonist, 59, 203
histology, prognostic impact, 178
homogeneity, statistical, 44, 55, 60
hormonal therapy, treatment option for recurrent ovarian cancer, 215
hospitalization. *See* toxicity, hospitalization
Hycamtin. *See* topotecan
hydration regimens: cyclophosphamide+cisplatin (CP), 81; GICOG trials, 11; paclitaxel+cisplatin (TP), 82
hypersensitivity. *See* toxicity, hypersensitivity
hypertension. *See* toxicity, hypertension
Hy's law, 241

ICON. *See* International Collaborative Ovarian Neoplasm
ICON1 (Colombo 2003), 1, 19, 23, 24, 32–37
ICON1/ACTION combined analysis (Trimbos 2003a), 1, 19–24, 42, 193, 197
ICON2 (Lancet 1998), 36, 46, 66–70, 91
ICON3 (Lancet 2002), 46, 70, 90–95, 185
ICON4/AGO-OVAR 2.2 (Parmar 2003), 200, 216, 217–221, 222, 242, 243, 246, 249, 255–256
ICON7 (Perrin 2011, Oza 2015), 46, 145–151, 156, 262
ifosfamide: response rates, 215; second-line therapy, 201
immunologically active subtype of ovarian cancer, ICON7, 151
inclusion criteria, more than one prior chemotherapy regimen allowed: CALYPSO, 244; gemcitabine versus PLD trial, 229; ICON4/AGO-OVAR 2.2, 218
inclusion criteria, one prior chemotherapy regimen allowed: Doxil Study 30–49, 209; ICON4/AGO-OVAR 2.2, 218; OVA-301, 236; topotecan versus paclitaxel trial, 202
inclusion criteria, stage I ovarian cancer: AGO-OVAR9, 133; GOG 175, 195; ICON2, 69; high-risk, 2, 6; ICON7, 146; low-risk, 2, 6; MITO-2, 127; MITO-7, 158; SCOTROC, 106

inclusion criteria, stage II ovarian cancer: AGO-OVAR-3, 101; AGO-OVAR9, 133; Danish Netherlands Trial, 75; EORTC-GCG 55865, 164; GOG 175, 195; ICON2, 69; ICON7, 146; JGOG 3016, 120; MITO-2, 127; MITO-7, 158; OV-10, 80; OV16, 138; SCOTROC, 106

inclusion criteria, stage III ovarian cancer: AGO-OVAR-3, 101; AGO-OVAR9, 133; CHORUS, 179; Danish Netherlands Trial, 75; EORTC 55971, 174; EORTC-GCG 55865, 164; GOG 47, 47; GOG 52, 50; GOG 97, 54; GOG 104, 62; GOG 111, 58; GOG 114, 86; GOG 132, 71; GOG 152, 168; GOG 158, 96; GOG 172, 110; GOG 178/SWOG 9701, 187; GOG 182/ICON5, 115; GOG 218, 151; ICON2, 69; ICON7, 146; JGOG 3016, 120; MITO-2, 127; MITO-7, 158; OV-10, 80; OV16, 138; SCOTROC, 106; topotecan versus paclitaxel study, 202

inclusion criteria, stage IV ovarian cancer: AGO-OVAR-3, 101; AGO-OVAR9, 133; CHORUS, 179; Danish Netherlands Trial, 75; EORTC 55971, 174; EORTC-GCG 55865, 164; GOG 47, 47; GOG 97, 54; GOG 111, 58; GOG 132, 71; GOG 152, 168; GOG 178/SWOG 9701, 187; GOG 182/ICON5, 115; GOG 218, 151; ICON2, 69; ICON7, 146; JGOG 3016, 120; MITO-2, 127; MITO-7, 158; OV-10, 80; OV16, 138; SCOTROC, 106; topotecan versus paclitaxel study, 202

Independent Data Monitoring Committee (IDMC), AURELIA, 260

Independent Review Committee (IRC), OCEANS, 255

induction chemotherapy: EORTC-GCG 55865, 167; impact on survival unclear, 163

infection. *See* toxicity, infection

Integrated Therapeutics Group (ITG), 126

intention-to-treat analysis: ICON1/ACTION, 21; OCEANS, 253

interaction analyses, ICON7, 148

interim analysis: Doxil Study 30–49, 212; EORTC-GCG 55865, 165; GOG 152, 171; GOG 175, 197; GOG 178/SWOG 9701, 189, 191; GOG 182/ICON5, 117, 119

interleukin-6, 79

International Collaborative Ovarian Neoplasm (ICON), 19, 66, 114, 145

interval cytoreduction: CHORUS, 180; Danish Netherlands Trial, 77; EORTC 55971, 175; EORTC-GCG 55865, 162–168; JGOG 3016, 122; OV-10, 82; GOG 182/ICON5, 117; MITO-7, 159; OV16, 140; SCOTROC, 107; surgical complications, 167t, 172t, 177t, 185t

intestinal obstruction: bevacizumab, 153; GOG 218, 153

intraperitoneal ^{32}P: complications with, 17–18, 19; dosing, 11, 16; GICOG trials, 11; GOG 7602, 6; GOG 95, 16; shortage of, 11; superiority of, 9

intraperitoneal catheter: GOG 114, 88; GOG 172, 114

intraperitoneal cisplatin: after bowel resection, 114; capillary uptake, 112–114; GOG 104, 63, 110; GOG 114, 110; GOG 172, 111; greater concentrations, 62, 110; improved survival, 112, 145; lower systemic exposure, 114; superiority over intravenous cisplatin, 64, 90; toxicity, 110, 112, 114; tumor penetration, 64

intraperitoneal paclitaxel: GOG 172, 111; intraperitoneal clearance, 114; toxicity, 114

intravenous pyelography, 3, 6, 11

Istituto Mario Negri, 32, 66, 90, 115, 217

Japanese Gynecologic Oncology Group (JGOG), 119

Jelliffe method: AGO-OVAR-3, 101; AGO-OVAR9, 133; GOG 114, 87; GOG 158, 96; GOG 175, 195; JGOG 3016, 120

JGOG. *See* Japanese Gynecologic Oncology Group

JGOG 3016 (Katsumata 2009, Katsumata 2013), 46, 119–126, 159, 194

Johnson & Johnson, 235

Kaplan and Meier test: ACTION, 21, 27; ACTION/ICON1 combined analysis, 23; AGO-OVAR9, 135; AGO-OVAR/NCIC/EORTC trial, 227; CALYPSO, 246; Danish Netherlands Trial, 77; Doxil Study 30–49, 212; EORTC 55971, 176; EORTC-GCG 55865, 165; gemcitabine versus PLD trial, 231; GICOG trials, 12;

GOG 95, 17; GOG 97, 55; GOG 111, 60; GOG 114, 88; GOG 158, 97; GOG 172, 112; GOG 7601, 4; GOG 7602, 7; ICON4/AGO-OVAR 2.2, 220; inverted, 129; JGOG 3016, 123; ICON1, 21, 34; ICON2, 68; ICON3, 92; MITO-2, 129; OCEANS, 253; OV-10, 83; OVA-301, 239; topotecan versus paclitaxel trial, 204
Karnofsky index, 101
Kruskal-Wallis rank test: GOG 97, 57; GOG 111, 60; GOG 158, 97; OV-10, 83

left ventricular ejection fraction: CALYPSO, 245; Doxil Study 30–49, 209, 210, 211, 214; OVA-301, 236, 238
leukemia, 42, 48, 193
leukopenia. *See* toxicity, leukopenia
likelihood ratio test, 53
linear models: GOG 172, 112; GOG 218, 154
liposomes, 127, 208
liver function. *See* hepatic function
log-rank test: ACTION, 21, 27; AGO-OVAR9, 135; AGO-OVAR/NCIC/EORTC trial, 227; AURELIA, 260; CHORUS, 183; Danish Netherlands Trial, 77; Doxil Study 30–49, 212; EORTC 55971, 176; EORTC-GCG 55865, 165; gemcitabine versus PLD trial, 231; GICOG trials, 12; GOG 95, 55; GOG 111, 60; GOG 114, 88; GOG 152, 170; GOG 175, 197; GOG 7601, 4; GOG 7602, 7; ICON1, 21; ICON2, 68; ICON3, 92; ICON7, 147, 148; Mantel-Cox version, 34, 68, 92; MITO-2, 131; OCEANS, 253; OV-10, 83; OV16, 142; OVA-301, 239; stratified, 34, 92, 117, 142, 183, 212, 239, 253, 260; unstratified, 83, 147, 260. *See also* Mantel-Cox log-rank test
low-grade serous ovarian cancer, poor response to chemotherapy, 199
luteinizing hormone-releasing hormone analogues, 234
lymphadenectomy: CHORUS, 181; prognostic impact, 14
lymphangiography, 3, 6, 11

magnesium sulfate, GOG 104, 63
magnetic resonance imaging (MRI): AGO-OVAR-3, 103; AURELIA, 259; CALYPSO, 245; CHORUS, 181; Doxil Study 30–49, 209, 211; GOG 218, 153; ICON7, 147; MITO-2, 129; OV16, 140; topotecan versus paclitaxel study, 202
maintenance therapy: accelerated recurrence after discontinuation, 192; definition, 186; data in non-ovarian malignancies, 187; optimal duration, 193
mammogram, EORTC 55971, 174
MaNGO. *See* Mario Negri Gynecologic Oncology
mannitol, GOG 104, 63
Mann-Whitney U test: GOG 114, 88; ICON4/AGO-OVAR 2.2, 220
Mantel-Cox log-rank test: ICON1, 34; ICON2, 68; ICON4/AGO-OVAR 2.2, 220. *See also* log-rank test
Mantel-Haenszel Chi-square test: GOG 52, 52; GOG 97, 57
Mario Negri Gynecologic Oncology (MaNGO), 243
measurable ovarian cancer: AGO-OVAR/NCIC/EORTC trial, 223; AURELIA, 257; bidimensional, 209; CALYPSO, 244; Doxil Study 30–49, 209; gemcitabine versus PLD trial, 229, 230; GOG 97, 54, 55; OCEANS, 250; OVA-301, 236; prognostic factor, 248; topotecan versus paclitaxel study, 202
Medical Research Council (MRC), 32, 66, 91, 114, 145, 179, 217
melphalan: aplastic anemia, 4t; GOG 7601, 3, 20; GOG 7602, 6; secondary cancers, 5, 9
mesenchymal subtype of ovarian cancer, ICON7, 151
metabolic toxicity. *See* toxicity, metabolic
methoxypolyethylene glycol, 127
metoclopramide, 11
MITO. *See* Multicentre Italian Trials in Ovarian Cancer
MITO-2 (Pignata 2009, Pignata 2011), 46, 126–132
MITO-7 (Pignata 2014), 46, 126, 157–161
MITO16MANGO2b trial, 151
mixed effects model, 241
MRC. *See* Medical Research Council
mucinous histology: no benefit with dose-dense paclitaxel administration, 123; poor response to chemotherapy, 199

mucositis. *See* toxicity, mucositis
Multicentre Italian Trials in Ovarian Cancer (MITO), 126, 157, 243
multidrug resistance, 215
multigated angiography, 245
multiple comparisons, GOG 218, 154
multiple gated acquisition scan, 211
myalgia. *See* toxicity, myalgia
myelodysplastic syndrome, 42
myelotoxicity. *See* toxicity, myelotoxicity

nail changes. *See* toxicity, nail changes
National Cancer Institute (NCI), 115
National Cancer Institute of Canada Clinical Trials Group (NCI-C-CTG), 80, 138, 145, 174, 222, 243
nausea. *See* toxicity, nausea
NCCTG. *See* North Central Cancer Treatment Group
NCI. *See* National Cancer Institute
NCI-C-CTG. *See* National Cancer Institute of Canada Clinical Trials Group
negative second look in advanced-stage ovarian cancer. *See* advanced-stage ovarian cancer, negative second look
neoadjuvant chemotherapy: CHORUS, 178–185; EORTC 55971, 174–178; fibrosis, 178; meta-analysis, 174, 179; worse outcome, 174
neuropathy. *See* toxicity, neurotoxicity
neurotoxicity. *See* toxicity, neurotoxicity
neutropenia. *See* toxicity, neutropenia
New York State Heart Association Classification System, Doxil Study 30–49, 209
NOCOVA. *See* Nordic Gynecological Cancer Study Group
nonassessable disease, topotecan versus paclitaxel trial, 204
non-inferiority study: AGO-OVAR-3, 103; CALYPSO, 246; CHORUS, 182; GOG 158, 96, 99
non-measurable ovarian cancer: GOG 97, 54; no benefit to adding cisplatin, 49; topotecan versus paclitaxel trial, 204
Nonprofit Italian Association for Cancer Research, 126
non-proportional hazards, ICON7, 148
Nordic Gynecological Cancer Study Group (NOCOVA), 80

Nordic Society for Gynecologic Oncology (NSGO), 90, 132, 145, 243
North Central Cancer Treatment Group (NCCTG), 15
Nscore neurotoxicity assessment, SCOTROC, 109
NSGO. *See* Nordic Society for Gynecologic Oncology
nuclear magnetic resonance (NMR), MITO-7, 159
number of treatment cycles: AGO-OVAR-3, 102; AGO-OVAR9, 134; AGO-OVAR/NCIC/EORTC trial, 224; CALYPSO, 244; Danish Netherlands Trial, 76–77, 79; Doxil Study 30–49, 210; EORTC-GCG 55865, 164; gemcitabine versus PLD trial, 230; GOG 157, 40; GOG 218, 156; JGOG 3016, 122; non-serous histology, 44–45; OCEANS, 251; OV-10, 82, 85; optimal duration unknown, 38; OV16, 139; OVA-301, 237; pegylated liposomal doxorubicin, 210; SCOTROC, 107; serous histology, 44–45; topotecan, 210; topotecan versus paclitaxel trial, 203

observation in early-stage ovarian cancer: trials advocating, 5, 24, 25, 29, 30–31, 32, 37, 42–43; trials including, 3, 11, 21, 23–24, 25, 26, 33, 36
occult stage III ovarian cancer: impact of chemotherapy in non-optimally-staged patients, 30; rate in early-stage ovarian cancer, 25
OCEANS (Aghajanian 2012), 156, 200, 249–256, 262
optimal cytoreduction: definition, 50; GOG 52, 50; GOG 104, 62; GOG 111, 86; GOG 158, 96; GOG 172, 110; GOG 178/SWOG 9701, 187; GOG 182/ICON5, 115; GOG 218, 152; JGOG 3016, 124; OV-10, 80; rate in CHORUS, 183; rate in EORTC 55971, 178; survival benefit, 163
ototoxicity. *See* toxicity, ototoxicity
OV-10 (Piccart 2000), 46, 74, 80–86, 90, 91, 95, 100, 105, 191, 201
OV16 (Hoskins 2010), 46, 120, 137–144
OVA-301 (Monk 2010), 200, 235–242
Ovarian Cancer Study Group, 1, 5
overall response rate, OVA-301, 239, 241
overall survival, 225

Index   309

overall survival as primary endpoint:
  ACTION, 27; AGO-OVAR9, 134;
  CHORUS, 182; EORTC 55971, 175;
  GOG 218, 153; ICON1, 34; ICON1/
  ACTION, 21; ICON4/AGO-OVAR 2.2,
  219
overall survival in advanced-stage ovarian
  cancer. *See* advanced-stage ovarian
  cancer, overall survival
overall survival in high-risk early-stage
  ovarian cancer. *See* early-stage ovarian
  cancer, high-risk, overall survival
overall survival in low-risk early-stage
  ovarian cancer. *See* early-stage ovarian
  cancer, low-risk, overall survival
overall survival in recurrent ovarian cancer.
  See recurrent ovarian cancer, overall
  survival
overall survival in stage I ovarian cancer.
  See stage I ovarian cancer, overall survival

paclitaxel: 3 vs. 24-hour infusion, 75, 80,
  99, 201, 206–207; activity in platinum-
  resistant ovarian cancer, 256; antiangiogenic effect, 157, 191, 193, 194;
  AURELIA, 258; cardiac effects, 60;
  combination-treatment efficacy, 60, 86;
  combined with bevacizumab, 258; data
  supporting extended use, 187, 191;
  discontinuation, 82; dose-dense
  administration, 120, 161; dose escalation,
  81; dose modifications, 59, 71, 169, 188;
  FDA approval, 235; GOG 132, 70–71;
  GOG 178/SWOG 9701, 186–193; higher
  dose in GOG 132, 71; hypersensitivity
  reaction, 106, 152; ICON4/AGO-OVAR
  2.2, 219; impact of duration versus dose,
  192; inferiority to platinum, 72;
  maintenance therapy, 186–193, 193–199,
  194, 195; maximum dose, 196; maximum
  tolerated dose, 101; methoxypolyethylene
  glycol, 127; myeloprotective effect, 220;
  not mandatory in upfront treatment,
  90–95, 185; premedication regimen, 39,
  59, 76, 81, 88, 96, 106, 169, 196; prolonged
  circulation, 127; recurrent ovarian cancer,
  243; response rates, 201, 206–207, 217;
  single-agent efficacy, 58, 201; therapeutic
  ratio, 192; timing of administration, 95;
  topotecan versus paclitaxel study,
  200–207, 234, 242; toxicity, 197; weekly
  administration, 157, 158, 195
paclitaxel + carboplatin (TC): AGO-
  OVAR-3, 99, 101; AGO-OVAR9, 133;
  CALYPSO, 244; Danish Netherlands
  Trial, 79, 99; EORTC 55971, 175;
  equivalence to paclitaxel + cisplatin (TP),
  99; GOG 157, 39; GOG 158, 96, 99; GOG
  175, 193–199; GOG 182/ICON5, 116;
  GOG 218, 152; ICON3, 91, 92, 100;
  ICON7, 146; JGOG 3016, 120; less
  toxicity than paclitaxel + cisplatin, 79;
  maximum tolerated dose, 101–102;
  MITO-7, 157–161, myelosuppression,
  105; number of cycles, 38, 40; OV16, 139;
  quality of life, 103; platinum-sensitive
  recurrent ovarian cancer, 217–221, 243,
  246; residual neurotoxicity rate, 132;
  response rate, 96, 105; SCOTROC, 106;
  standard therapy for advanced ovarian
  cancer, 38, 100, 119, 187, 194; toxicities,
  157, 161; weekly administration, 157–161;
  with third chemotherapy drug, 114–119,
  120, 132–137, 137–144
paclitaxel + cisplatin (TP): 24-hour
  paclitaxel infusion, 58; 3-hour paclitaxel
  infusion, 76, 80; AGO-OVAR-3, 99, 101;
  better toxicity profile than high-dose
  monotherapy, 72; CHORUS, 180; Danish
  Netherlands Trial, 79, 99; dose adjustment, 71, 82; equivalence to non-taxane
  platinum regimen, 95; GOG 111, 59–60,
  80, 100; GOG 114, 87; GOG 132, 70, 71;
  GOG 152, 168–173; GOG 158, 96, 99;
  GOG 172, 110; MITO-2, 128; neurotoxicity, 91; OV-10, 80, 81, 100; overall
  survival, 105; quality of life, 103;
  response rates, 105; sequential therapy,
  74; standard of care, 75, 86, 91, 201;
  superiority over cyclophosphamide + cisplatin (CP) regimen, 60, 74, 83, 90;
  toxicity, 95
pain. *See* toxicity, pain
paired T-test, AGO-OVAR/NCIC/EORTC
  trial, 227
palliation, goal of therapy for recurrent
  ovarian cancer, 233
palmar-plantar erythrodysesthesia (PPE).
  See toxicity, palmar-plantar
  erythrodysesthesia

paracentesis, AURELIA, 261t
partial response (PR): Doxil Study 30–49, 211; GOG 47, 48; topotecan versus paclitaxel trial, 203
pathologic response in advanced-stage ovarian cancer. *See* advanced-stage ovarian cancer, pathologic complete response
pathologic response rate: GOG 97, 55, 57; GOG 104, 63, 64; with intraperitoneal cisplatin, 64
patient-reported outcomes, 262
Pearson's Chi-square test: GOG 104, 64; GOG 111, 60; GOG 114, 88
pegylated liposomal doxorubicin (PLD): approved agent, 208, 235; area under the curve, 208; AURELIA, 258; cardiac monitoring, 211, 214; clearance, 116, 208; combined with bevacizumab, 258; combined with carboplatin, 127, 243–244; combined with paclitaxel and carboplatin, 116; cumulative dose, 211, 214, 230, 238, 245; dose modifications, 208, 210; dosing every 3 weeks, 127, 237; dosing every 4 weeks, 116, 210, 230, 237, 244; Doxil study, 207–217, 242; elimination half-life, 208; equivalent to topotecan, 200–207, 229, 234; FDA approval, 235; gemcitabine versus PLD trial, 228–234; OVA-301, 235–242; pegylated liposomes, 127, 208; platinum-resistant ovarian cancer, 22, 256; platinum-sensitive ovarian cancer, 215, 217; prevention of multidrug resistance, 215; recurrent ovarian cancer, 115, 127, 132, 243; response rates, 208; safety profile, 216, 217; synergy with trabectedin, 236; therapeutic benefit, 208; toxicities, 208, 210, 215, 234; volume of distribution, 208
pegylated liposomal doxorubicin + carboplatin. *See* carboplatin + pegylated liposomal doxorubicin (PLD)
pelvic ultrasonography, 3, 6, 11
performance status: ECOG, 101, 106, 120, 127, 133, 139, 146, 158, 202, 223, 236, 244, 250, 257; GOG, 54, 58, 71, 87, 96, 110, 115, 152, 169, 195; Karnofsky, 209; prognostic factor, 233; World Health Organization (WHO), 76, 81, 174; Zubrod, 230

peripheral edema. *See* toxicity, peripheral edema
PharmaMar, 235
platelet count, prognostic impact, 79
platelet toxicity. *See* toxicity, platelet
platinum, efficacy in ovarian cancer: ACTION, 23; GICOG trials, 15; GOG 95, 9; ICON1, 23, 35; meta-analysis, 36, 66
platinum-free interval, impact on probability of response to treatment, 217
platinum-resistant ovarian cancer: AURELIA, 257, 260; bevacizumab activity, 250, 260; definition, 217, 256; choice of chemotherapy agents, 217, 229, 242, 256; gemcitabine, 228–234; gemcitabine versus PLD trial, 229; OVA-301, 236; overall survival, 256; paclitaxel activity, 58, 70; pegylated liposomal doxorubicin activity, 228–234, 242; progression-free survival, 260; topotecan activity, 138; topotecan versus paclitaxel trial, 204
platinum-sensitive ovarian cancer: AGO-OVAR/NCIC/EORTC trial, 223, 249; CALYPSO, 24, 2464; choice of chemotherapy agents, 217, 222, 242, 249, 255–256; definition, 217; gemcitabine activity, 133; ICON4/AGO-OVAR 2.2, 218; OCEANS, 253; OVA-301, 236; overall survival, 127; paclitaxel activity, 70; paclitaxel plus platinum activity, 220; pegylated liposomal doxorubicin (PLD) activity, 127, 214, 242; pegylated liposomal doxorubicin (PLD) + carboplatin activity, 127, 246; progression-free survival, 127, 249; response rate, 127; topotecan activity, 127
PLD. *See* pegylated liposomal doxorubicin
posterior reversible encephalopathy syndrome (PRES). *See* toxicity, posterior reversible encephalopathy syndrome
postoperative mortality, CHORUS, 185
power analysis. *See* sample size
primary cytoreduction: CHORUS, 180; EORTC 55971, 175; standard of care, 174, 179
proctosigmoidoscopy, 3, 6, 11
progression: AGO-OVAR/NCIC/EORTC trial, 225; GOG 152, 171; GOG 178/SWOG 9701, 191; greater hazard for

Index

progression after maintenance paclitaxel, 191; OCEANS, 252
progression-free interval in advanced-stage ovarian cancer. *See* advanced-stage ovarian cancer, progression-free interval
progression-free survival, 225
progression-free survival as primary endpoint: AGO-OVAR/NCIC/EORTC trial, 225; AURELIA, 259; CALYPSO, 246; Danish Netherlands Trial, 77; determined by investigators, 252, 259; endorsed by AACR ASCO and FDA, 235, 239; endorsed by GCIG, 157; gemcitabine versus PLD trial, 231; GOG 52, 52; GOG 111, 60; GOG 132, 72; GOG 178/SWOG 9701, 189, 192; GOG 218, 153; ICON7, 147; JGOG 3016, 122; median, 144; MITO-2, 129; MITO-7, 159; OCEANS, 252; OV-10, 83; OV16, 141; OVA-301, 238; rationale, 192, 228, 248; SCOTROC, 109
progression-free survival in advanced-stage ovarian cancer. *See* advanced-stage ovarian cancer, progression-free survival
progression-free survival in recurrent ovarian cancer. *See* recurrent ovarian cancer, progression-free survival
progressive disease: Doxil Study 30–49, 211; MITO-2, 129; OV16, 141; topotecan versus paclitaxel trial, 204
proportional hazards model: CHORUS, 183; Grambsch-Therneau test, 183; GOG 95, 17; GOG 97, 55; GOG 111, 60; GOG 152, 171; GOG 157, 40
proportion without progression as primary endpoint, AGO-OVAR-3, 103
proteinuria. *See* toxicity, proteinuria
pulmonary toxicity. *See* toxicity, pulmonary

QLQ-C30 questionnaire: AGO-OVAR-3, 102; AGO-OVAR9, 134; AGO-OVAR/NCIC/EORTC trial, 224, 227; CALYPSO, 245; CHORUS, 181; domains, 140, 211; Doxil Study 30–49, 211; EORTC 55971, 175; ICON7, 147; OV16, 140; OVA-301, 238; SCOTROC, 107; symptom scales, 211
QLQ-OV28 questionnaire: AGO-OVAR9, 134; AGO-OVAR/NCIC/EORTC trial, 224, 227; CALYPSO, 245; CHORUS, 181; EORTC 55971, 175; ICON7, 147; OV16, 140; OVA-301, 238; questions related to ovarian cancer symptoms and treatments, 141; SCOTROC, 107
quality of life: AGO-OVAR9, 134; AGO-OVAR/NCIC/EORTC trial, 224, 227; CALYPSO, 245; CHORUS, 181, 183; Doxil Study 30–49, 211; endpoint, 83, 100, 102; EORTC 55971, 175; Functional Assessment of Cancer Therapy—Ovarian (FACT-O) questionnaire, 111, 153, 159, 231; gemcitabine versus PLD trial, 231, 233; goal in recurrent ovarian cancer, 215, 242; GOG 172, 111, 114; GOG 218, 153, 157; ICON4/AGO-OVAR 2.2, 219, 222; ICON7, 147; MITO-2, 129; MITO-7, 159; OV16, 140; OVA-301, 238, 241; prognostic factor, 233; QLQ-C30 questionnaire, 102, 107, 129, 134, 140–141, 147, 175, 181, 211, 224, 238, 245; QLQ-OV28 questionnaire, 107, 134, 140, 147, 175, 181, 224, 238, 245; SCOTROC, 107; treatment toxicities, 126

radiotherapy: treatment option for early-stage ovarian cancer, 10; treatment option for recurrent ovarian cancer, 215
ranitidine, 81, 88, 106
RECIST (Response Evaluation Criteria in Solid Tumors): AGO-OVAR9, 134; AURELIA, 257; CALYPSO, 244, 245; gemcitabine versus PLD trial, 230; GOG 218, 153; ICON7, 147; MITO-2, 129; MITO-7, 159; OCEANS, 250, 252; OV16, 141; OVA-301, 236; SCOTROC, 107
RECIST response in advanced-stage ovarian cancer. *See* advanced-stage ovarian cancer, RECIST response
RECIST response in recurrent ovarian cancer. *See* recurrent ovarian cancer, RECIST response
recurrence definition, GOG 178/SWOG 9701, 189
recurrence-free survival: definition, 29, 34; suboptimal staging, 43
recurrence-free survival in high-risk early-stage ovarian cancer. *See* early-stage ovarian cancer, high-risk, recurrence-free survival

recurrence patterns: ACTION, 28t; GICOG trials, 13t, 14t; GOG 7602, 9
recurrence rate as primary endpoint: GOG 157, 40; GOG 175, 196
recurrence rate in high-risk early-stage ovarian cancer. *See* early-stage ovarian cancer, high-risk, recurrence rate
recurrent ovarian cancer, disease-control rate: gemcitabine, 231t; gemcitabine versus PLD trial, 231, 231t; pegylated liposomal doxorubicin, 231t
recurrent ovarian cancer, duration of response: AGO-OVAR/NCIC/EORTC trial, 225, 226t; carboplatin, 226t; carboplatin+gemcitabine, 226t, 254t; carboplatin+gemcitabine+bevacizumab, 254t; OCEANS, 254t; OVA-301, 239; paclitaxel, 205t; topotecan, 205t; topotecan versus paclitaxel trial, 205–206t
recurrent ovarian cancer, overall survival: AGO-OVAR/NCIC/EORTC trial, 226t; AURELIA, 261t; carboplatin, 226t; carboplatin+gemcitabine, 226t, 254t; carboplatin+gemcitabine+bevacizumab, 254t; chemotherapy alone, 261t; chemotherapy+bevacizumab, 261t; Doxil study 30–49, 213t; gemcitabine, 231t; gemcitabine versus PLD trial, 231t; ICON4/AGO-OVAR 2.2, 221t; OCEANS, 254t; paclitaxel, 205t; pegylated liposomal doxorubicin, 213t, 231t; platinum chemotherapy, 221t; platinum+paclitaxel, 221t; platinum-resistant, 213t, 214t; platinum-sensitive, 213t; topotecan, 205t, 213t; topotecan versus paclitaxel trial, 205–206t
recurrent ovarian cancer, progression by CA125: CALYPSO, 247t; carboplatin+pegylated liposomal doxorubicin (C-PLD), 247t; paclitaxel+carboplatin (TC), 247t
recurrent ovarian cancer, progression-free survival: AGO-OVAR/NCIC/EORTC trial, 226t; AURELIA, 261t; CALYPSO, 247t; carboplatin, 226t; carboplatin+gemcitabine, 226t, 254t; carboplatin+gemcitabine+bevacizumab, 254t; carboplatin+pegylated liposomal doxorubicin (C-PLD), 247t; chemotherapy alone, 261t; chemotherapy+bevacizumab, 261t; Doxil study 30–49, 213t; gemcitabine, 231t; gemcitabine versus PLD trial, 231t; ICON4/AGO-OVAR 2.2, 221t; OCEANS, 254t; OVA-301, 240t; paclitaxel+carboplatin (TC), 247t; pegylated liposomal doxorubicin, 213t, 231t, 240t; pegylated liposomal doxorubicin+trabectedin, 240t; platinum chemotherapy, 221t; platinum+paclitaxel, 221t; platinum-resistant, 213t, 240t; platinum-sensitive, 213t, 240t; topotecan, 213t
recurrent ovarian cancer, RECIST response: AGO-OVAR/NCIC/EORTC trial, 226t; AURLEIA, 261t; CALYPSO, 247t; carboplatin, 226t; carboplatin+gemcitabine, 226t; carboplatin+pegylated liposomal doxorubicin (C-PLD), 247t; chemotherapy alone, 261t; chemotherapy+bevacizumab, 261t; Doxil study 30–49, 213t; gemcitabine, 231t; gemcitabine versus PLD trial, 231t; ICON4/AGO-OVAR 2.2, 221t; paclitaxel, 205–206t; paclitaxel+carboplatin (TC), 247t; pegylated liposomal doxorubicin, 213t, 231t; platinum chemotherapy, 221t; platinum+paclitaxel, 221t; topotecan, 205–206t, 213t; topotecan versus paclitaxel trial, 205–206t
recurrent ovarian cancer, response by CA125 criteria: AURELIA, 261t; chemotherapy alone, 261t; chemotherapy+bevacizumab, 261t
recurrent ovarian cancer, response rate: AGO-OVAR/NCIC/EORTC trial, 226t; AURELIA, 261t; carboplatin, 226t; carboplatin+gemcitabine, 226t, 254t; carboplatin+gemcitabine+bevacizumab, 254t; chemotherapy alone, 261t; chemotherapy+bevacizumab, 261t; gemcitabine, 231t; gemcitabine versus PLD trial, 231t; OCEANS, 254t; pegylated liposomal doxorubicin, 231t
recurrent ovarian cancer, time to failure: gemcitabine, 231t; gemcitabine versus PLD trial, 231t; pegylated liposomal doxorubicin, 231t
recurrent ovarian cancer, time to progression: paclitaxel, 205–206t; topotecan, 205–206t; topotecan versus paclitaxel trial, 205–206t

Index

recurrent ovarian cancer, time to response: paclitaxel, 205–206t; topotecan, 205–206t; topotecan versus paclitaxel trial, 205–206t

relapse: early relapse, 204; interim relapse, 204; late relapse, 204; resistant disease, 204

relapse-free survival, 12

renal function: AGO-OVAR-3, 101; AGO-OVAR9, 133; AGO-OVAR/NCIC/EORTC trial, 223; Danish Netherlands Trial, 75–76; Doxil Study 30–49, 209; GOG 97, 54; GOG 104, 62; GOG 111, 58; GOG 114, 87; GOG 132, 71; GOG 152, 169; GOG 158, 96; GOG 182/ICON5, 115; JGOG 3016, 120; OV16, 138; OVA-301, 236; topotecan versus paclitaxel study, 202

renal toxicity. *See* toxicity, renal

residual disease status, prognostic impact, 52, 64, 79, 119, 131, 178, 179, 183

response duration, GOG 97, 57

response duration in advanced-stage ovarian cancer. *See* advanced-stage ovarian cancer, response duration

Response Evaluation Criteria in Solid Tumors (RECIST). *See* RECIST

response rate: Cochran-Mantel Haenszel test, 253; lack of correlation with survival, 137; phase II endpoint, 137

response rate as primary endpoint, GOG 47, 48

response rate in advanced-stage ovarian cancer. *See* advanced-stage ovarian cancer, response rate

response rate in recurrent ovarian cancer. *See* recurrent ovarian cancer, response rate

restricted maximum likelihood, GOG 172, 112

restricted mean difference, ICON7, 148

reversible posterior leukoencephalopathy syndrome. *See* toxicity, reversible posterior leukoencephalopathy syndrome (RPLS)

RPLS. *See* toxicity, reversible posterior leukoencephalopathy syndrome

SAAK. *See* Swiss Group for Clinical Cancer Research

salvage therapy: better treatments needed, 52; early-stage ovarian cancer, 25, 30; intraperitoneal, 62; paclitaxel activity, 58; timing of initiation, 74

sample size: ACTION, 27; AGO-OVAR-3, 103; AGO-OVAR9, 135; AGO-OVAR/NCIC/EORTC trial, 225; AURELIA, 260; CHORUS, 182; Danish Netherlands Trial, 77; Doxil Study 30–49, 211; EORTC 55971, 176; EORTC-GCG 55865, 165; Freedman's method, 231; gemcitabine versus PLD trial, 231; GOG 47, 48; GOG 52, 52; GOG 95, 17; GOG 104, 64; GOG 132, 72; GOG 152, 171; GOG 157, 40; GOG 158, 97; GOG 172, 112; GOG 175, 196; GOG 178/SWOG 9701, 189; GOG 182/ICON5, 117; GOG 218, 154; GOG 7601, 3; GOG 7602, 7; ICON1, 34; ICON2, 68; ICON3, 92; ICON4/AGO-OVAR 2.2, 220; ICON7, 147; JGOG 3016, 123; MITO-2, 129; MITO-7, 159; OCEANS, 252; OV-10, 83; OV16, 141; OVA-301, 239; SCOTROC, 109

Schering-Plough Italy, 126

Schoenfeld residuals, OV16, 142

SCOTROC (Vasey 2004), 46, 105–109

Scottish Group, 80

Scottish Gynaecological Cancer Trials Group, 105

secondary debulking surgery: difficulty in assessing efficacy, 173; EORTC-GCG 55865, 162–168; GOG 152, 168–173; JGOG 3016, 122; timing after chemotherapy, 170

secondary malignancy. *See* toxicity, secondary malignancy

second-line chemotherapy: impact on overall survival, 192; non-curative, 191

second-look surgery: AGO-OVAR-3, 103; does not influence survival, 52; EORTC 55971, 175; EORTC-GCG 55865, 164; GOG 47, 47; GOG 52, 51; GOG 97, 55; GOG 104, 63, 64; GOG 111, 60; GOG 114, 88, 90; GOG 158, 97; GOG 172, 111; JGOG 3016, 122; no clinical benefit, 117; OV-10, 82

sepsis. *See* toxicity, sepsis

serous histology: number of chemotherapy cycles, 44–45; response to chemotherapy, 44–45

SIAK. *See* Swiss Institute for Cancer Research

skin toxicity. *See* toxicity, skin
small bowel perforation. *See* gastrointestinal perforation
SmithKline Beecham Pharmaceuticals, 200
Southwest Oncology Group (SWOG), 15, 86, 115, 187
splenectomy, CHORUS, 181
stable disease: Doxil Study 30–49, 211; topotecan versus paclitaxel trial, 204
stage, prognostic impact, 79, 131, 178
stage I ovarian cancer, disease-free survival: cisplatin, 13t; GICOG trials, 13t; GOG 7601, 4t; melphalan, 4t; no further treatment, 4t, 13t
stage I ovarian cancer, overall survival: GOG 7601, 4t; melphalan, 4t; no further treatment, 4t
stem cell support, treatment option for recurrent ovarian cancer, 215
stomatitis. *See* toxicity, stomatitis
stratification factors: age, 141, 189, 204; ascites, 204; bulky disease, 212; cell type, 3, 7; center, 129, 141, 182, 219, 246; chemotherapy regimen, 182, 260; clinical response, 165; differentiation, 34; first-line therapy, 225; GCIG group, 147; grade, 27; histologic grade, 3, 7; institution, 27, 34, 165, 176; intended platinum treatment, 219; interval between surgery and chemotherapy, 147; largest preoperative tumor size, 176; last chemotherapy received, 219; measurable disease, 171, 225, 246; method of biopsy, 176; minimization technique, 165; optimal versus suboptimal, 189; performance status, 129, 154, 165, 237; platinum-free interval, 225, 252, 260; platinum sensitivity, 212, 237; prior antiangiogenic therapy, 260; prior treatment with paclitaxel, 189; radiologic tumor size, 182; residual disease, 112, 129, 141, 154; residual tumor size, 103, 135, 147; response to chemotherapy, 171, 204; secondary debulking surgery, 220; second-look surgery, 112; stage, 7, 27, 34, 103, 129, 135, 147, 154, 176, 182; surgery for recurrence, 252; therapy-free interval, 246; time since completion of last chemotherapy, 219, 220
subgroup analysis, 21

suboptimal debulking: EORTC-GCG 55865, 164, 168; GOG 47, 47; GOG 97, 54; GOG 111, 58; GOG 132, 71; GOG 152, 168–169; GOG 178/SWOG 9701, 187; GOG 182/ICON5, 115; GOG 218, 152; ICON7, 146; JGOG 3016, 124; OV-10, 80; overall survival, 43
surgical morbidities, CHORUS, 185
surgical re-exploration: GOG 7601, 3; GOG 7602, 7
surgical staging: description, 2, 6, 11, 16, 20, 26, 39, 195; improved survival, 30; incomplete documentation, 42; prognostic factor, 2, 30; trials including comprehensive staging, 2, 16, 20, 39, 195; trials lacking comprehensive staging, 24, 26, 33
survival as endpoint: ACTION, 21, 27; GOG 104, 63; GOG 7601, 3; GOG 7602, 7; GICOG trials, 12; ICON1, 21, 34; ICON2, 68
survival in advanced-stage ovarian cancer: bulky disease with complete response to chemotherapy, 173; gross optimal, 119; microscopic residual, 119; not otherwise specified, 100, 115; optimal, 176; platinum-sensitive, 216, 220; suboptimal, 119; suboptimal primary debulking and interval debulking, 176
survival in early-stage ovarian cancer, 2, 10, 15, 19, 20, 36, 193, 197
survival in high-risk early-stage ovarian cancer: GOG 7602, 9, 38; GOG 95, 17, 19; ICON1, 36
survival in low-risk early-stage ovarian cancer: GOG 7601, 5, 15, 37; stage I, 197; stage Ia$_1$ (GOG 7601), 5; stage Ib$_1$ ovarian cancer (GOG 7601), 5; stage II, 197
survival in stage III ovarian cancer: GOG 158, 99; GOG 172, 114
Swiss Group for Clinical Cancer Research (SAAK), 32, 90
Swiss Institute for Cancer Research (SIAK), 66
SWOG. *See* Southwest Oncology Group

Taxol. *See* paclitaxel
TC. *See* paclitaxel+carboplatin
Tenckhoff catheter, 88
therapeutic ratio, 192

Index

therapy-free interval, prognostic factor, 248
thrombocytopenia. *See* toxicity, platelet
thromboembolism. *See* toxicity, thromboembolism
time to failure in recurrent ovarian cancer. *See* recurrent ovarian cancer, time to failure
time to progression as primary endpoint, Doxil Study 30–49, 212
time to progression in recurrent ovarian cancer. *See* recurrent ovarian cancer, time to progression
time to response in recurrent ovarian cancer. *See* recurrent ovarian cancer, time to response
timing of chemotherapy initiation, no prognostic impact, 52
tinnitus. *See* toxicity, tinnitus
topoisomerase inhibitor, topotecan, 201
topotecan (Hycamtin): 3-day dosing, 142; 5-day dosing, 144, 202–203, 210, 258; approved agent, 208, 235; AURELIA, 258; camptothecin analogue, 138, 201; combined with bevacizumab, 258; combined with paclitaxel and carboplatin, 116, 137, 137–144; dose escalation, 203; dose-limiting toxicity, 202, 207; dose reduction, 203; Doxil study, 207–217, 242; equivalent to pegylated liposomal doxorubicin, 200–207, 234; FDA approval, 235; GOG182/ICON5, 142; intermittent daily dosing, 202; lack of cross-resistance to platinum and taxanes, 208; maximum tolerated dose, 202; platinum-resistant ovarian cancer, 229, 256; recurrent ovarian cancer, 115; refractory ovarian cancer, 144; response rates, 208; sequential doublets, 138, 139; topoisomerase inhibitor, 201; topotecan versus paclitaxel study, 200–207, 234, 242; treatment discontinuation, 203; toxicities, 210, 215; weekly dosing, 258
Topotecan versus paclitaxel (ten Bokkel 1997), 115, 200, 200–207, 229, 234, 242, 243
toxicity, abdominal pain: cyclophosphamide+cisplatin (CP), 65t; GOG 104, 66, 65t; GOG 172, 111; GOG 7602, 8t; intraperitoneal ^{32}P, 8t; intraperitoneal cisplatin-based chemotherapy, 65t; paclitaxel+carboplatin (TC), 108t; SCOTROC, 108t
toxicity, allergic reaction: CALYPSO, 248t; carboplatin+pegylated liposomal doxorubicin (C-PLD), 248t; cyclophosphamide+cisplatin (CP), 61t; Danish Netherlands Trial, 79; docetaxel+carboplatin, 108t; GOG 111, 59, 61t; OV16, 145t; paclitaxel+carboplatin (TC), 145t, 248t; paclitaxel+cisplatin (TP), 61t; SCOTROC, 108t
toxicity, alopecia: AGO-OVAR/NCIC/EORTC trial, 227t, 228; CALYPSO, 246, 248t; carboplatin, 69t, 94t, 227t; carboplatin+gemcitabine, 227t, 228; carboplatin+pegylated liposomal doxorubicin (C-PLD), 130t, 248t; cyclophosphamide+cisplatin (CP), 61t, 85t; cyclophosphamide+doxorubicin+cisplatin (CAP), 69t, 94t; Danish Netherlands Trial, 79; Doxil study 30–49, 214t; GOG 111, 61t; GOG 132, 72; GOG 178/SWOG 9701, 193; ICON2, 69t, 70, ICON3, 94t, 95; ICON4/AGO-OVAR 2.2, 221t; MITO-2, 130t, 131, 161; MITO-7, 160t, 161; OV-10, 85t; paclitaxel, 206t; paclitaxel+carboplatin (TC), 94t, 95, 108t, 130t, 157, 160t, 161, 243, 248t; paclitaxel+cisplatin (TP), 61t, 85t; pegylated liposomal doxorubicin (PLD), 127, 214t; platinum chemotherapy, 221t; platinum+paclitaxel, 221t; SCOTROC, 108t; topotecan, 206t, 214t; topotecan versus paclitaxel trial, 206t; weekly paclitaxel+carboplatin, 160t
toxicity, anaphylaxis, OV16, 140
toxicity, anemia: AGO-OVAR/NCIC/EORTC trial, 226t; AGO/OVAR-3, 104t; AGO-OVAR9, 136t; carboplatin, 226t; carboplatin+gemcitabine, 226t; carboplatin+pegylated liposomal doxorubicin (C-PLD), 130t; cisplatin, 73t; cyclophosphamide+cisplatin (CP), 56t, 61t, 65t; Danish Netherlands Trial, 78t; docetaxel+carboplatin, 108t; dose-dense paclitaxel+carboplatin, 125t; Doxil study 30–49, 214t; gemcitabine, 233t; gemcitabine versus PLD trial, 233t; GOG 97, 56t; GOG 104, 65t; GOG 111, 61t; GOG 132, 73t, 74; GOG 157, 41t;

toxicity, anemia (*cont.*)
GOG 182/ICON5, 118t; intraperitoneal cisplatin-based chemotherapy, 65t; JGOG 3016, 125t, 161; MITO-2, 130t; MITO-7, 161; OCEANS, 252; paclitaxel, 73t, 206t; paclitaxel+carboplatin (TC), 41t, 104t, 108t, 118t, 136t, 161; paclitaxel+carboplatin (TC), 78t, 104t, 125t, 130t; paclitaxel+cisplatin (TP), 61t, 73t, 78t; pegylated liposomal doxorubicin (PLD), 214t, 233t; SCOTROC, 108t; topotecan, 206t, 214t; topotecan versus paclitaxel trial, 206t

toxicity, anorexia, MITO-2, 131

toxicity, arterial thrombosis: AURELIA, 261t; bevacizumab, 153; chemotherapy alone, 261t; chemotherapy+bevacizumab, 261t; GOG 218, 153, 156t; paclitaxel+carboplatin (TC), 156t; paclitaxel+carboplatin+bevacizumab (PCB), 156t

toxicity, arthralgia: CALYPSO, 248t; carboplatin+pegylated liposomal doxorubicin (C-PLD), 248t; cyclophosphamide+cisplatin (CP), 85t; Danish Netherlands Trial, 79; OV-10, 85t; OV16, 140; paclitaxel, 206t; paclitaxel+carboplatin (TC), 108t, 248t; paclitaxel+cisplatin (TP), 85t; SCOTROC, 108t; topotecan, 206t; topotecan versus paclitaxel trial, 206t

toxicity, bilirubin, Doxil Study 30–49, 210

toxicity, bleeding: carboplatin+pegylated liposomal doxorubicin (C-PLD), 131t; GOG 218, 156t; ICON7, 150t; MITO-2, 131t; paclitaxel+carboplatin (TC), 131t, 150t, 156t; paclitaxel+carboplatin+bevacizumab (PCB), 150t, 156t

toxicity, cardiac: Danish Netherlands Trial, 79; doxorubicin, 208; GOG 111, 59–60; GOG 114, 89t; GOG 172, 113t; GOG 175, 197, 198t; intraperitoneal cisplatin-based chemotherapy, 89t, 113t; maintenance chemotherapy, 198t; maintenance paclitaxel, 197; OV-10, 82; paclitaxel+cisplatin (TP), 89t, 113t; pegylated liposomal doxorubicin (PLD), 127

toxicity, cardiac ischemia, GOG 111, 60

toxicity, central nervous system bleeding: GOG 218, 156t; paclitaxel+carboplatin (TC), 156t; paclitaxel+carboplatin+bevacizumab (PCB), 156t

toxicity, congestive heart failure: OVA-301, 240t; pegylated liposomal doxorubicin (PLD), 240t; pegylated liposomal doxorubicin+trabectedin, 240t

toxicity, constipation: Danish Netherlands Trial, 79; gemcitabine, 231t; gemcitabine versus PLD trial, 231t; pegylated liposomal doxorubicin, 231t

toxicity, cutaneous. *See* toxicity, skin

toxicity, death due to treatment: CALYPSO, 248t; carboplatin+pegylated liposomal doxorubicin (C-PLD), 130t, 248t; cyclophosphamide+cisplatin (CP), 61t, 65t; docetaxel+carboplatin, 108t; GOG 104, 65t; GOG 111, 61t; Doxil study 30–49, 214t; GOG 114, 89t; GOG 172, 113t; GOG 218, 155t; ICON7, 150t; intraperitoneal cisplatin-based chemotherapy, 65t, 89t, 113t; MITO-2, 130t; MITO-7, 160t; OV16, 143t; OVA-301, 241t; paclitaxel+carboplatin (TC), 108t, 130t, 143t, 150t, 155t, 160t, 248t; paclitaxel+carboplatin+bevacizumab (PCB), 150t, 155t; paclitaxel+cisplatin (TP), 61t, 89t, 113t; pegylated liposomal doxorubicin (PLD), 214t, 241t; pegylated liposomal doxorubicin+trabectedin, 241t; SCOTROC, 108t; topotecan, 214t, 215; weekly paclitaxel+carboplatin, 160t

toxicity, dermatologic. *See* toxicity, skin

toxicity, diarrhea: carboplatin+pegylated liposomal doxorubicin (C-PLD), 130t; Danish Netherlands Trial, 79; MITO-2, 130t, 131; paclitaxel+carboplatin (TC), 130t; paclitaxel+cisplatin (TP), 169; topotecan versus paclitaxel trial, 207

toxicity, dyspnea: gemcitabine, 233t; gemcitabine versus PLD trial, 233t; GOG 104, 66; pegylated liposomal doxorubicin (PLD), 233t

toxicity, fatigue: AGO-OVAR9, 137; GOG 172, 112, 113t; gemcitabine, 231t, 233t; gemcitabine versus PLD trial, 231t, 233t; intraperitoneal cisplatin-based chemotherapy, 113t; paclitaxel+carboplatin (TC), 157; paclitaxel+cisplatin (TP), 113t; pegylated liposomal doxorubicin (PLD), 231t, 233t

Index

toxicity, febrile neutropenia: AGO-OVAR/ NCIC/EORTC trial, 227t; AGO/OVAR-3, 104t; AGO-OVAR9, 136t; AGO-OVAR/ NCIC/EORTC trial, 224; carboplatin, 227t; carboplatin+gemcitabine, 227t; carboplatin+pegylated liposomal doxorubicin (C-PLD), 131t; cyclophosphamide+cisplatin (CP), 56t, 84t; docetaxel+carboplatin, 108t; Doxil Study 30–49, 210; gemcitabine, 233t; gemcitabine versus PLD trial, 230, 233t; GOG 97, 56t; GOG 175, 196; GOG 218, 152; JGOG 3016, 121; MITO-2, 131t; MITO-7, 160t; OCEANS, 255; OV-10, 82, 84t; OV16, 139, 143t; OVA-301, 237; paclitaxel+carboplatin, 104t, 108t, 131t, 136t, 143t, 160t; paclitaxel+cisplatin (TP), 84t, 104t; pegylated liposomal doxorubicin, 233t; SCOTROC, 108t; weekly paclitaxel+carboplatin, 160t

toxicity, fever: carboplatin, 94t; cyclophosphamide+cisplatin (CP), 61t; cyclophosphamide+doxorubicin+ cisplatin (CAP), 94t; Danish Netherlands Trial, 78t, 79; GOG 111, 61t; GOG 132, 72; GOG 172, 113t; GOG 182/ICON5, 118t; ICON3, 94t, 95; intraperitoneal cisplatin-based chemotherapy, 113t; paclitaxel, 206t; paclitaxel+carboplatin (TC), 78t, 94t, 95, 118t; paclitaxel+ cisplatin (TP), 61t, 78t, 113t; pegylated liposomal doxorubicin (PLD)+carboplatin, 127; topotecan, 206t; topotecan versus paclitaxel trial, 203. 206t

toxicity, fistula: AURELIA, 261t; bevacizumab, 250; chemotherapy alone, 261t; chemotherapy+bevacizumab, 261t; GOG 218, 155t; paclitaxel+carboplatin (TC), 155t; paclitaxel+carboplatin+ bevacizumab (PCB), 155t

toxicity, gastrointestinal: AGO-OVAR-3, 105; cisplatin, 73t; cyclophosphamide+ cisplatin (CP), 56t, 61t; cyclophosphamide+doxorubicin (CA), 49t; cyclophosphamide+doxorubicin+ cisplatin (CAP), 49t; cyclophosphamide+ cisplatin (CP), 18t; docetaxel+carboplatin, 108t; GOG 47, 49t; GOG 95, 18t; GOG 97, 55, 56t; GOG 111, 59, 61t; GOG 114, 89t; GOG 132, 73t, 74; GOG 158, 97, 98t, 99; GOG 172, 112, 113t; GOG 182/ ICON5, 118t; GOG 7602, 8t; intraperitoneal ^{32}P, 18t; intraperitoneal cisplatin-based chemotherapy, 89t, 113t; melphalan, 8t; paclitaxel, 73t; paclitaxel+carboplatin (TC), 98t, 118t; paclitaxel+cisplatin (TP), 61t, 73t, 89t, 98t, 113t; SCOTROC, 108t

toxicity, gastrointestinal perforation: AURELIA, 257, 259, 261t, 262; bevacizumab, 153, 250; chemotherapy alone, 261t; chemotherapy+bevacizumab, 261t; GOG 95, 18; GOG 218, 153, 155t, 156; ICON7, 150t; intraperitoneal ^{32}P, 18; OCEANS, 255; paclitaxel+carboplatin (TC), 150t, 155t; paclitaxel+carboplatin+ bevacizumab (PCB), 150t, 155t; risk-factors, 257–258

toxicity, genitourinary: GOG 158, 98t; paclitaxel+carboplatin (TC), 98t; paclitaxel+cisplatin (TP), 98t

toxicity, granulocyte: cisplatin, 73t; cyclophosphamide+cisplatin (CP), 18t, 65t; Danish Netherlands Trial, 78t; GOG 47, 47–48; GOG 52, 51; GOG 95, 18t; GOG 104, 65t; GOG 132, 73t; GOG 157, 41t; GOG 158, 98t; intraperitoneal ^{32}P, 18t; intraperitoneal cisplatin-based chemotherapy, 65t; OV16, 143t; paclitaxel, 73t; paclitaxel+carboplatin (TC), 41t, 78t, 98t, 143t; paclitaxel+cisplatin (TP), 73t, 78t, 98t

toxicity, hearing loss. See toxicity, ototoxicity

toxicity, heart block: GOG 111, 60; paclitaxel, 60

toxicity, hematologic: AGO-OVAR9, 137; AGO-OVAR/NCIC/EORTC trial, 228; carboplatin, 94t; carboplatin+ gemcitabine, 228, 243; cyclophosphamide+doxorubicin+cisplatin (CAP), 94t; GOG 114, 89t; GOG 172, 112; ICON3, 94t; ICON4/AGO-OVAR 2.2, 221t; intraperitoneal cisplatin-based chemotherapy, 89t; JGOG 3016, 121, 123; MITO-2, 131–132; MITO-7, 161; paclitaxel+carboplatin (TC), 94t, 157, 161; paclitaxel+cisplatin (TP), 89t; pegylated liposomal doxorubicin, 116, 210; platinum chemotherapy, 221t; platinum+paclitaxel, 221t; topotecan, 215, 234

toxicity, hemorrhagic cystitis, GOG 97, 55
toxicity, hepatic: GOG 172, 113t; GOG 182/ICON5, 118t; intraperitoneal cisplatin-based chemotherapy, 113t; Hy's law, 241; OVA-301, 238, 240t, 241; paclitaxel+carboplatin (TC), 118t; paclitaxel+cisplatin (TP), 113t; pegylated liposomal doxorubicin (PLD), 240t; pegylated liposomal doxorubicin+trabectedin, 240t, 241; SCOTROC, 106
toxicity, hospitalization: OV16, 145t; paclitaxel+carboplatin (TC), 145t
toxicity, hypersensitivity: bevacizumab, 153; CALYPSO, 246, 248, 248t; carboplatin+pegylated liposomal doxorubicin (C-PLD), 248t; cyclophosphamide+cisplatin (CP), 85t; dose-dense paclitaxel+carboplatin, 125t; GOG 218, 152, 153; JGOG 3016, 125t; OV-10, 82, 85t; paclitaxel, 106, 152; paclitaxel+carboplatin (TC), 125t, 248t; paclitaxel+cisplatin (TP), 85t; SCOTROC, 106
toxicity, hypertension: AURELIA, 257, 261t, 262; bevacizumab, 153, 157; carboplatin+gemcitabine, 254t; carboplatin+gemcitabine+bevacizumab, 254t; chemotherapy alone, 261t; chemotherapy+bevacizumab, 261t; GOG 218, 153, 155t, 156, 157; ICON7, 150t; OCEANS, 254t; paclitaxel+carboplatin (TC), 150t, 155t; paclitaxel+carboplatin+bevacizumab (PCB), 150t, 155t
toxicity, infection: AGO/OVAR-3, 104t; carboplatin+pegylated liposomal doxorubicin (C-PLD), 131t; cyclophosphamide+cisplatin (CP), 56t; GOG 97, 56t; GOG 114, 89t; GOG 172, 113t; GOG 175, 197, 198t; ICON4/AGO-OVAR 2.2, 221t; intraperitoneal cisplatin-based chemotherapy, 89t, 113t; maintenance chemotherapy, 198t; maintenance paclitaxel, 197; MITO-2, 131t; OV16, 139; OVA-301, 237; paclitaxel, 206t; paclitaxel+carboplatin (TC), 104t, 131t; paclitaxel+cisplatin (TP), 89t, 104t, 113t; platinum chemotherapy, 221t; platinum+paclitaxel, 221t; topotecan, 206t; topotecan versus paclitaxel trial, 203, 206t

toxicity, leukopenia: AGO/OVAR-3, 104t; AGO-OVAR9, 136t; carboplatin, 69t; carboplatin+pegylated liposomal doxorubicin (C-PLD), 131t; cyclophosphamide+cisplatin (CP), 18t, 52t, 56t, 65t; cyclophosphamide+doxorubicin+cisplatin (CAP), 52t, 69t; Doxil study 30–49, 214t; GOG 95, 18t; GOG 97, 56t; GOG 104, 65t; GOG 114, 89t; GOG 158, 98t; GOG 172, 113t; ICON2, 69t, 70; intraperitoneal ^{32}P, 18t; intraperitoneal cisplatin-based chemotherapy, 65t, 89t, 113t; MITO-2, 131t; paclitaxel+carboplatin (TC), 98t, 104t, 131t, 136t; paclitaxel+cisplatin (TP), 89t, 98t, 104t, 113t; pegylated liposomal doxorubicin (PLD), 214t; topotecan, 214t
toxicity, metabolic: GOG 114, 89t; GOG 158, 98t, 99; GOG 172, 112, 113t; intraperitoneal cisplatin-based chemotherapy, 89t, 113t; paclitaxel+carboplatin (TC), 98t; paclitaxel+cisplatin (TP), 89t, 98t, 113t
toxicity, mucositis: CALYPSO, 248, 248t; carboplatin+pegylated liposomal doxorubicin (C-PLD), 248t; Danish Netherlands Trial, 79; gemcitabine, 231t; gemcitabine versus PLD trial, 231t; ICON4/AGO-OVAR 2.2, 221t; MITO-2, 131; OV16, 140; OVA-301, 240t; paclitaxel+carboplatin (TC), 248t; paclitaxel+cisplatin (TP), 169; pegylated liposomal doxorubicin (PLD), 116, 127, 231t, 240t; pegylated liposomal doxorubicin+trabectedin, 240t; platinum chemotherapy, 221t; platinum+paclitaxel, 221t; SCOTROC, 107
toxicity, myalgia: CALYPSO, 248t; carboplatin+pegylated liposomal doxorubicin (C-PLD), 248t; cyclophosphamide+cisplatin (CP), 85t; Danish Netherlands Trial, 79; OV-10, 85t; OV16, 140; paclitaxel, 206t; paclitaxel+carboplatin (TC), 108t, 248t; paclitaxel+cisplatin (TP), 85t; SCOTROC, 108t; topotecan, 206t; topotecan versus paclitaxel trial, 206t
toxicity, myelotoxicity: AGO-OVAR-3, 105; carboplatin, 75; cyclophosphamide+doxorubicin (CA), 49t; cyclophospha-

Index

mide+doxorubicin+cisplatin (CAP), 49t; GOG 47, 49t; GOG 7601, 4t; GOG 7602, 8t; ICON4/AGO-OVAR 2.2, 220; limits intravenous chemotherapy intensity, 111; melphalan, 4t, 8t; OV-10, 82; pegylated liposomal doxorubicin (PLD), 127; SCOTROC, 109; topotecan, 202; topotecan combination therapy, 138
toxicity, nail changes: docetaxel+carboplatin, 108t; SCOTROC, 108t
toxicity, nausea: AGO/OVAR-3, 104t; CALYPSO, 248, 248t; carboplatin, 69t, 94t; carboplatin+pegylated liposomal doxorubicin (C-PLD), 248t; cisplatin, 13t, 14t; cyclophosphamide+cisplatin (CP), 52t, 85t; cyclophosphamide+doxorubicin+cisplatin (CAP), 52t, 69t, 94t; Danish Netherlands Trial, 78t; doxorubicin, 208; gemcitabine, 231t; gemcitabine versus PLD trial, 231t; GICOG trials, 13t, 14t; ICON2, 69t, 70; ICON3, 94t; ICON4/AGO-OVAR 2.2, 221t; OV-10, 85t; OV16, 143t; OVA-301, 237; paclitaxel, 206t; paclitaxel+carboplatin (TC), 78t, 94t, 104t, 143t, 248t; paclitaxel+cisplatin (TP), 78t, 85t, 104t; pegylated liposomal doxorubicin (PLD), 127, 231t; platinum chemotherapy, 221t; platinum+paclitaxel, 221t; topotecan, 206t; topotecan versus paclitaxel trial, 206t
toxicity, neuropathy. *See* toxicity, neurotoxicity
toxicity, neurotoxicity: AGO-OVAR/NCIC/EORTC trial, 227t; AGO/OVAR-3, 104t, 105, 223; AGO-OVAR/NCIC/EORTC trial, 228; AURELIA, 262; CALYPSO, 244, 246, 248t; carboplatin, 94t, 227t; carboplatin+gemcitabine, 117t, 228; carboplatin+pegylated liposomal doxorubicin (C-PLD), 130t, 248t; cisplatin, 73t, 75; cyclophosphamide+cisplatin (CP), 61t, 65t, 85t; cyclophosphamide+doxorubicin+cisplatin (CAP), 94t; cumulative, 243; Danish Netherlands Trial, 78t, 79; docetaxel+carboplatin, 108t; dose-dense paclitaxel+carboplatin, 125t; gemcitabine, 233t; gemcitabine versus PLD trial, 233t; GOG 97, 55; GOG 104, 63, 65t; GOG 111, 59, 61t, 85; GOG 114, 88, 89t; GOG 132, 71, 73t;

GOG 152, 173; GOG 158, 97, 98t, 99; GOG 157, 41t, 194; GOG 172, 111, 112, 113t; GOG 175, 197, 198t; GOG 178/SWOG 9701, 188, 190t, 191, 192, 193; GOG 182/ICON5, 118t; GOG 218, 152; ICON3, 94t, 95; ICON4/AGO-OVAR 2.2, 221t, 222; intraperitoneal cisplatin-based chemotherapy, 65t, 89t, 113t; JGOG 3016, 121, 125t, 125; maintenance chemotherapy, 198t; maintenance paclitaxel, 190t, 191, 197; MITO-2, 128, 130t, 131; MITO-7, 158, 159, 160t, 161; OV-10, 82, 85, 85t; OV16, 140, 145t; paclitaxel, 73t, 206t; paclitaxel+carboplatin (TC), 41t, 78t, 79, 93, 94t, 98t, 104t, 108t, 118t, 125t, 130t, 145t, 57, 160t, 161, 243, 248t; paclitaxel+cisplatin (TP), 61t, 73t, 78t, 79, 85t, 85, 89t, 98t, 104t, 113t, 170; pegylated liposomal doxorubicin (PLD), 233t; pegylated liposomal doxorubicin (PLD)+carboplatin, 127; platinum chemotherapy, 221t; platinum+paclitaxel, 221t; SCOTROC, 106, 108t, 109; topotecan, 206t; topotecan versus paclitaxel trial, 206t; weekly paclitaxel+carboplatin, 160t
toxicity, neutropenia: AGO-OVAR/NCIC/EORTC trial, 226t; AGO/OVAR-3, 104t; AGO-OVAR9, 136t; AGO-OVAR/NCIC/EORTC trial, 224; CALYPSO, 248t; carboplatin, 226t; carboplatin+gemcitabine, 224, 226t; carboplatin+pegylated liposomal doxorubicin (C-PLD), 131t, 248t; CHORUS, 185t; cyclophosphamide+cisplatin (CP), 61t, 84t; docetaxel+carboplatin, 108t; dose-dense paclitaxel+carboplatin, 125t; Doxil Study 30-49, 210, 214t; gemcitabine, 231t, 233t; gemcitabine versus PLD trial, 230, 231t, 233t; GOG 104, 66; GOG 111, 61t; GOG 132, 71, 72; GOG 178/SWOG 9701, 188, 190t; GOG 182/ICON5, 118t; GOG 218, 152, 155t; JGOG 3016, 121, 125t, 161; maintenance paclitaxel, 190t; MITO-2, 131t; MITO-7, 158, 160t, 161; neoadjuvant chemotherapy, 185t; OCEANS, 252, 255; OV-10, 82, 84t; OV16, 139; OVA-301, 237, 240t, 241; paclitaxel, 206t; paclitaxel+carboplatin (TC), 104t, 108t, 118t, 125t,

toxicity, neutropenia (*cont.*)
  131t, 136t, 155t, 160t, 161, 248t;
  paclitaxel + carboplatin + bevacizumab
  (PCB), 155t; paclitaxel + cisplatin (TP),
  61t, 84t, 104t, 169; pegylated liposomal
  doxorubicin (PLD), 214t, 231t, 233t, 240t;
  pegylated liposomal doxorubicin
  (PLD) + carboplatin, 127; pegylated
  liposomal doxorubicin (PLD) + trabectedin, 240t, 241; primary debulking
  surgery, 185t; SCOTROC, 106, 107, 108t;
  topotecan, 206t, 210, 214t, 215; topotecan
  versus paclitaxel trial, 203, 206t, 207;
  weekly paclitaxel + carboplatin, 160t
toxicity, ototoxicity: AGO/OVAR-3, 104t;
  cisplatin, 75; cyclophosphamide +
  cisplatin (CP), 65t, 85t; GOG 97, 55;
  GOG 104, 65t, 66; GOG 111, 59; GOG
  132, 74; intraperitoneal cisplatin-based
  chemotherapy, 65t; OV-10, 82, 85t;
  paclitaxel + carboplatin (TC), 104t;
  paclitaxel + cisplatin (TP), 85t, 104t,
  170
toxicity, pain: GOG 158, 98t; GOG 172,
  112, 113t; GOG 218, 155t, 156; intraperitoneal cisplatin-based chemotherapy,
  113t; paclitaxel + carboplatin (TC), 98t,
  155t; paclitaxel + carboplatin + bevacizumab (PCB), 155t; paclitaxel + cisplatin
  (TP), 98t, 113t
toxicity, palmar-plantar erythrodysesthesia
  (PPE): AURELIA, 262; CALYPSO, 248,
  248t; carboplatin + pegylated liposomal
  doxorubicin (C-PLD), 127, 248t;
  description, 216; dimethyl sulfoxide, 216;
  Doxil study 30–49, 214t; dose modifications, 216; gemcitabine, 231t, 233t;
  gemcitabine versus PLD trial, 231t, 233t,
  234; OVA-301, 238, 241; OVA-301, 240t;
  paclitaxel + carboplatin (TC), 248t;
  pegylated liposomal doxorubicin (PLD),
  127, 208, 210, 214t, 215, 216, 231t, 233t,
  234, 240t, 241; pegylated liposomal
  doxorubicin + trabectedin, 240t;
  pyridoxine, 216; treatment, 216;
  topotecan, 214t
toxicity, peripheral edema: docetaxel +
  carboplatin, 108t; SCOTROC, 108t
toxicity, platelet: AGO-OVAR/NCIC/
  EORTC trial, 226t; AGO/OVAR-3, 104t;
  AGO-OVAR9, 136t; AGO-OVAR/NCIC/
  EORTC trial, 224; CALYPSO, 248t;
  carboplatin, 69t, 226t; carboplatin +
  gemcitabine, 224, 226t; carboplatin +
  pegylated liposomal doxorubicin
  (C-PLD), 130t, 248t; cyclophosphamide +
  cisplatin (CP), 56t, 61t, 65t; cyclophosphamide + doxorubicin (CA), 49t;
  cyclophosphamide + doxorubicin +
  cisplatin (CAP), 49t, 52t, 69t;
  cyclophosphamide + cisplatin (CP), 18t,
  52t, 85t; Danish Netherlands Trial, 78t;
  docetaxel + carboplatin, 108t; dose-dense
  paclitaxel + carboplatin, 125t; Doxil study
  30–49, 214t; gemcitabine, 233t;
  gemcitabine versus PLD trial, 230, 233t;
  GOG 47, 47–48, 49t; GOG 52, 51; GOG
  95, 18t; GOG 97, 56t; GOG 104, 65t;
  GOG 111, 61t; GOG 114, 89t; GOG 132,
  71, 74; GOG 158, 98t; GOG 172, 113t;
  GOG 175, 196; GOG 178/SWOG 9701,
  188; GOG 182/ICON5, 118t; ICON2, 69t;
  intraperitoneal ^{32}P, 18t; intraperitoneal
  cisplatin-based chemotherapy, 65t, 89t,
  113t; JGOG 3016, 121, 125t, 161; ICON2,
  70; MITO-2, 130t; MITO-7, 158, 161;
  OCEANS, 252; OV-10, 82, 85t; OV16,
  139, 143t; OVA-301, 237; paclitaxel, 206t;
  paclitaxel + carboplatin (TC), 78t, 89t,
  104t, 108t, 118t, 125t, 130t, 136t, 143t;
  161, 248t; paclitaxel + cisplatin (TP), 61t,
  78t, 85t, 89t, 98t, 104t, 113t, 169;
  pegylated liposomal doxorubicin (PLD),
  214t, 233t; SCOTROC, 107, 108t;
  topotecan, 206t, 214t; topotecan versus
  paclitaxel trial, 206t, 207
toxicity, posterior reversible encephalopathy syndrome (PRES): GOG 218, 156t;
  paclitaxel + carboplatin (TC), 156t;
  paclitaxel + carboplatin + bevacizumab
  (PCB), 156t
toxicity, proteinuria: AURELIA, 261t, 262;
  bevacizumab, 153; chemotherapy alone,
  261t; chemotherapy + bevacizumab, 261t;
  GOG 218, 153, 155t, 156; carboplatin +
  gemcitabine, 254t; carboplatin + gemcitabine + bevacizumab, 254t; OCEANS,
  254t, 255; paclitaxel + carboplatin (TC),
  155t; paclitaxel + carboplatin + bevacizumab (PCB), 155t

Index

toxicity, pulmonary: cyclophosphamide+ cisplatin (CP), 65t; Danish Netherlands Trial, 79; GOG 104, 65t; GOG 182/ICON5, 118t; intraperitoneal cisplatin-based chemotherapy, 65t; MITO-7, 160t; paclitaxel+carboplatin (TC), 118t, 160t; weekly paclitaxel+carboplatin, 160t

toxicity, renal: AGO/OVAR-3, 104t; cisplatin, 73t, 75; cyclophosphamide+ cisplatin (CP), 18t, 56t, 61t; Danish Netherlands Trial, 79; GOG 95, 18t; GOG 97, 55, 56t; GOG 104, 63; GOG 111, 59, 61t; GOG 132, 71, 73t, 74; GOG 158, 97; GOG 172, 111, 113t; ICON4/AGO-OVAR 2.2, 221t; intraperitoneal ^{32}P, 18t; intraperitoneal cisplatin-based chemotherapy, 113t; MITO-2, 128; OV-10, 82; OV16, 140; paclitaxel, 73t; paclitaxel+carboplatin, 104t; paclitaxel+cisplatin (TP), 61t, 73t, 104t, 113t, 170; platinum chemotherapy, 221t; platinum+paclitaxel, 221t; topotecan, 210

toxicity, reversible posterior leukoencephalopathy syndrome (RPLS): bevacizumab, 153; carboplatin+gemcitabine, 254t; carboplatin+gemcitabine+bevacizumab, 254t; GOG 218, 153; OCEANS, 254t, 255

toxicity, RPLS. See toxicity, reversible posterior leukoencephalopathy syndrome

toxicity, secondary malignancy: GOG 175, 198t; maintenance chemotherapy, 198t

toxicity, sepsis: Doxil study 30–49, 214t; paclitaxel, 206t; pegylated liposomal doxorubicin (PLD), 214t; topotecan, 206t, 214t; topotecan versus paclitaxel trial, 206t

toxicity, skin: carboplatin+pegylated liposomal doxorubicin (C-PLD), 130t; Danish Netherlands Trial, 79; gemcitabine, 233t; gemcitabine versus PLD trial, 233t; GOG 175, 197, 198t; maintenance chemotherapy, 198t; MITO-2, 128, 130t, 131; paclitaxel+carboplatin (TC), 130t; pegylated liposomal doxorubicin (PLD), 116, 127, 208, 233t; SCOTROC, 107

toxicity, stomatitis: carboplatin+pegylated liposomal doxorubicin (C-PLD), 130t; cyclophosphamide+cisplatin (CP), 85t; Doxil study 30–49, 214t; MITO-2, 130t; OV-10, 85t; OVA-301, 238, 240t; paclitaxel+carboplatin (TC), 130t; paclitaxel+cisplatin (TP), 85t; pegylated liposomal doxorubicin (PLD), 127, 208, 210, 214t, 215, 240t; pegylated liposomal doxorubicin+trabectedin, 240t; topotecan, 214t

toxicity, thrombocytopenia. See toxicity, platelet

toxicity, thromboembolism: AURELIA, 261t; bevacizumab, 153; chemotherapy alone, 261t; chemotherapy+bevacizumab, 261t; GOG 218, 153, 155t; ICON7, 150t; OV16, 143t; paclitaxel+carboplatin (TC), 143t, 150t, 155t; paclitaxel+carboplatin+bevacizumab (PCB), 150t, 155t

toxicity, tinnitus: cyclophosphamide+ cisplatin (CP), 65t; GOG 104, 65t, 66; GOG 132, 71; intraperitoneal cisplatin-based chemotherapy, 65t; paclitaxel+ cisplatin (TP), 170

toxicity, venous thrombosis. See toxicity, thromboembolism

toxicity, vomiting: AGO/OVAR-3, 104t; CALYPSO, 248, 248t; carboplatin, 69t, 94t; carboplatin+pegylated liposomal doxorubicin (C-PLD), 248t; cisplatin, 13t, 14t; cyclophosphamide+cisplatin (CP), 52t, 56t, 85t; cyclophosphamide+doxorubicin+cisplatin (CAP), 52t, 69t, 94t; doxorubicin, 208; gemcitabine, 231t; gemcitabine versus PLD trial, 231t; GICOG trials, 13t, 14t; GOG 97, 56t; ICON2, 69t, 70; ICON3, 94t; ICON4/AGO-OVAR 2.2, 221t; MITO-7, 161; OV-10, 85t; OV16, 145t; OVA-301, 237; paclitaxel, 206t; paclitaxel+carboplatin (TC), 94t, 104t, 145t, 161, 248t; paclitaxel+cisplatin (TP), 85t, 104t; pegylated liposomal doxorubicin (PLD), 127, 231t; platinum chemotherapy, 221t; platinum+paclitaxel, 221t; topotecan, 206t; topotecan versus paclitaxel trial, 206t

toxicity, wound disruption: bevacizumab, 153, 156; GOG 218, 153, 156, 156t; paclitaxel+carboplatin (TC), 156t; paclitaxel+carboplatin+bevacizumab (PCB), 156t

toxicity assessments: GICOG trials, 12; GOG 111, 59; GOG 157, 39; SCOTROC, 107
toxicity bowel obstruction: GOG 7602, 8t; intraperitoneal ^{32}P, 8t
TP. See paclitaxel+cisplatin
trabectedin: activity in ovarian cancer, 236; dosing, 237; Ecteinascidia turbinata, 235; mechanism of antineoplastic effect, 235; OVA-310, 235–242; synergy with pegylated liposomal doxorubicin, 236; transcription-coupled nucleotide excision repair, 235
transcription-coupled nucleotide excision repair, 235
transfusion, blood: Doxil study 30–49, 214t; topotecan versus paclitaxel trial, 206t
transfusion, platelets, topotecan versus paclitaxel trial, 206t
treatment discontinuation: AGO-OVAR-3, 102; AGO-OVAR9, 134; AURELIA, 259; Doxil Study 30–49, 210; GOG 97, 55; GOG 104, 63; GOG 111, 59; GOG 152, 170; GOG 158, 97; GOG 178/SWOG 9701, 188; GOG 218, 152; MITO-2, 128; topotecan versus paclitaxel trial, 203
treatment modifications: GOG 97, 54, 57; GOG 111, 59; GOG 157, 39; GOG 158, 96–97; OV-10, 82
treosulfan, 234
tumor kinetics, 137
tumor size, prognostic impact, 79, 173, 178

ultra-radical procedures, CHORUS, 181
ultrasound: AGO/OVAR-3, 103; GICOG trials, 12; topotecan versus paclitaxel study, 202

vascular endothelial growth factor (VEGF), 145, 151, 249, 257
venous thromboembolism. See toxicity, thromboembolism
ventricular irritability, 60
vinorelbine, response rates, 215
vomiting. See toxicity, vomiting

weekly paclitaxel. See dose-dense paclitaxel
whole abdominal radiation, 20
Wilcoxon Mann-Whitney test, AGO-OVAR9, 135
Wilcoxon rank-sum test: CALYPSO, 246; GOG 172, 112; OV16, 142
World Health Organization, response criteria: CHORUS, 181; EORTC 55971, 175; EORTC-GCG 55865, 165; topotecan versus paclitaxel trial, 203
World Health Organization toxicity assessment, GICOG trials, 12
wound disruption. See toxicity, wound disruption

X-ray: AGO/OVAR-3, 103; Doxil Study 30–49, 209

Zelens exact test, AGO-OVAR9, 135

About the Author

CHRISTINE S. WALSH, MD, MS, is an attending physician in gynecologic oncology and a research scientist with the Department of Obstetrics and Gynecology at Cedars-Sinai Medical Center and an associate professor of obstetrics and gynecology at Cedars-Sinai Medical Center and the Geffen School of Medicine at the University of California, Los Angeles (UCLA). Dr. Walsh received her bachelor's degree from Stanford University and her medical degree from the Columbia College of Physicians and Surgeons. She completed a residency in obstetrics and gynecology at the Brigham and Women's Hospital and Massachusetts General Hospital combined program in Boston, Massachusetts. She completed her fellowship in Gynecologic Oncology at the UCLA and Cedars-Sinai Medical Center combined program in Los Angeles, California. She received a Master of Science in Clinical Research from the Geffen School of Medicine at UCLA. Dr. Walsh has been the fellowship program director for the gynecologic oncology training program at UCLA and Cedars-Sinai Medical Center since 2011.

CPSIA information can be obtained
at www.ICGtesting.com
Printed in the USA
LVOW04s0127101216
516634LV00013B/165/P